# The New York Academy of Medicine, 1947–1997

ENHANCING THE HEALTH OF THE PUBLIC

Marvin Lieberman
and
Leon J. Warshaw

KRIEGER PUBLISHING COMPANY
MALABAR, FLORIDA
1998

Original Edition 1998

Printed and Published by
**KRIEGER PUBLISHING COMPANY**
**KRIEGER DRIVE**
**MALABAR, FLORIDA 32950**

**Library of Congress Cataloging-In-Publication Data**

Lieberman, Marvin.
    The New York Academy of Medicine, 1947-1997: enhancing the health
of the public / Marvin Lieberman and Leon J. Warshaw.—Original
ed.
      p.  cm.
    Includes bibliographical references and index.
    ISBN 0-89464-984-1 (hard cover: alk. paper)
    1. New York Academy of Medicine—History.  2. Medicine—New York
(State)—Societies, etc.—History.  I. Warshaw, Leon J.  II. Title.
    [DNLM:  1. New York Academy of Medicine.  2. Societies, Medical—
history—United States.  3. Societies, Scientific—history—United
States.  4. Research—history—United States.  5. History of
Medicine, 20th Cent.—United States.  WB 1 AA1 L7n 1998]
R291.L54   1998
610'.6'0747—dc21
DNLM/DLC
for Library of Congress                        97-29698
                                         CIP

10   9   8   7   6   5   4   3   2

already the largest medical library in the United States but for that of the Surgeon General.

The committee structure related activities at the Academy to the City and State Departments of Health, the City Department of Hospitals, and the Medical Examiner's Office. In addition, issues in graduate medical education were engaged, "Graduate Fortnights" were presented as contributions to the continuing education of physicians, and research symposia for scientists in the New York metropolitan area were conducted. Abstracts of papers delivered were published in the *Bulletin of the New York Academy of Medicine*. Eleven clinical Sections met regularly under the aegis of the Committee on Sections and the Committee on Medical Information sought to keep the public informed about matters medical.

After World War II the environment in which the Academy worked changed radically and at an increasing pace. Biomedical research expanded exponentially under the stimulus of the National Institutes of Health, and scientific advance was quickly and widely translated into alterations in practice, which quickly became subspecialized. Diagnosis and treatment came to include an expanding technology, and new and effective therapies started to appear in numbers.

Health care delivery systems changed more slowly at first, and then with rapidly increasing extent and impact. In the past decade rising concern with health care costs has moved the system in the direction of managed care, a sea change by any definition, one that continues to redefine not only the organization and fiscal structure of American health care, but in the process the fiduciary responsibilities of physicians and hospitals.

These changes, continuing through the 1980s and 1990s, altered the field in which the Academy was seeking to service its responsibilities; as examples, a great deal of continuing medical education moved to the medical schools and hospitals in and around New York, with a resultant diminution in interest in Academy Sections identified with the larger clinical specialties; health policy matters in New York City were increasingly tied to discussions at the state and federal levels; and information management

# Foreword

THE NEW YORK ACADEMY OF MEDICINE, 150 years old in 1997, has a long and distinguished history in pursuit of its mission, "To Enhance the Health of the Public." At the end of its first hundred years a detailed history was written by Philip Van Ingen, and published by the Columbia University Press in 1949.

In concluding his history, Van Ingen noted the following: "From a small group of 185 men, a number of whom were influenced by motives of self-advancement; without an official home and with little immediate prospect of obtaining one; torn by internal rivalries and jealousies; originally administered by ten officers, a President, four Vice Presidents, a Recording Secretary, Domestic and Foreign Corresponding Secretaries, a Treasurer, a Librarian, and five Standing Committees, all elected for one year only; without paid assistance, except for a professional collector of dues; with a hoped for annual income of only $555; but with a full measure of determination and boundless optimism—from these beginnings has developed the present New York Academy of Medicine."

At the time Van Ingen was writing, the Academy had some 2,400 Fellows and an endowment of $4.5 million. Its governance structure, which had served well for a century, consisted of a Board of Trustees charged with managing the finances and real estate of the institution, and a Council, which transacted the general executive business of the Academy and determined its policy. The Council supervised Academy activities fairly closely, and appointed the Director of the Academy as well as the Executive Secretaries of Standing Committees. The President served for two years and, Van Ingen noted, ". . . cannot commit the Academy to any course of action without the approval of the Council." The Director was responsible for the administration of the institution.

The Library in 1947 contained some 252,000 volumes, and was

# Table of Contents

came increasingly to rely on electronics, rather than the printed page.

As these changes progressed, along with many others, internal discussions came to focus increasingly on maintaining the usefulness, and even the viability, of the Academy. As was the case with most institutions in biomedicine and health care, it became clear that the Academy had to adapt to a rapidly changing environment with a close examination, and to some extent reorientation, of its programs.

In the past decade, led by seasoned and devoted leadership at the Board and Council levels, the governance and management structure of the Academy has been radically revamped. Increasingly, as it has pursued its traditional mission, the Academy has moved to modernize and fortify programs related to enhancing the care delivered to the sick individual and, at the same time, understanding and addressing major issues in the health of populations. With this refocusing, with the assembly of an outstanding senior executive and professional staff, and with a commitment to producing Academy programs at the highest possible level of quality, has come a renewed appreciation of the usefulness and of the unique opportunity availability to this old, and at the same time new, pro bono, private sector institution. In contrast to 1947, the Academy now counts nearly 3,000 Fellows; its Library holds more than 700,000 volumes, and its endowment is more than $70 million. Most important, in the course of its reinvigoration, and building on the programs and accomplishments of years past, the Academy has found new opportunities, new avenues to act through, in behalf of the society the biomedical and health care establishments must serve.

The present volume documents the events of the past fifty years. The uses of history are, of course, many; in presenting this extension of the story of the New York Academy of Medicine we are hopeful that we are offering a source of interest to the Fellows and friends of the Academy, a compilation for the use of social and medical historians, and a benchmark against which the future trajectories of this and similarly oriented institutions can be measured.

Particular thanks go to doctors Marvin Lieberman and Leon J. Warshaw for their labors in writing this history, to the Library and Archival staffs of the New York Academy of Medicine, to those who gave of their time and recollections so as to add to the richness of the story, and to the Board of Trustees of the Academy for its support of this important element in the Sesquicentennial celebration of the institution.

Jeremiah A. Barondess, M.D.

# Preface

To CELEBRATE THE CENTENNIAL of the New York Academy of Medicine, Philip Van Ingen, a long-time Fellow, undertook the formidable task of tracing the history of the Academy from its founding in 1847 to the end of its first hundred years. A highly regarded New York physician who had been President of the American Academy of Pediatrics as well as the American Pediatric Society, Dr. Van Ingen was an excellent choice for this assignment having been active in Academy affairs for over forty years while pursuing his special interest in medical history as a member of the New York Historical Society.

Starting in the fall of 1945, he sifted through a huge mass of documentary material which included minutes of meetings, reports, annals and publications in medical and lay journals, to compile the fascinating history of the trials and tribulations of the Academy as an organization, and the problems that it confronted,. Not published until 1949, his book presents a year-by-year account of its activities under the leadership of the chain of successive presidents against the backdrop of advances in medical art and science and the health-related issues of the day.[1]

In 1995, in anticipation of the Academy's 150th anniversary, Dr. Marvin Lieberman, who was retiring after thirty-one years in a variety of staff positions, accepted the challenge of bringing the history up-to-date. After more than a year of delving through the many drawers and boxes to which the voluminous records of Academy activities had been consigned, searching the archival collections of the Library, and interviewing many of the people who had been directly involved, he produced the framework for this volume. At

---

[1]Van Ingen, P. 1949 *The New York Academy of Medicine: Its First Hundred Years.* New York: Columbia University Press.

that point, Dr. Leon J. Warshaw, an Academy Fellow, who was completing a three-year stint as Associate Editor of the International Labor Organization's *Encyclopaedia of Occupational Health and Safety*, was recruited to conduct additional research and to edit the preliminary draft.

The authors are greatly indebted to the many Fellows and staff members who provided assistance, information and encouragement: to President Jeremiah Barondess who conceived and authorized this activity; Senior Vice President Alan R. Fleischman; Senior Vice President Patricia J. Volland; Leslie Goldman, Director of the Office of School Health Programs; and Arthur Downing, Director of the Library. We are indebted to Chris McKee, Catherine Graber and Michael North of the Library staff for their help in unearthing hard-to-find materials and, especially, for verifying the completeness and accuracy of the many references.

In addition, for graciousness in granting interviews in connection with research on the book, we are grateful to Thomas Basler, Alfred N. Brandon, Martin Cherkasky, Duncan W. Clark, Daniel J. Ehrlich, Tova Friedler, Julie A. Hantman, Brett A. Kirkpatrick, Margaret E. Mahoney, Jacqueline Messite, Michael C. McGarvey, David McNutt, Richard C. Menschel, Lynn Krasner Morgan, Thomas Q. Morris, Anne M. Pascarelli, Mary Ann Payne, Peter Rogatz, Robert Schiffler, JoAnn Silberstein, William C. Stubing, and Wendy Wisbaum.

We also wish to thank Kristen Flansburg and Carol Gonzalez-Barrett of the Executive Office; Antonio Aponte, manager of Building Operations, and his staff; Luciano Otero and Eric Richardson of Central Services. Others in the Library to whom we are grateful include Lois Fischer Black of the Rare Book Room; Rhonna Goodman, Peter Wansor and Linda Gardin of Library Administration; Marsha Suer Clark of Serials and Acquisitions; Mary Mylenki of the Regional Medical Library; Russell Humphries of Access Services; Stephen Chiaffone of Document Delivery; Dixon Berry, Michael Minichino, Joel Beard, Luis Gonzalez and Michael McClung of Information Systems, and Patricia Gallagher, Kathel Dunn and Timothy Roberts of the Reference Deparment.

Other staff members who provided valuable assistance include Maureen Leness and Maureen O'Connor of the Development Office; Merlie C. Elizes, Jacqueline Gibbons, Lawrence Coppola and Siui-Ping Fung of the Business Office; Adelaida Jama and Ilya Speranza of the Office Medical Affairs; Denise Copper of the Office of Finance and Administration; James Spellos, Adam Margolis, Beth Schwartz and Sherry Williams of the Office of Medical Education; Ilvan Burgos, Carolyn Cox McDonald, Ed Diller, Joanne Eichel and Freya Kaufman of the Office of School Health Programs; Ellen Parish and Theresa Jackson of the Office of Special Populations; and Gary Stein and Rosemary Alcantara of the HIV Professional Development Project.

We are greatly indebted to Elaine S. Rudd, editor at Krieger Publishing Company, for her skill, diligence and patience in shepherding our manuscript through the travail of publication.

We also wish to express deep gratitude to our wives, Purlaine Lieberman and Mona Warshaw, for their unfailing support and forbearance.

Having observed and/or participated in most of the events in this history, and having enjoyed working more or less closely with many of those whose names are mentioned in it, producing this volume has been a source of gratification that more than made up for the labor it entailed. We hope that it will provide similar gratification to the Fellows and others who will read it.

Marvin Lieberman
Leon J. Warshaw

# Chapter 1
## 1847–1947
## The First Hundred Years

## THE ORIGIN AND DEVELOPMENT OF THE NEW YORK
## ACADEMY OF MEDICINE

During the early decades of the nineteenth century, New York City experienced a remarkable economic expansion, spurred primarily by the opening of the Erie Canal in 1825. The concentration of trade that made the City the dominant port on the Eastern seaboard was accompanied by diversification of its economic base. The growth was primarily in maritime trade, manufacturing and transportation, while banking and finance grew to a new prominence that has never been relinquished. In all, except for the financial crisis of 1837, it was an era of unprecedented growth and prosperity.[1]

The city grew geographically with the area of settlement enlarging northward from its origins at the tip of Manhattan reaching to what is now Union Square by the time the New York Academy of Medicine was founded. By that time, the population had reached approximately 300,000 largely due to a surge in immigration, which included over a million people from Ireland fleeing the great Potato Famine of 1845–1851, many of whom settled in New York City. This growth was seen by many members of the "upper classes" as a source of instability and a threat to the fabric of the community. Rapid urbanization was taking place; crowded and unhealthy tenements were becoming a prominent feature of the New York scene. The wealthy colonial landholders were pushed aside as the new breed of entrepreneurs gained economic, social and political power, and the gap between rich and poor in the City widened. There was a general perception that a distressing decline in values had occurred. It was a time of religious revival and reform, and many organizations were created to contend with the "evils" of urban life.[2]

Many of these organizations were devoted to enhancing the cultural landscape of the City, mimicking those already established in Boston and Philadelphia. While many of those prominent in them were members of the faculties of Columbia University and New York University, between which there was great rivalry, they also gave time, energy and, in some instances, money to the creation and support of new independent institutions. These included the New York Literary and Philosophical Society, the New York Historical Society, and the American Academy of Fine Arts. In 1817, two physicians on the faculty at the College of Physicians and Surgeons, Samuel Latham Mitchell and David Hosack, along with DeWitt Clinton, then the Mayor of New York City and a strong supporter of cultural activities, led the way in organizing the Lyceum of Natural History which provided the hall for the organizing meetings of the New York Academy of

Medicine in 1847 and which later became the New York Academy of Sciences.¹

Medical practice at that time was chaotic and disorganized. It was led by "regular" physicians, graduates of orthodox university education featuring the study of anatomy, chemistry and other basic sciences, often coupled with a preceptorship or other semi-formal training. The treatments they offered were often extremely drastic featuring bleeding and purging the efficacy of which were especially problematic. There was little or no scientific basis for most medical procedures, which were either ineffective or dangerous.

Almost as a reaction, there was a broad range of alternative forms of treatment which included homeopathy, perhaps the most popular, a variety of sectarian practices, and quackery of all types.

The regular practitioners felt greatly threatened by the rise of homeopathy and the development of parallel groups by practitioners who scoffed at their reliance on purging and bleeding. All were permitted to practice by New York State resulting in great competition for patients and the income they represented. In 1834, when efforts to persuade the New York State to bar them from practice failed, the regular physicians persuaded the Legislature, as a compromise, to deny access to the courts by botanical physicians and other "irregulars" who sought to sue for unpaid fees.³

The situation at the time was aptly described by a medical historian as follows: "The chaotic state of the profession, the rampant and defiant air of quackery, and its contaminating and demoralizing influence by association upon professional morals was keenly felt. There was no public medical society in New York City the proceedings of which were reported, nor was there anything added to the common stock of scientific literature of the profession. The New York County Medical Society had a mere organic existence; nothing was done in scientific work, and the society had little influence on the ethical condition of the profession."⁴ This, then, was the environment into which the New York Academy of Medicine was born.

THE BIRTH OF THE ACADEMY

The Academy was conceived at a dinner on November 18, 1846 celebrating the fourth anniversary of the Society for the Relief of Widows and Orphans of Medical Men that was attended by eighty of the most prominent regular physicians of the City. Responding to a toast, Dr. Alexander H. Stevens, President of the College of Physicians and Surgeons, the older of the two medical schools then in the City, congratulated the assembled physicians for setting aside their antagonism for one another and demonstrating a spirit that would enhance their dignity and command respect for the profession. He concluded by expressing the hope that they would be brought together in a "body corporate" that would move to the "establishment of a medical hall, unconnected with hospitals or colleges, to contain meeting rooms, a library, etc., and be a place of general resort, both for ourselves and brethren from abroad."[5]

The response was immediate. About half of the physicians present remained after the dinner for a meeting in which they confirmed the desirability of establishing "a local medical voluntary association" and appointed a committee to undertake its organization. On December 8, 1846, several New York newspapers published a notice calling the regular practitioners of the city to cooperate "in an undertaking to elevate the character of our profession and to advance its interests and increase its usefulness by furnishing facilities for medical intercourse, promoting harmony among its members, and offering means of mutual improvement therein. In prosecution of these objects it is proposed to establish an Academy of Medicine and Surgery and to provide a permanent place for its meetings."[6]

The notice called for a meeting on December 12, 1846 at the Lyceum of Natural History and was signed by the leaders of medicine in New York City at the time: Dr. Valentine Mott, President and Professor of Surgery at New York University Medical College, Dr. Isaac Wood, President of the Medical Society of the City and County of New York, and Dr. Stevens whose toast had inspired the undertaking.

At that meeting, it was acknowledged that the major reason for the formation of the Academy was the desire of the regular physicians to distinguish themselves from the "irregular practitioners," primarily the homeopaths, even if they were graduates of a regular medical school. Dr. Mott said that the "least flavor or tincture of homeopathy would not be recognized by those of the old school," and, he declared, "We must alter our generation and be educated anew before we can believe in the doctrine of the infinitesimal."[7] Dr. Wood expressed a wish to exclude not only the irregular practitioners but also any regular physicians who "met and consulted with them."

The need for a new organization for this purpose was dictated by the fact that the articles of incorporation of the Medical Society of the City and County of New York, as it was then called, did not permit the exclusion of homeopaths. "The concerns of elite societies had not changed since the beginning of the century," notes medical historian William G. Rothstein, "they still wanted to separate themselves from the rank and file of the profession and to develop some mechanism for sharing prestige and the emoluments to be gained from intervention among themselves."[8]

### The First Constitution and By-laws

With a harmony that was notable for gatherings of physicians in those days, the meeting agreed unanimously to form the new organization and, after some discussion of who its members should be, appointed a committee of fourteen, including the three who had signed the public notice, that was charged to draw up a constitution and by-laws. This was accomplished and presented at a second meeting held on January 6, 1847, an achievement that established a speed record for such formal Academy action that virtually remains unbroken to this day.

The name selected for the new organization was "The New York Academy of Medicine" and its stated objectives were as follows:

- "First. The separation of the irregular practitioners.
- Second. The association of the profession proper for purposes of mutual recognition and fellowship.
- Third. The promotion of the character, interests and honor of the fraternity, by maintaining the union and harmony of the regular profession of the city and its vicinity, and aiming to elevate the standard of medical education.
- Fourth. The cultivation and advancement of the sciences, by our united exertions for mutual improvement, and our contributions to the medical literature."[9]

The members were to comprise Resident Fellows, "regular physicians, resident for three years in the City, State or Region," and Corresponding Fellows. The By-laws stipulated that "no proprietor or vendor of any patent or secret remedy or medicine, nor any empirical or irregular practitioner" could be admitted or retain his membership. (This stricture was later relaxed somewhat when it was recognized that most of the physicians had been prescribing such "secret" remedies as "McCunn's Elixir of Opium" and "Henry's Magnesia," and it became known that Valentine Mott, then already a world-famous surgeon, had used ether as an anesthetic just months after Richard Morton had demonstrated its effectiveness in a surgical procedure at the Massachusetts General Hospital in Boston and attempted to patent it under the name of "lethion."[10])

Officers of the Academy were to include a President, four Vice Presidents, a Recording Secretary, two Corresponding Secretaries, one for domestic and the other for foreign correspondence, a Treasurer and a Librarian, all to be elected annually by ballot at the January meeting of each year. The Librarian was to take charge of "all books, pamphlets, manuscripts, anatomical or pathological specimens, apparatus, instruments, medals, coins or scientific property of whatever kind," each item to be inscribed with the name of its donor and to be listed in a catalogue. The Archives were to include a copy of "every oration, memoir or medical paper presented before the Academy."[11]

The President was to appoint four Standing Committees and a

Council of Appeal, each comprising five Resident Fellows. The committees included the following:

- Committee on Admissions—charged to supervise the election of new Fellows and, especially, to guard against admitting irregular or unqualified practitioners to membership.
- Committee on Finance—charged to collect an "annual tax not to exceed $3.00," payment of which was to be considered "a point of honor," and to provide quarters for the Library and Museum.
- Committee on Medical Ethics — charged to "hear and decide" all complaints of breach of etiquette or violations of medical ethics and to rule on all questions of medical ethics submitted to it.
- Committee on Publications—charged to superintend the publication of all orations, memoirs or papers under the title of *Transactions of the New York Academy of Medicine*.

The Council of Appeal was charged to decide all questions of violation of the Constitution and could summon any Fellow to appear before it.

The Constitution and By-laws were approved by all but one dissenting Fellow, and it was decided that all those involved in this and the prior meetings would sign the document as Founding Fellows. After much discussion of the order of signing, 132 names were affixed to the document. Dr. Stephen Hasbrouck, Sr., the lone dissenter, did not sign the document although he apparently remained a Fellow. The meeting was then adjourned for a week during which a specially-appointed Nominating Committee was to draw up a list of three candidates for each of the designated offices.

When the meeting was resumed on the afternoon of January 13, 1847, it was voted unanimously that, since the Academy was not yet organized, "any person who decided to enroll, against whom nobody spoke, could sign [the Constitution] as a Founder."[12] Accordingly, fifty-three additional signatures were entered bringing the total number of Founders to 185 and then the list was closed. This document has been preserved in what is now the Rare Book Room of the Academy Library. Also, before the candidates for the offices were presented, a Treasurer pro tem was appointed and ordered to collect at once a tax of $1.00 to defray the expenses of organization from each person who had signed. Thereupon, Dr. John Stearns was elected the first President of the Academy. The others elected to office are as follows:

- Vice Presidents: Drs. F.U. Johnston, Thomas Cock, John B. Beck and John W. Francis
- Recording Secretary: Dr. F. Campbell Stewart
- Domestic Corresponding Secretary: Dr. William C. Roberts
- Foreign Corresponding Secretary: Dr. Benjamin Drake
- Treasurer: Dr. Robert Watts, Jr.
- Librarian: Dr. Thomas M. Markoe

Dr. Isaac Wood, who had joined Drs. Mott and Stevens in declining nomination for the office of Vice President, officially founded the Library by donating his three-volume set of Paine's Commentaries, a compendium of essays on "vital powers," the philosophy of bloodletting, the pathology of venous congestion and humoral pathology, a gift that is still preserved in the Rare Book Room of the Academy Library. The author, Dr. Martyn Paine, who was one of the founders of the medical college affiliated with the University of the City of New York, was best known for his successful efforts to repeal the law that made dissection of the human body a criminal offense.

Dr. Stearns was well qualified for his new office. Then seventy-seven years old, he had graduated from Yale "with distinguished honors" and attended medical lectures at the University of Pennsylvania from 1789 to 1793 after which, without taking a degree as was the custom in those days (Later, in 1812, he received the honorary degree of Doctor of Medicine from the Regents of the State of New York), he entered medical practice in Watertown, New York. After election to the State Senate in 1809 in which he served through 1813, he practiced in Albany and, finally, moved to New York City in 1819. He was instrumental in forming the New York State Medical Society in 1806, serving as its first Secretary and later, commencing in 1818, served three consecutive one-year terms as its President.

The last of the organizing meetings was held approximately two weeks later on January 20, 1847. It was attended by 159 of the enrolled Fellows who had a "long and animated" discussion of an issue presented by the Committee on Membership which had twenty-five names under consideration and was seeking a more precise distinction between "regularity" and "irregularity." Finally, unanimous approval was won by a motion proposed by Dr. James Manley which excluded "all homeopathic, hydropathic, chrono-thermal and botanical physicians and also all mesmeric and clair-voyant pretenders to the healing art, and all others who at any time or on any pretext claimed peculiar merits for their mixed practices not founded on the best system of physiology and pathology as taught in the best schools in Europe and America, and shall be deemed to exclude also all such persons as associate with them in consultation."[13]

The founding of the Academy was met with acclaim. It was welcomed by the Medical Society of the State of New York and a number of the county societies. *The New York Medical and Surgical Reporter* reported details of the meetings, and the *Annalist* of January 15, 1847 stated: "The sixth of January last was a proud day for the profession of this city and one which is destined, we fondly believe, to be commemorated hereafter as the commencement of a new era in our science. It witnessed, we trust, the founding of the first great barrier between quackery and medical integrity; the desire of standing well among one's fellows; and the first step toward a professional harmony of purpose and sentiment, the suppression of roguery and the elevation of the standard of professional qualifications."[14]

## The First Stated Meeting

The activities of the Academy were formally launched at the first stated meeting which was held on February 3, 1847 with eighty-seven Fellows attending. It opened with President Stearn's Inaugural Address which concluded with the following restatement of the Academy's mission: "To elevate the standard of medical education, to exclude from our profession all ignorant pretenders, to enlighten the public mind on the subject of medicine and its collateral branches of science, and to take all necessary measures to promote the honor, the dignity, the respectability and the usefulness of the medical profession . . ."[15]

The activities of that meeting and the ensuing year followed Dr. Stearn's outline, setting a pattern that the Academy has more or less followed to this day. For example, professional matters were addressed by electing a delegation of fifteen Fellows to attend the National Convention in Philadelphia at which the American Medical Association was organized. Apparently, this too was motivated by the same concerns that had prompted the forming of the Academy, namely the fact that "competition from homeopaths and other sects was having severe economic repercussions and was also affecting the pride of well-trained physicians."[16] The Code of Ethics adopted by the American Medical Association and formally endorsed by the Academy in October, 1847 and published jointly in 1848, also imposed a ban on consultations between homeopaths and regular physicians.

Medical education was addressed by presentation of a scientific paper at each meeting. The topics covered in that first year included: treatment of ununited fractures; *Revelations of the Microscope;* history of institutions for the insane; signs, symptoms and causes of inflammation; and placenta praevia. Because of the cost, publication of these papers was delayed until 1851 when the Academy began publishing its *Transactions.*

Issues of public health were addressed by the formation of a number of special committees:

- The first investigated and reported on "the use of Sulphuric Ether in mitigating pain in surgical operations." After review of the report, an enlarged committee was appointed and instructed to conduct experiments on animals but, since the Academy never acted on a series of resolutions calling for the establishment of a laboratory for "chemical, physiological and pathological research," they were not undertaken.
- A second committee visited local hospitals to investigate the prevalence and treatment of typhus fever which was endemic in New York City at

that time. Its report was printed both in medical journals and the daily newspapers.

- A third committee was appointed to "examine into the effects, proximate and remote, upon the general health of the City caused by the numerous distilleries, gas works, slaughter houses, milk establishments, lead manufactories, tanneries and all other manufactories, and establishments which are, or may be styled nuisances from their deleterious effects on the health, and particularly to report the effects on the human economy of milk taken from kine tuberculously or otherwise diseased from improper food or confined situations in these milk establishments."[17] A detailed report of its exploration of the milk industry was subsequently reported in the *Transactions,* but the other environmental concerns apparently were never addressed.
- Another committee was appointed in response to a request from the Common Council of the City to investigate sewerage and the "present and prospective sanitary condition of the city" but after two years, it was disbanded without making a report.
- A final committee was appointed to collaborate with the College of Pharmacy in exploring the possibility of restricting the importation of adulterated and impure drugs. It culminated in a memorandum to the Congress endorsing legislation proposed by the College of Pharmacy to control the importation of drugs.

In addition, governmental activities were addressed by two "memorials" addressed to the State legislature: one endorsed a proposed law requiring registration of births, deaths and marriages; and the other urged State action for the care of "youthful idiots."

Academy finances were a cause of concern, prophetically for financial difficulties were to hinder the Academy's activities repeatedly in the years and decades that followed. A "collector" had to be appointed to get Fellows to pay their dues but, even with that, lack of funds proved to be a problem and a number of activities, including establishing the Academy's publications, had to be postponed.

Governance of the Academy was also addressed, particularly at the end of the year when a revision of the Constitution and By-laws was presented for consideration. By that time, membership had grown to 265 Fellows.

### The First Anniversary

In all, it was a most auspicious beginning, with a number of significant accomplishments and a number of activities that were engaged but never completed. The year closed with the first anniversary oration, a two hour presentation, delivered to an audience of more than 2,500 people at the Broadway Tabernacle on November 10, 1847 by John W. Francis, who was subsequently elected to serve as the second President of the Academy. Prior to the meeting, the Fellows gathered at the home of President Stearns and then marched the two and a half blocks to the Tabernacle as a body. According to the *Annalist,* "every part of the room was filled, literally filled to the very walls, with well-dressed persons of both sexes. Scarcely was standing room afforded either upon the floor or in the galleries. . . . Hundreds must have gone away disappointed at being unable to obtain places . . . The forceful manner in which, at the close of his discourse, the subject of legislative support of indigenous quackery, the bill of pains and penalties inflicted by its sects on the community was adverted to, will not soon be forgotten."[18]

In addition to that powerful peroration on the evils of the "irregular" physicians, Dr. Francis called attention to the disagreement among the "regular" physicians about the remedies they prescribed, noting that "given the desire for economic advantage through self-promotion, there was a need for physicians to subordinate their individuality. . . . They feared that, not just that persons already secessionist would grow in public favor, but also that respectable physicians might decide intellectual issues on an irrational basis, that they would let confusion or social and economic motives become the deciding forces in the intellectual sphere."[19]

## THE NEXT NINETY-NINE YEARS

The saga of the Academy's next ninety-nine years is admirably detailed in Dr. Philip Van Ingen's centennial volume. Dividing the years into the terms of the succession of presidents, he enumerated the Academy's major activities and undertakings against the backdrop of changes in medical practice and the health-related problems of the City.

In 1851, the Academy was able to secure an Act of Incorporation from the legislature of the State of New York.

In 1854, because of the lack of effectiveness of the scientific committees, the Academy was officially divided into sections, each of which was devoted to a medical specialty or a basic scientific discipline, an arrangement that has persisted to this day. The first sections were devoted to Theory and Practice, Obstetrics and Diseases of Women and Children, Anatomy, Surgery, and Chemistry. Each section was required to appoint two or more of its members each year, each to present original papers before the entire Academy.[20]

The leaders of the Academy were deeply involved in the civic reform movements of the time. They were particularly troubled by the plight of the poor and the threat to the public's health from the terrible sanitary conditions in housing. In 1852, the Committee on Public Health and Legal Medicine chaired by Dr. John Griscom, one of the founders of the Academy, issued a lengthy report citing the inadequacy of the current dispensary system for providing care to the sick poor, noting that inadequate remuneration of the physicians made it impossible for them to perform faithfully (A century later, similar statements were to be made with respect to Medicaid!). The report recommended that one or more physicians be appointed for each Ward in the City who were to be paid adequately and were to be required to live in their districts. In addition to providing medical care to the poor "living in their cellars and garrets," they were to act as "sanitary police being empowered to note and command the removal of nuisances and hazards to health."[21] This was the beginning of a persistent campaign of public information and lobbying of the State Legislature in Albany, led primarily by Dr. Griscom, that culminated in 1866 in the creation of the Metropolitan Board of Health, the precursor of the current Department of Health.[22]

So ardent and persistent was Dr. Griscom's campaign that it drew frowns from some of the Fellows and was the basis for the following thinly-veiled attack, entitled *Puffery and the Academy of Medicine,* which appeared in the *American Medical Gazette* for April 1961:

The attention of the Academy of Medicine has, by some of the morning papers, been called to the fact that, contrary to its standing rules, and in defiance of its recent resolutions forbidding any of its Fellows to report its meetings for the daily press, or to do anything akin to puffery or advertising, one of the most prominent of these gentlemen has lately been running about from one city editor to another, trying to get them to endorse and advertise a certain health bill which he has concocted, and by which, if passed at Albany, he hopes to get money. Now, as no member of so respectable, learned and influential a body as the Academy of Medicine can, under penalty of expulsion, "advertise his health pills, or puff his health bills," in the public press, we hope proper action will without delay be taken by the Academy to prevent a repetition of such forbidden manoeuvers, and to put an end to such unprofessional and reprehensible practices by everyone over whom it has jurisdiction or control.[23]

There is no record of any action having been taken against Dr. Griscom for his lobbying efforts.

From its very beginnings, the Academy has played a major role in establishing the norms of medical ethics. Starting with its endorsement and publication of the Code of Ethics articulated by the fledgling American Medical Association, to which the Academy's delegates contributed significantly, to the present day, the Academy has been quite explicit in setting standards for professional conduct. Originally focused on such matters as relationships with "fringe" practitioners, use and promotion of patent medicines, and self-aggrandizement, advertising and publicity, its statements on such broad issues as the 1996 position on participation of physicians in capital punishment have influenced the actions of both medical and nonmedical organizations as well as the City and State governments.

## The First Academy Building

Early Academy meetings were held in the "small chapel" of New York University and, from 1868 through 1875, in a lecture room rented from the College of Physicians and Surgeons, then located at 23rd Street and Fourth Avenue. The move to have its own building was initiated in 1866 when Dr. Samuel S. Purple, a founding member of the Academy who later served as President from 1875–1878, offered to donate his collection of several thousand volumes of medical references to the Library as soon as the Academy would erect a "fire proof building sufficiently commodious to contain said library with its prospective additions and which building shall also be suitable for the purposes of a museum and a Hall in which the meetings of the Academy and the profession can be held."[24] He also offered a pledge of $2,000 toward the construction of the proposed building, but it took almost twelve years to accumulate sufficient funds to purchase the 28' by 60' four-story brownstone building at 12 West 31st Street to be the first home of the Academy. Two large rooms on an upper floor of this building were assigned to the Library and represented its real beginning. In 1878, the Academy voted to open the Library to the public and, in 1880, the first full-time librarian, Mr. John S. Brownne, was hired. (He was also required to live in the building and act as a superintendent, monitoring the performance of the succession of janitors and seeing that the building and its contents were properly maintained.)

Despite the strictures against consorting with homeopathic physicians, the chasm between them and the regular physicians was being bridged. By 1882, a growing proportion of the local physicians were homeopaths: 10 percent of the physicians practicing in New York City and 17 percent of those practicing in Brooklyn, then an independent city. These even included some graduates of the regular medical schools. Dr. Abraham Jacobi, one of the major figures in the Academy and a leader in American medicine, told a meeting of the New York State Medical Society that, "if they as regular physicians believed medicine was 'one and indivisible,'

then they should relate to homeopaths in a spirit of conciliation."
Cooperation between the homeopaths and regular physicians was,
he said, "absolutely necessary if higher standards of medical education were to be realized."[25]

In December 1888, thanks to an extended fund raising campaign
which produced a number of large bequests, the Academy was able
to purchase a 75' by 100' plot on the north side of West 43rd Street
between Fifth and Sixth Avenues on which the second home of the
Academy was constructed. It was a most impressive building containing meeting rooms, the Fellows Room, the Collation Room, a
smoking room and, in addition to an elevator, the reading rooms
and stacks of the Library. The first meeting in the new building was
held on October 2, 1890 in Hosack Hall, the majestic lecture hall
named in gratitude for the earmarked $70,000 bequest from the
estate of Celine B. Hosack, the widow of David Hosack, the editor
of the *American Medical and Philosophical Register* and "in his day,
the best known practitioner in New York City."[26] Mrs. Hosack also
left $10,000 for an endowed bed at Roosevelt Hospital the occu-
pant of which was to be designated by the President and Trustees of
the Academy.

### The Fiftieth Anniversary

The fiftieth anniversary of the Academy was celebrated at Carnegie Hall on January 29, 1897 with President Grover Cleveland
delivering the closing address in which he urged the Academy
"never to forget its duty was not only, as highly intelligent members of the community, to develop the science of medicine, but to
use its tremendous influence in the cause of true citizenship."[27]

The Library continued to grow apace thanks to gifts and purchases. It began to publish two lists of the medical periodicals it
received, one of *English Journals* and the other of *Foreign Journals*.
In 1892, a full-time Assistant Librarian was hired and, later that
year, A. L. Northrup, D.D.S., a prominent dentist, donated 18,000
issues of dental journals, 60 pamphlets, and 517 volumes most of

which were added to the Academy's reference library making it "one of the most valuable dental libraries in the United States." By 1897, the Library contained 38,320 volumes along with thousands of duplicates and when, in 1898, the Governors of the New York Hospital donated its library of 23,000 volumes, many of which were given to twenty-one other libraries and institutions, the Academy could rightfully claim having the largest private medical library in the Unites States, second only to the Library of the Surgeon General in Washington, D.C., a rank that it has held to this day.[28]

Such growth was not without problems. Just about every year, the Library Committee complained about lack of space and the fact that the budget allocations for the Library were inadequate. In fact, in his uplifting, scholarly Oration at the 1897 semicentennial celebration at Carnegie Hall, Dr. Abraham Jacobi, the eminent pediatrician who was then President of the Academy, had included a plea for financial help to make the Library self-supporting.

By the close of the nineteenth century, the Academy had become a center for medical education. Papers presented at its meetings included original reports of new discoveries in the structure and physiology of the major organs of the body, of innovations in surgical procedures and other medical technology, and of advances in the treatment of a variety of diseases. The meetings were supplemented by the growing value of the Library as a resource available without charge to both the profession and the public. In addition, the Academy took leading positions in the continuing struggle for improvements in the training and licensure of physicians and other health professionals.

The Academy had also become a center for activism on matters important to the health of the City and its citizens, both on its own and in consort with other professional and civic organizations. It had addressed such diverse issues as the quality of milk available to New Yorkers, factory laws, clean streets, the formation of the Metropolitan Board of Health, quarantine regulations, the establishment of free public baths, eye examinations for children, the organization of dispensaries, and the elimination of corruption in municipal government.

The Academy's concern over the health of the public continued after the turn of the century. In 1905, it began the first of a series of lectures on health matters aimed at the general public. In 1911, the Section on Public Health was replaced by the formation of a formal Committee on Public Health, Hospitals and Budget (in 1926, the name was changed to the Committee on Public Health Relations and later to the Committee on Public Health), the members of which were to be appointed annually. With the initial support of annual contributions from Mrs. Edward H. Harriman, the Committee was charged "to collect information on public health, sanitation and hygiene including comparative studies of the methods and results of public health activities in other cities in this country and abroad, to cooperate actively with all public health agencies and activities in the City, to monitor municipal budget allocations for public health agencies and hospitals, and to study the performance of the City's public and private hospitals with respect to construction, equipment, administration and medical efficiency." Among its early successes was the endorsement of legislation, which it had helped to draft, that in 1918 replaced the inefficient system of coroners with the Office of the Chief Medical Examiner.[29]

## The New Building

A recurrent theme at the Academy was anxiety about its marginal financial status (on a number of occasions money had to be borrowed to pay bills remaining unpaid at the end of the year), about the inadequacy of the meeting facilities, and about the need for additional space for the Library and its collections. By 1909, it was recognized that something needed to be done about the inadequacy of the 43rd Street building and, in 1910, financed by a mortgage on the property, two adjacent buildings were purchased, one next door at 15 West 43rd Street, and the other behind it at 10 West 44th Street. But, for a variety of reasons, including World War I, only makeshift rearrangements like increasing the number of seats in Hosack Hall and storing some of the Library's books in the unused adjacent buildings were undertaken. In 1921, when the proposal for expansion at this site was eroded by dissatisfaction with several successive plans submitted by architects, a consensus emerged, sparked primarily by the ideas and energy of Dr. D. Bryson Delevan, a member of the Council, in favor of a move to an entirely new building to be erected when sufficient funds would become available.

In addition to the funds for the building, it was decided to seek endowments that would support a "greater" Academy as an educational institution. These efforts were successful: the Carnegie Corporation promised a grant of one million dollars for the building provided the Academy furnished the site, and the Rockefeller Foundation promised an endowment grant of approximately one and a quarter million dollars. Ivy Lee, the Rockefeller family's public relations advisor, was hired to lead an intensive fund-raising campaign featuring theater parties and appeals not only to the Fellows, but also to the members of medical societies in the area. This effort succeeded in raising almost another half million dollars, not quite double the original objective.

A 100' by 120' site at the corner of Park Avenue and 60th Street was purchased in 1923 but on the advice of the architects, contractors and both Foundations, based primarily on the high cost of building materials at the time, actual construction was deferred. Meanwhile, because it was not much larger than the West 43rd Street site and the elevated cost of the high-rise building required to provide the needed additional space, disfavor with the plan began to mount. In 1924, a much less expensive and more practicable site at Fifth Avenue and 103rd Street was purchased, and on October 30, 1925, the cornerstone was laid for the impressive Byzantine/Romanesque building designed by the architects York and Sawyer that is the present home of the Academy. In 1929, the Academy purchased three adjoining buildings which were used for a time for overflow Library books and other materials and later were demolished to create the current parking lot. In 1933, without halting Academy activities, the building was extensively remodeled and enlarged in accord with a new design by York and Sawyer, the original architects.

The Library transferred its 133,000 volumes to the building on
August 2, 1926, many others having been donated to other libraries and disposed of as "waste paper" and, on November 18, 1926,
with much fanfare, the new building was officially opened.

At a festive dinner held on the preceding evening, twenty-two
distinguished physicians, surgeons and scientists from around the
world were elected as Honorary Fellows of the Academy. Among
them were such legendary figures as Sir Charles Sherrington from
Oxford, Georges F. I. Widal from Paris, Carlos Chagas from Bra-
zil, Frank Billings from Chicago, Harvey W. Cushing from Boston,
George Dock from Los Angeles, Chevalier Jackson from Philadelphia, and Theobald Smith from the Rockefeller Institute. Dr. Harvey Cushing spoke on *Books and the Doctor;* Mayor Jimmy
Walker who, like so many political figures, had to leave for another engagement, "spoke lightly, as usual, without saying much";
and Dr. William S. Thayer, Professor of Medicine at Johns Hopkins University, who had also been elected an Honorary Fellow,
facetiously described his findings after having been sent to inspect
medical circles in New York by the Angel Ithuriel who was "dis-
turbed by the reports of the press and Sinclair Lewis's novels."[30]

The opening ceremonies, which took place on November 18,
1926, included a number of speeches following a dedicatory
prayer by the Rev. Henry Sloane Coffin, President of the Union
Theological Seminary. These were followed by a tour of the building, including an exhibition of *Early and Later Medical Americana*
presented by the Library. Then, after the serving of refreshments,
Professor M. I. Pupin of Columbia University delivered the Carpen-
ter Lecture on *Ionization and Chemical Reactions.* In all, it was a
magnificent celebration.[31]

## The First Director

From the beginning, the Academy had been blessed by the quality
of its leadership. With a very few exceptions, its Presidents, Trustees and Committee Chairmen, despite ongoing responsibilities to

their practices and other commitments and the lack of remuneration, served with great distinction. It had become clear, however, that managing the increasingly complex operations of the Academy required a full-time commitment. Accordingly, in 1924, Dr. Linsly R. Williams was appointed as the first full-time Director of the Academy. His credentials were impressive. He had been a Fellow of the Academy since 1904 and had served as chairman of the Section on Medicine. He had been Deputy Commissioner of Health of the State of New York, an executive with the Rockefeller Foundation, and, at the time of his appointment, was Managing Director of the National Tuberculosis Association. His first challenge was the plan to move the Academy from the now overcrowded buildings on West 43rd Street. It was he who had selected the site on 103rd Street, a lower cost site than the one on 60th Street that had already been purchased. Actually, he was so sure of the desirability of that site that he took the responsibility of buying and holding it until the formal approval of the Trustees could be obtained, an action that was revealed only after his death.[32]

Dr. Williams's assumption of his position as Director on January 1, 1924 ushered in a new era for the Academy. No time was lost in referring to him the kinds of questions that previously would have required consideration by a slow-moving special committee. These not only related to details of operational administration, but also matters of organization, finance and policy. Included among the actions he originated were resumption of the publication of the *Bulletin* after a lapse of twenty-three years, and creation of the Committee on Medical Education and the Bureau of Medical Information which, together with the Committee on Public Health, became standing committees each staffed by a salaried secretary.

Many noteworthy events occurred during Dr. Williams's tenure as Director which lasted until his death in January 1934. One was the establishment in 1928 of the Graduate Fortnight, a very popular annual series of a two week sequence of lectures, demonstrations, exhibits and clinics devoted to a particular subject in medical science.

The Medical Information Bureau

In the same year, the Medical Information Bureau was organized with Dr. Iago Galdston, who later achieved worldwide renown as a medical journalist, as its Executive Secretary. Initially serving both the Academy and the New York County Medical Society, this Bureau provided information to the media about medical discoveries and events. It inaugurated a daily health column that was syndicated to several hundred newspapers by the Associated Press, and, in 1932, it produced the *Academy Radio Hour*, a weekly talk on health by an Academy Fellow that was broadcast locally over WABC and relayed to radio stations in every part of the country. In addition, it arranged and supervised each year several hundred radio programs on health for a large number of health-related organizations, including the American Red Cross, the National Tuberculosis Association, the Society for the Control of Cancer, and the Children's Welfare Association.[33]

In 1925, on the retirement of John S. Brownne who had served as Librarian since 1880, Dr. Archibald Malloch, a Canadian physician on the faculty at McGill University who had catalogued William Osler's library, was appointed to succeed him. In addition to managing the continuing growth of the Library as the full-time Librarian, Mr. Brownne and his family lived on the top floor of the building on East 30th Street and again in the building at West 43rd Street where he was also made responsible for attending to repairs, supervising the succession of janitors, and acting as Superintendent.[34]

Dr. Malloch was ably assisted by Ms. Janet Doe who was appointed Assistant Librarian in 1929 and made responsible for the Rare Book Room and its increasingly valuable collection of incunabula, manuscripts, photographs and medical instruments, a responsibility given later to Ms. Gertrude Annan. Dr. Malloch brought the library into the modern era. Repairing and preservation of books, long neglected, was started in 1929. Bibliographic and photoduplication services, singularly valuable to physicians, scientists and commercial organizations involved in research and a significant source of revenue to the Academy, were introduced. In 1932, thanks largely to the efforts of Dr. Samuel W. Lambert, a revolving "publication fund" was established. One of the first efforts of that fund was the reprinting of the *Icones Anatomicae* of Andreas Vesalius, a magnificent, prize-winning volume, published in 1934 conjointly with the Library of the University of Munich, using the original wood blocks created for the first edition printed in 1543.

Under Dr. Williams, the Academy's contributions to medical education, public health, the social aspects of medicine, and public health education grew and became widely acknowledged. A major achievement was the establishment of new relationships between the Academy and the local medical societies. Although many of their leaders were Fellows of the Academy, these relationships were "none too cordial" when he assumed the role of Director in 1924. Thanks to his patience and diplomatic skill, he succeeded in establishing the concept that organized medicine had its "own distinct field" in which the Academy should not intrude while the Academy also had its field in which organized medicine should not interfere.

Although never far from financial difficulty, Dr. Williams's success in obtaining grants and bequests provided support adequate to sustain the Academy's increasing activities. To a very large extent, he achieved his ambition to make the Academy "the place to which anybody and everybody in search of information and advice on all matters which had a medical angle, however slight, would instinctively turn."[35]

In a tribute recalling his life, Dr. Iago Galdston, the long-time Executive Secretary of the Committee on Medical Information, credited Dr. Williams with being the founder of the "present-day" Academy of Medicine. He wrote, "Its operating structure, its location, its physical magnitude all bear witness to his far-reaching understanding. . . . Linsly Williams helped convert the Academy from what it was for near to eighty years, that is, a club for the medical elite and reputable, into an institution dedicated to the promotion of science and discipline of medicine for the public good."[36]

The characterization of the early Academy as "a club for the medical elite" which Dr. Williams changed to "an instrument de-

voted to the science of medicine and to the public good" is undoubtedly too sharply drawn and may be considered an example
of Dr. Galdston's well-known journalistic hyperbole. Over the
years, while the Fellows were indeed the "elite" of the medical
profession who maintained the collegiality characteristic of such
"learned societies," their contributions to the "public good" were
no less notable in their time than those that came later. If anything,
the change may be attributed to the role played so well by Dr.
Williams as a full-time Director in organizing, expediting and facilitating the activities of the Fellows as volunteers who had other
commitments and responsibilities, and in managing the never-
ending stream of mundane problems inherent in the operations of
so complex an organization.

In 1934, Dr. John A. Hartwell, who had been the twenty-third
President of the Academy from 1929 to 1932, was appointed to
succeed Dr. Williams as Director. In 1939, he was succeeded in
turn by Dr. Herbert B. Wilcox, a prominent pediatrician whose
contributions to the Academy included a 1935–1937 term as Vice
President; he served until 1946. Under their direction, the "good
works" continued.

In 1934, the Medical Information Bureau inaugurated the very
popular series of *Lectures to the Laity* which continued each year
until 1943, attracting large audiences and much favorable attention when they were subsequently published.

In 1935, seven years of work was completed on the preparation
of *A Standard Classified Nomenclature of Disease,* which was
given over to the Council on Medical Education of the American
Medical Association for further promulgation and revision. This
publication was the forerunner of the *International Classification
of Diseases* which is extensively used around the world by hospitals, medical schools and organizations to standardize their medical record-keeping and reporting.

In 1937, the Academy successfully withstood a challenge of its
tax status from the Internal Revenue Service precipitated by provisions of the recently enacted Federal Social Security Act. In response
to the comprehensive brief prepared for the hearing by the Acad-

emy's Counsel that reviewed its activities and their significance, the Commissioner of Internal Revenue affirmed the Academy's tax-exempt status. This not only freed it from the potential burden of paying income taxes but, perhaps equally important, made contributions to the Academy tax-deductible to the donors.[37]

With the help of a grant from the Rockefeller Foundation, a critical study was undertaken of the handling of health information by the media. The results were made public at a Health Education Conference held in October 1940, which was attended by representatives of the medical profession, public and voluntary health agencies and the media. They affirmed the value of the Committee on Medical Information as a resource for verifying the significance and accuracy of medical information purveyed to the public.[38]

## The Academy during World War II

At the outset of America's entry into World War II in 1941, the admittedly remote, but nevertheless widely entertained, threat of a "token bombing" of New York City by German aircraft (On Thanksgiving Day 1943, a report that the German battleship *Emden,* which carried catapult-launched planes, had been sighted a hundred miles offshore in the Atlantic actually triggered the mobilization of emergency defense measures) led to the authorization of the Library to microfilm its "shelf list" while the rare books were boxed and stored in an inside area on one of the lower floors of the building. The expense of this effort created a burden for the chronically-marginal budget of the Library, and it caused considerable inconvenience to its staff.[39]

A *cause celebre* arose in 1943 when the Morland Act Commission, appointed by New York State to investigate misconduct in the administration of workers' compensation cases, accused a group of physicians, including twenty Fellows of the Academy, of such irregularities as improper billing, rebates for referrals and fee-splitting. The Committee on Professional Conduct promptly investigated. After interviewing all but the four Fellows then on active duty with the armed forces, the Committee was convinced that seven were innocent of the charges and so informed them with the admonition that, as Fellows, they must "avoid any appearance of participation in activities that might reflect unfavorably upon the standing of the Academy and the profession." There was satisfactory proof of the guilt of only two of the nine other Fellows who had been named but, nevertheless, the resignation from the Academy was requested of all of the nine who could not be cleared.[40]

Academy activities continued without interruption during the war years although meetings were difficult to arrange and attendance diminished. The 1944 Lectures to the Laity, this time a series of six sessions at two-week intervals devoted to Psychiatry in Clinical Practice, attracted an average attendance of 650. The Library continued to grow both in new books and journals and in usage, and in 1946, the Friends of the Rare Book Room was organized to promote support for new acquisitions.

In 1942, the Council authorized the creation of a standing committee, later named the Committee on Medicine and the Changing Order, to study how medicine would be affected by and respond to the "economic and social changes that are taking place now and that are clearly forecast for the immediate future." In preparation for its more than 120 meetings, it commissioned and published (with funding from the Commonwealth Fund) a dozen valuable monographs on various aspects and fields of medical services. Its report, which appeared in 1947, just in time for the centennial of the Academy, cited the futility of viewing medical care as an isolated phenomenon, emphasizing instead the importance of considering it as a part of everyday living. It offered a large number of far-reaching recommendations on "a multiplicity of problems of varying geographical, social, economic and educational circumstances."[41]


## THE FIRST HUNDRED YEARS

In its first hundred years (1847 to 1946), the Academy may be said to have experienced three major organizational task and structural orientations. The first orientation was in place from 1847 to 1890. During this period, the environment in which the Academy was founded, and in which it played a major role, had the following features: the scientific basis of medicine was minimal but on the verge of transformation, while the medical elite waged a battle both against medical sectarians and for sanitary and public health reforms in New York City. This period saw the beginning of the Library, and the first efforts to establish a permanent physical home for the Academy. There was no salaried staff, all activities being carried out by the purely voluntary participation of the members. The Academy served as an instrument of elite physicians and by encouraging the pooling of library resources, by sharing and transmitting new medical information, and by participating in addressing such public health-related problems as housing, milk supplies and sanitation, it made important contributions toward improving the status of physicians and, at the same time, was a major force for civic betterment in the City.

The second orientation, which lasted from 1890 to 1925, coincided with the flowering of modern medical science and the reform and expansion of medical education. Thanks to support from private philanthropy, the Academy was able to supplement its reliance on the participation of Fellows as unpaid volunteers with the hiring of full-time employees to serve as Librarian and as Executive Secretary of the newly-formed Committee on Public Health. The creation of this Committee was significant in that it served as an effective mechanism to transmit information and recommendations on public health problems to public officials and the public at large, thus enhancing the visibility of the Academy. And its organization as a standing committee with a permanent, salaried staff person as Executive Secretary provided a model for facilitating the participation of the Fellows in an expanding range of activities that continued to grow more significant and far-reaching.

The third orientation began in 1925 with the appointment of Linsly R. Williams as the first full-time Director and the move to the Academy's current home on Fifth Avenue and 103rd Street, the construction of which he had so largely engineered. This move and the rapid growth of Academy activities in range and importance was made possible by large gifts from the Rockefeller, Carnegie and other foundations, which not only paid for the building, but also created the endowment whose income has covered a major portion of the Academy's operating budget. Continuing support in the form of contributions, grants and bequests has made it possible for the Academy to achieve its mission as a force for improvements in medical education, public health and the provision of health care. And, as in the very beginning, it has been the interest, devotion and hard work of the Fellows in the various committees and sections, now with the help of the staff, that solidified the reputation of the Academy locally in New York City and its environs, nationally and abroad.

## NOTES

1 Baatz S. 1990 *Knowledge, Culture, and Science: The New York Academy of Sciences.* New York: The New York Academy of Sciences pp. 4–5.
2 Homburger E. 1994 *Scenes from the Life of a City: Corruption and Conscience in Old New York.* New Haven: Yale University Press.
3 Haller JS, Jr. 1994 *Medical Protestants: The Eclectics in American Medicine.* Carbondale, IL: Southern Illinois University Press. pp. 56–57.
4 Walsh JJ. 1919 *History of Medicine in New York: Three Centuries of Medical Progress.* New York: National Americana Society. Vol. 3, p. 676.
5 Van Ingen P. 1949 *The New York Academy of Medicine: Its First Hundred Years.* New York: Columbia University Press. p. 4.
6 ibid. p. 5.
7 ibid. p. 6.
8 Rothstein WG. 1972 *American Physicians in the Nineteenth Century: From Sects to Science.* Baltimore: Johns Hopkins University Press. p. 202.
9 Van Ingen, P. op. cit. pp. 7–8.
10 ibid. p. 10.
11 ibid. p. 9.
12 ibid. p. 11.

13 ibid. p. 13.

14 ibid. p. 10.

15 ibid. p. 14.

16 King, LS. 1991 *Transformations in American Medicine. Baltimore: Johns Hopkins University Press.* p. 210.

17 Van Ingen, P. op. cit. p. 17.

18 ibid. p. 22.

19 Calhoun DH. 1965 *Professional Lives in America.* Cambridge, MA: Harvard University Press. p. 46.

20 Van Ingen, P. op. cit. pp. 75–76.

21 ibid. pp. 58–59.

22 Homburger. op. cit. pp. 57ff.

23 Van Ingen, P. op. cit. pp. 115–116.

24 ibid. pp. 155–161.

25 Rothstein. op. cit. p. 302.

26 Garrison FH. 1929 *An Introduction to the History of Medicine, 4th Edition.* Philadelphia: WB Saunders Company. p. 443.

27 Van Ingen, P. op. cit. p. 261.

28 ibid. pp. 272–273.

29 ibid. pp. 333–339.

30 ibid. pp. 408–411.

31 ibid. pp. 411–412.

32 ibid. p. 383.

33 ibid. pp. 434–435.

34 ibid. pp. 394–395.

35 ibid. p. 452.

36 Galdston I. 1985 Memorial tribute to Linsly R. Williams, MD, 1875–1934. *Bulletin of the New York Academy of Medicine.* 61:393–394.

37 Van Ingen, P. op. cit. p.485.

38 ibid. pp. 493–494.

39 ibid. p. 505.

40 ibid. pp. 510–511.

41 ibid. pp. 529–533.

# Chapter 2
## 1947–1956
# The Centennial Through the 1950s

At the end of World War II, the people of the United States, relatively untouched by the effects of war, looked forward to the challenge of moving to a peacetime economy. Stimulating this effort were the many scientific and technological innovations that could be considered by-products of the war. On the medical front, there were such great advances as the development of sulfa drugs, the production and use of antibiotics such as penicillin, blood storage and transfusion techniques and the treatment of burns.[1] Collective bargaining during the wartime wage freeze and the strikes after the war resulted in a remarkable expansion of fringe benefits connected with employment which included a substantial expansion of employer-sponsored and, for the most part, paid-for health insurance coverage of American workers and their dependents. These benefits fueled the increase in funding for health care services, especially in hospitals.

The war solved the problem of unemployment and low personal income growth that had dogged the US economy in the 1930s. Starting in 1938, however, a conservative coalition dominated the Congress and maintained the long-lasting stalemate that prevailed in American public life. The postwar period continued the paralysis in American domestic public policy. One historian has suggested that: "From 1945 to the latter 1950s, the nation worried about the Russians and about Communists at home but was fundamentally complacent about the nature of its own society. Problems rumbled under the surface—urban decay, festering race relations, tragically costly health crises among the poor—but they were largely ignored."[2] But the postwar period would also see major transformations in the American health care establishment as a consequence of the massive infusion of resources for health services, education and research.

In this period, President Truman and his Congressional allies sought to enact a system of national health insurance to be funded under the Social Security System through the imposition of payroll taxes paid both by employers and employees. But this attempt to establish universal health insurance as a national policy could not

overcome the opposition in the Congress. At the same time, however, a bipartisan consensus was achieved on a related proposal by
President Truman that authorized federal support for the burgeon-
ing programs in hospital construction, professional training and
biomedical research.

The growth of research funding and the generous subsidization
of medical education fostered the expansion of specialty training.
This, in turn, led to remarkable developments in medical technology. The frequent changes in undergraduate and graduate medical
education and in the research arena were to have profound influences on organizations, like the Academy, which play significant
roles in providing postgraduate training and continuing medical
education programs outside the walls of hospitals and medical
schools.


## INNOVATION AND ORGANIZATIONAL BEHAVIOR

The historian, Henry Adams, said: "Innovation was the most useful purpose which New York could serve in human interests, and
never was a city better fitted for its work."[3] In their classic study of
New York politics, Sayre and Kaufman echoed Adams' comment
about innovation in New York City suggesting that "change continues to be a hallmark of the city. The rapidity and extent of
change helps to keep the diversity of the city from declining."[4]

The Academy is a unique organization in the health field, the
existence of which is an embodiment of Adams's tribute to the
innovative spirit of New York City. Its creation and continued
existence were made possible only by the wealth of talent and the
richness and diversity of material resources in the City. Repeatedly,
when changes in the environment confronted the Academy with
threats to its meaningful survival, its energetic and talented leadership was able to develop new strategies that would renew its vitality while mustering the material resources needed to implement
them, thus enabling the organization to stay the course.

While other institutions in New York City and elsewhere began to undertake roles that the Academy had filled in the past, the Academy met the challenge by venturing onto new paths that would renovate its spirit and energize its programs. However, it never diminished its commitment to contribute to human betterment through education of health professionals and the public about public health, medical practice and health-related affairs, through advocacy that would advance the public weal, and through preserving and strengthening medical ethics. Without question, health-related institutions and organizations, supplemented by the knowledge and skills of the health professions, have had great potential for contributing to the enhancement of human well-being. From its inception, the Academy has been well-positioned to provide the leadership in transforming that potential into human betterment.

In responding to its changing environment, The Academy has had to periodically reexamine what James Q. Wilson, the noted student of politics and bureaucracy, has labeled "its critical organizational tasks" which he has defined as "behaviors which, if successfully performed by key organizational members, would enable the organization to manage its critical environmental problem."[5]

Wilson focused on public bureaucracies, but his analysis is also useful in the study of nongovernmental organizations such as businesses and not-for-profit entities like the Academy. In explaining why he uses the term, "tasks," rather than "goals," he commented that organizations "are likely to have general, vague, or inconsistent goals about which clarity and agreement can only occasionally be obtained."[6] To attempt to define goals specifically may result either in "meaningless verbiage or deep disagreements."

While acknowledging that tasks must often be defined in terms of goals, Wilson noted that the latter are usually not connected in the straightforward way that is implied by the notion that tasks denote "means" logically related to "ends."[7]

It is not enough to define an organization's critical tasks appropriately, Wilson said. To be successful, there must be a widespread endorsement of that definition. When that can be achieved, the organization may be described as having a "sense of mission."

Obtaining such an endorsement from the Academy's members

and staff is not always easy. All of the Fellows are affiliated with other institutions, agencies and organizations, some of which may have overlapping or even competing objectives. Many are too preoccupied with their daily activities to be able to devote the requisite time and energy to the areas on which the Academy is focusing. As a result, as in most voluntary organizations, virtually every issue is debated by a larger or smaller cadre of proponents and an even smaller number of dissenters, while the majority of the members remain silent. Involving that majority in the debate is a major challenge to the skills in communication and statesmanship of the leadership group; failure to do so risks engendering a sense of alienation and the divisive feeling that a small group of "insiders" among the members and staff is "running the show."

Obtaining endorsement of the definition of the critical tasks from outside the organization is also critical. This must be obtained from the other organizations and agencies with which the Academy must work to accomplish these tasks and, perhaps even more important, from the potential sources of the requisite financial support. Dues payments, contributions and bequests from the Academy's Fellows and friends provide a significant level of support but, even when supplemented by the income from the Academy's endowment, they have never been enough. Fortunately, dating from the grants in 1926 from the Carnegie and Rockefeller Foundations that subsidized the construction of the Academy building and created its endowment fund, the Academy's activities have won the favor of many of the philanthropic foundations interested in medical and health care issues.


CONFLICTS IN MEDICINE: SELF-ADVANCEMENT AND
THE PUBLIC GOOD

Although many of its programs benefit the entire community, it must be recalled that a substantial impetus to the creation and maintenance of organizations such as the Academy is the goal of professional success, or what Dr. Philip Van Ingen described as "motives of self-advancement not directly tied to human welfare."[8] In the late nineteenth century and well into the twentieth, new occupational specialties were emerging, a trend that was also true in medicine and health, with goals that included "modernizing their professions and enjoying newly acquired prestige."[9] .... "In the postwar period one answer in defining the role of the individual in American society was for the individual to learn the rules of the modern occupational system, abide by them and succeed."[10] The Academy played a role in helping physicians do precisely that.

The cleavages in medicine at the time the Academy was founded in 1847 were based on battles between regular physicians and irregular practitioners, and within the ranks of the regulars between those who had established practices and those who sought to compete through publicity about their "cures" or public quarreling about the efficacy of particular remedies. In the post–World War II period, there were also divisions in medicine. As a result of changes in technology, knowledge and social organization, a variety of cleavages emerged within the profession, including differences between surgeons and cognitive physicians (physicians who talk with their patients rather than performing procedures), between doctors working in group practices and salaried positions and those in solo fee-for-service practice, and between full-time and part-time practitioners in academic institutions. These cleavages were reflected in differing views on the role of government, on national health insurance, and on the organization of medical services.

Most physicians in the late 1940s and 1950s were suspicious of big organizations, whether public or private. They welcomed the growth in private individual and group health insurance which helped a large proportion of the population to pay its health care bills, but they looked with dismay on efforts to design a government program that would provide universal coverage. But, there were some physicians who differed from organized medicine in their views of the role of government with respect to those without financial protection against the costs of health care. The health care financing proposal of Senator Robert Wagner of New York, Senator

James Murray of Montana and Representative John Dingell of Michigan, which was endorsed by President Truman, called for the federal government to use the Social Security System to provide a package of hospital and medical benefits comparable to those provided by the most generous Blue Cross and Blue Shield plans. It would be funded by payroll taxes, and there would be freedom of choice of physicians who would continue to be paid on a fee-for-service basis. Thus, the federal government would play a major role in paying for health services.

This expanded role of government was similar to those that had been emerging in varying patterns in the western democracies since World War II in which, in effect, the population is guaranteed health care as a right of citizenship. The medical profession would continue to have a major say in how they would be paid and regulated, and would participate through their professional organizations in negotiations about the level of payment and other material issues. Under the Truman proposal, fee-for-service practice would be preserved and physicians who participated in the program would have been assured a continuing flow of income.

While the Academy's leadership has taken justifiable pride in the fact that its influence is more than local, the major arena for the Academy's activities has been New York City. The pattern of the relationships with the City agencies was characterized, especially in the 1940s and 1950s by heavy reliance of these agencies on the support of a variety of non-governmental groups in which the Academy figured prominently. The Academy participated as part of all three of the clientele groups delineated by Sayre and Kaufman: "associations" of persons served or regulated by the given agency; "professional groups" from whose ranks the agency's dominant professional personnel are drawn; and "functional groups" whose social or economic activities parallel those of the agency."[11]

During the 1940s, the Academy played a particularly important role in providing assistance to the two City agencies primarily involved in health care: the Department of Health and the Department of Hospitals. This relationship which, as noted earlier, began with the role of the Academy in forming the Metropolitan Health

Board, the precursor of the Department of Health, became somewhat tenuous during the 1950s and 1960s but began to revive somewhat in the 1980s and really burgeoned in the 1990s. While relationships with the State's health-related agencies were never as intense as those with the City agencies, the Academy has provided a warm and productive collaboration over the last fifty years.

## THE ACADEMY AT THE TIME OF ITS CENTENNIAL

To commemorate the Academy's hundredth birthday, the *New York Times* said in an editorial: "To the city as a whole, this centenary assumes the character of a public celebration. And with reason. From the day of its creation, the Academy has been more than a body of physicians who meet periodically to discuss questions of purely professional importance. There has never been a lack of science at these meetings, but what endears the Academy to citizens is the sense of social responsibility it has always manifested. The health of the community has been a major concern, and that concern has been expressed not only in giving advice during epidemics and other emergencies but in educating the public and the medical profession on which that public relies for service."[12]

At the time of its centennial in 1947, the Academy, located in the beautiful building on Fifth Avenue and 103rd Street that had been erected in 1926, had an active membership of 2,463 Fellows (1,846 Resident Fellows, including 200 who had paid dues for thirty years and were now exempt, 516 Non-resident, Associate and Research Fellows, 81 Corresponding Fellows, and 20 Honorary Fellows). Its constitution, which had been last revised in 1940, stated that its purpose was the "advancement of the science and art of medicine, the maintenance of a public medical library, and the promotion of public health and medical education."[13]

The officers included a President elected for two years, three Vice Presidents whose three year terms were staggered so that one retired each year, and a Secretary and Treasurer each elected for three years. There were two governing bodies: a Board of Trustees and a Council (this bicameral structure was to be scrapped in 1990). The Board of Trustees consisted of the President, Secretary and Treasurer and ten Trustees, each serving five years with two retiring each year. The Trustees were responsible for the finances, invested funds, personal and real estate property of the Academy, and had to approve all expenditures.[14]

The Council, composed of the six officers, the ten Trustees, and the chairs of the six standing committees, was responsible for overseeing the management of the Academy, for the formulation of its policies, and for approval of its formal position statements. The Board of Trustees and the Council often met jointly.

The day-to-day administration was the responsibility of the Director, a full-time salaried position established in 1924. The Director reported to the Council and to the Board of Trustees.

The Academy's endowment had reached $4.5 million by the end of 1946 and was producing an annual income of approximately $336,000, almost four times the revenue from membership dues which totaled $88,750.[15]

There were six statutory standing committees. The Committee on Library, established in 1875, provides oversight of the operations of the Library. Like the Committees on Public Health, Medical Education, Sections, and Medical Information, its members are recommended by the Director and appointed by the President with the concurrence of the Council. The members of the Committee on Admissions are elected by the Academy Fellowship; they investigate the ethical, personal and professional qualifications of candidates for Fellowship who have been nominated by an active Fellow and endorsed by two others. When the Committee approves the application, the election is made by the Council.

The Director at the time of the centennial was Dr. Howard Reid Craig who had assumed that position just a few months earlier and was to hold it for twenty years. He was a pediatrician affiliated with Babies Hospital where Dr. Herbert B. Wilcox, his predecessor as Director, had been his Chief of Service and had recommended him for the Academy position. Dr. Craig had been active in Academy activities since his election as a Fellow in 1927 having served as a

Section Secretary and Section Chairman and, since 1942, as Chairman of the Committee on Library.

Dr. Craig was a native New Yorker. While studying for the ministry as a postgraduate student at Wesleyan University, he obtained a job tending the furnace in the home of a local physician who became fond of him and took him on his rounds. This experience led Dr. Craig to change to a career in medicine. His graduation from Cornell University School of Medicine in 1919 was followed by an internship at Memorial Hospital and residencies at Bellevue and Babies Hospitals. In 1922, he entered the private practice of pediatrics on the east side of Manhattan. Through his successful practice and his extensive involvement in both professional and civic affairs, especially the Citizen's Committee for Children, he established relationships with the most affluent and influential New Yorkers, including several mayors and their Commissioners of both Health and Hospitals. It was the development of a painful arthritis that led him to give up his active practice and accept the appointment as Director of the Academy. The arthritis improved and, in 1966, in memorializing his twenty years of service in that position, Dr. Robert L. Levy, a former President of the Academy, suggested that "perhaps the quieter and more regular life at the Academy played a role in his cure."[16] The fact that Dr. Craig considered the Directorship of the Academy to be less stressful than practice as a pediatrician provides some indication of the pace and demands of the Academy operations at that time.

In October 1951, Dr. Craig summarized his views on the role of the Director. As the person responsible to the Council for administration, "He must know what every department is doing, what its problems are, and with what effectiveness it is operating. The work of each department must be coordinated with each of the others so that there is no duplication of effort or clashing of interests or enthusiasms. To accomplish this, he must attend every meeting of every committee. In other words, he must be part of every Academy activity without putting himself in the position of attempting to direct or control these activities. Initiative and imagination on the part of the Fellows of the Academy and the staff have been the most important factors in its growth and strength. Since the Director is concerned with expenditures and finances, he must have knowledge of programs to justify their expense and see to it that the Academy's capital is invested optimally. The second function of the Director is to develop relationships with medicine and with the world outside of medicine, ranging from government to industry, unions, philanthropic organizations and social agencies. The last function of the Director is to visualize the future and the Academy's needs."[17]

In his address, Dr. Craig saw the Academy as having three prime interests: "(1) medical education, aimed particularly at the practicing physician but covering other professional levels and the lay public; (2) a working library of the first magnitude; (3) public health and welfare of the community. These objectives were clearly stated by the founders of the Academy in 1847 and throughout the years, to the credit of the Fellows, they have remained and are today the fundamental objectives of the New York Academy of Medicine."[17]

The charge to the Director of coordinating Academy activities was not without problems. As the management consulting firm of Cresap, McCormick and Paget pointed out in 1957 when they studied the Academy's administration, while the By-laws specified that the Director is responsible for supervising and coordinating all activities, there was no clear-cut definition of that role. They reported that "the present organizational structure, which provides that certain administrative officers are primarily responsible to the standing committees, reduces the administrative authority of the Director and limits the effectiveness of his coordinating actions."[18]

In the first ten years of Dr. Craig's tenure as Director, a distinguished group had positions of leadership on the Academy's staff. It included: Edwin H. L. Corwin, Ph.D., long-time Executive Secretary of the Committee on Public Health who retired in 1952 after forty-one years of service, and Dr. Harold K. Kruse who succeeded him; Dr. Iago Galdston, who had been Executive Secretary of the Medical Information Bureau since its founding in 1928 and continued in that role when it became the standing Committee on Medical Information in 1938; and Dr. Mahlon Ashford who served simultaneously as Executive Secretary of the Committee on Medical Education and as Editor of the *Bulletin* from 1936 to 1951 and was followed in both of these positions by Dr. Robert L. Craig, the brother of Dr. Howard Reid Craig. Dr. Archibald Malloch, who retired in 1949 after serving for more than twenty years as Librarian, was followed in that position by Ms. Janet Doe who, in 1956, was succeeded in turn by Ms. Gertrude Annan, all three of whom had international reputations as leading medical librarians.

## THE LIBRARY

In 1947, the Library with over 252,000 bound volumes and occupying a good part of the space in the Academy building, was the second largest medical library in the country, exceeded in size and influence only by the Surgeon General's Library, now known as the National Library of Medicine. With ample justification, Dr. Howard Reid Craig called it "our greatest material heritage and treasure."[19] It was also the most significant item in the Academy's budget. It was open to the public, although only Fellows and certain paid subscribers had borrowing privileges.

The Librarian was Dr. Archibald Malloch who had seen its collection of books almost double since his appointment in 1935. When forced to retire because of ill health in 1949, he was succeeded by Ms. Janet Doe who had joined the Library in 1926 and was formally appointed Assistant Librarian in 1929. A native of Vermont, Ms. Doe graduated from Wellesley College and after nurses' training at the Vassar Camp for Nurses and experience as a nurse at Presbyterian Hospital in New York City, she received certification as a librarian from the New York Public Library Training School.[20]

In 1936, Ms. Doe was succeeded by Ms. Gertrude L. Annan, a graduate of Brown University who had worked in the John Carter Brown Library. Ms. Annan had joined the Library staff in 1929 as Head of the Rare Book Room; she became Associate Librarian in 1933.[21]

It is well recognized that, in the sequence of Archibald Malloch, Janet Doe and Gertrude Annan, the Academy Library was led by persons regarded by their peers as giants in their field. Under their creative leadership, with support by the administration, staff and Fellows of the Academy and help from a number of public and private organizations and individuals, the Library became one of the great cultural institutions in New York and the nation. It is not only an important source of medical and scientific information that is particularly valuable to students of history, clinical medicine, public health and health policy, but its Rare Book Room is a veritable museum packed with rare bibliographic treasures and medical artifacts—it even has a remarkable collection of cookbooks.

Early in the nineteenth century, relying on the availability of the Academy Library to the public, the New York Public Library stopped adding to its own medical collection and, in 1949, turned over its collection of some 22,000 medical volumes to the Academy. Since that time, the Library has been the only medical reference source open to the public in the metropolitan area.

In 1946, in a move that has led to accelerated growth of the Library's historical collections, Dr. Malloch persuaded Drs. Alfred M. Hellman and Frederic D. Zeman to create the Friends of the Rare Book Room. The first President of the Friends, Dr. Fenwick Beekman, also served as President of the New York Historical Society which, in 1948, in conjunction with the Brooklyn Museum, presented the Edwin Smith Surgical Papyrus to the Academy. Dr. Malloch is credited as being "largely responsible for rousing the interest of Dr. Fenwick Beekman, through whose efforts that valuable accession was acquired."[22]

The Edwin Smith Papyrus, perhaps the most valuable medical relic from Ancient Egypt, had been acquired by Edwin Smith in Thebes in 1862 and was later presented by his daughter to the New York Historical Society whence it came to the Academy. A roll over fifteen feet long, dated 1600 BC, it was presumably copied from a treatise originally written a thousand years earlier. It is written on both sides in cursive script. The front presents forty-nine cases in clinical surgery including sword gashes, fractures and blunt injuries, each presented in a formalized style that is remarkable similar to the format used in modern medical journals. The back offers incantations against "pestilential winds" and for the rejuvenation of old men.[23] Its value is incalculable. It is only one of the treasures ensconced in the Library's collections.

### Growth of the Library

In retracing the growth of the Library, Ms. Doe said,

Seldom could a physician buy all the books he needed. The solution lay in a pooling of individual funds and libraries to form one good collection from which all could satisfy their needs. Growing slowly at first, the Academy's little group of volumes waxed from a few hundred volumes to a few thousand. Then, an occasional large gift stimulated others—the first such major gift was that of Dr. Samuel Purple Smith in 1875—and when once a sizable collection was established, it attracted further legacies and donations. The Medical Journal Association and the New York Hospital Library, one of the largest and best-stocked in the City, were deposited here. Innumerable physicians gave their large and small stocks to swell the total through the years. By the turn of the century, 50,000 volumes had been accumulated, and the New York Public Library began to rely on this institution to meet the needs of the public instead of building up its own collection, capping its trust in this respect two years ago [1950] by making over to the Academy Library all of its medical books. Thus, to all intents and purposes, the Academy Library serves as the public medical library of New York City. And it is glad to do so, for it has received much from New York citizens and institutions, even through it is privately supported and receives no public funds.[24]

Ms. Doe also said, "The possession of an outstanding accumulation of the scientific literature brings with it a certain obligation to see that its resources are available to those who need them. It has extended its general services as far as seems justifiable on a free basis, but some unavoidably on a paid non-profit basis. Further, it has believed wholeheartedly in the practice of mutual help among libraries as the surest way to advance the interests of all. By assistance to and from each other, the ability of libraries to give better service has been increased."[25]

The commitment to community service was not without costs. Ms. Annan pointed to the changed environment confronting the Library after the war. The support of medical education and the funding of hospital construction by the federal government encouraged the development of libraries in hospitals and medical schools. Libraries everywhere were confronted with an enormous increase in the number of books and journals, accompanied by escalation of their prices.[20] The need to maintain the quality of their collections forced librarians to press for increased budget allocations. The members of the Library Committee, committed as they were to maintaining the preeminence of the Library, had no choice but to endorse such requests, thereby creating problems for those forced to contend with the Academy's perennial fiscal constraints.[21] Years later, requests for larger Library allocations were to increase further when the Library staff sought to acquire computers and software for cataloguing the collection and tracking the movement of books.

An immediate problem facing the Library was the shortage of space for the increasing number of books and journals, a problem that has recurred ever since it was founded. In 1953, several major improvements were undertaken: a balcony was built in the Periodicals Room to provide additional space for journals and for staff; and stacks were installed in the east end of the building in space that had been used as a museum and other purposes. Unfortunately, the relief provided by these renovations was short-lived and, accordingly, in 1957, the Academy hosted a meeting of medical administrators and librarians in the area out of which grew a cooperative venture for storing and retrieving medical publications which became known as the Medical Library Center of New York (*vide infra*).

## COMMITTEE ON PUBLIC HEALTH

The Committee on Public Health was originally called the Committee on Public Health Hospitals and the Budget when it was founded in 1911 and in 1926, its name was changed to the Committee on Public Health Relations. Later, it became the Committee on Public Health. It then had thirty-five members who, as for all of the standing committees at that time, were appointed each year by the President subject to approval by the Council (five Committee members were designated as the official delegates of the five New York City county medical societies). A large measure of the success of this Committee may be credited to the work of Dr. Edward H. Lewinski-Corwin, who had been appointed as its salaried full-time Executive Secretary at the Committee's inception, immediately after earning a Ph.D. degree from Columbia University. Dr. Corwin had a staff of five including both professional and clerical personnel.[26] He served for forty-one years, being succeeded by Dr. Howard D. Kruse, a medical nutritionist who had earned a medical degree from Johns Hopkins University and a doctorate in chemistry from Dickinson College. Dr. Kruse served as Executive Secretary until 1968.

The Committee on Public Health functioned in three ways: first "in an advisory capacity to community representatives when guidance on a medical or public health issue is called for;" second, through "undertaking of surveys and inquiries into existing conditions;" and finally, as an "educational body which conducts conferences and issues papers for the medical profession and the community at large."[27] Dr. James Alexander Miller, the highly regarded physician who served on the Committee for more than thirty years, did not exaggerate when he said, "Largely through this Committee, the Academy has developed from a medical society to a powerful civic institution."[28]

During the course of its history, the Committee undertook numerous studies relating to public health and frequently acted as an advisor to public and private health agencies. The Committee's reports and recommendations contributed to the reform of the New York City Board of Health, the shift from a system of coroners to one featuring professionally qualified medical examiners, the reform of blood banking in the City, and the legitimization of the birth control movement. Perhaps its most important contribution was improving the welfare of mothers and children through a series of studies and recommendations on neonatal deaths and prenatal care that included, among others, *Infant and Maternal Care in New York City*, published in 1952 by the Columbia University Press. In no small measure, the acceptance of the Committee's recommendations over the years may be attributed to the participation in its activities of such internationally acclaimed leaders in public health as Dr. Hermann M. Biggs, the General Health Officer in the New York City Department of Health from 1902 to 1914 and New York State Health Commissioner from 1914 to 1923, Dr. S. S. Goldwater, the long-time Superintendent and Director of the Mt. Sinai Hospital who served the City as Commissioner of Health from 1914 to 1915 and as Commissioner of Hospitals from 1934 to 1940 (The Goldwater Memorial Hospital on Roosevelt Island in the East River is named after him), and Dr. Haven Emerson, Dean of the Columbia University School of Public Health and Administrative Medicine, who also served as the City's Commissioner of Health and as a member of the Board of Health.

Between 1947 and 1957, the Committee addressed the problem of drug abuse and addiction repeatedly. It sponsored well-attended conferences on this subject in 1951 and 1952 and, in a report issued in 1955, it emphasized the concept that drug addiction is an illness which deserves treatment by physicians. The Committee opposed a federal legislative proposal that would have imposed draconian penalties on persons supplying drugs to minors and second offenders. In place of this legislation, which was not enacted, it offered a six-point program which included a provision to take the profit out of illicit drug sales by furnishing addicts with drugs under federal control while the addict is encouraged to accept treatment, reliance on education to prevent addiction, the provision of medical treatment to addicts, epidemiological studies of addiction, and stringent punishment of nonaddict drug dealers.[29]

In 1943, and again in 1955, the Committee issued comprehensive reports on the abuse of barbiturates that included recommendations for stricter controls over the distribution and retail sales of these drugs. These were later embodied in legislation enacted by the State.[30]

In 1948, after the infamous smog emergency in Donora, Pennsylvania, which caused the severe illness of 43 percent of the inhabitants of that area, the Committee addressed the problem of air pollution. It supported a City Council measure proposing the creation of a Bureau of Smoke Control in the Department of Housing and Buildings, and it also urged the Department of Health to maintain control over noxious fumes in the City.[31]

The Committee also addressed problems presented by the blood supply in the City. In 1948, it issued recommendations supporting the creation of blood transfusion clinics in the City's hospitals and, in 1956, initiated a comprehensive study of all aspects of the problem of blood supply in New York City that led to the establishment of the Community Blood Council in 1958, which later became the New York City Blood Center.[32]

The problem of alcoholism was a perennial area of concern to the Committee. It sponsored a major conference on that topic in 1947 in which it emphasized that alcoholism is a medical problem and advocated the establishment of special clinics to deal with it. The Committee also collaborated with the Council on Problems in Alcoholism in urging the adoption of a comprehensive solution to this problem that would include developing an organized effort to treat this disease; persuading more voluntary hospitals and physicians to become involved in its treatment; and expanding treatment facilities, including psychiatric and social services.[33]

During this period, the Committee was well served by its Chairmen: Drs. James Alexander Miller (1942–1948), George Baehr (1949–1953), Harry S. Mustard (1954), and Frederick R. Bailey (1955–1958).

COMMITTEE ON MEDICAL EDUCATION

In 1949, Dr. George Baehr, then President of the Academy, summarized its role in medical education by noting that, "The Academy has endeavored to contribute to the continuing education of the physician through its Library, through the monthly meetings of its eleven clinical and scientific Sections, and through the work of its Committee on Medical Education."[34]

The Committee on Medical Education was created in 1924 by uniting two separate organizations concerned with promoting and publicizing opportunities for postgraduate medical education: the Society for Advancement of Clinical Study in New York, established in 1912 to publicize clinics and medical meetings in New York City; and the New York Association for Medical Education, a group concerned with postgraduate medical study that was formed in 1919. The Executive Secretary was Dr. Mahlon Ashford who came to the Academy in 1937 after retiring from the Army Medical Corps; he served through 1951. He also served as Editor of the *Bulletin*. He was succeeded in both positions by Dr. Robert L. Craig, an obstetrician and gynecologist who was the younger brother of Dr. Howard Reid Craig, and who served until 1959. Dr. Craig was succeeded in turn by Dr. Aims C. McGuiness, the former Dean of the University of Pennsylvania Graduate School of Medicine who had served in the US Department of Health, Education and Welfare during the Eisenhower administration. Dr. McGuiness served until 1966.

The Office of Medical Education, another name for the staff of the Committee, organized and coordinated lectures and conferences sponsored by the Academy, conducted studies of special problems relating to postgraduate medical education, and coordinated the large variety of educational programs developed by the specialty Sections. It also had administrative responsibility for the various scholarships, research fellowships and other grants provided by the Academy.[35]

The Academy's Centennial occurred during a critical era in medical education. The undergraduate curriculum was being overhauled in most of the nation's medical schools while internships and residencies were being revised and lengthened to accommodate the demand for more intensive training in the medical specialties and subspecialties. Advances in medical science and technology developed during the years of World War II were being introduced into daily use, while physicians returning from military service were seeking refresher courses and retraining as they returned to civilian practice. As part of the Centennial celebration, the Committee conducted a comprehensive three-day conference that examined medical education from the preparation of high school and college premedical students to postgraduate and continuing medical education.[36]

For some years, two features of the Committee's activities, the series of Friday Afternoon Lectures and the annual Graduate Fortnight, had enjoyed great popularity and attracted large audiences. The weekly lectures, inaugurated in 1927, included state-of-the-art reviews of clinical topics aimed at active practitioners and presented by prominent experts, many of whom came from out of town, while the Graduate Fortnights, inaugurated in the following year, offered more comprehensive reviews of significant discrete areas of medicine. For example, the Twentieth Graduate Fortnight in 1947 covered *Diseases of Metabolism and of the Endocrine Glands* while the Twenty-sixth Graduate Fortnight in 1951 reviewed *Disorders of the Circulatory System*. Six mornings during each of the two weeks were devoted to lectures and panel discussions presented in the Academy building where exhibits and displays were available for viewing, while the afternoons were devoted to a series of clinics held at cooperating hospitals.

These events drew large audiences until the early 1950s when competition from the local medical schools and the many teaching hospitals in the New York area resulted in a gradual decline in attendance. Accordingly, in 1952, the Friday Afternoon Lectures were replaced by a series of six monthly Panels on Therapeutics, and in 1957 the Graduate Fortnight was reduced to a one-week program called the Postgraduate Week.[37]

In 1952, the Academy discontinued publication of the bulletins which, since their inauguration in 1912 by the Bureau of Clinical Information of the Society for the Advancement of Clinical Study, had listed operative clinics and other programs at local hospitals for the benefit of physicians from the City and elsewhere who might wish to attend them.

## Academy Sections

From its very beginning, the Academy has been organized into Sections, each focusing on a particular medical specialty or discipline. Fellows are free to become members of as many Sections as they wish, and the Section meetings are usually open without a fee to all who may be interested in attending. Each Section elects a chairperson, a vice-chairperson, and members of an advisory council who provide the leadership in organizing its activities. Originally, the Sections were coordinated by the Committee on Sections but this was given over to the Committee on Medical Education. The eleven Sections active in 1947 were Dermatology and Syphilology, Genito-Urinary Surgery (now Urology), Historical and Cultural Medicine (now Historical Medicine), Medicine, Neurology and Psychiatry, Obstetrics and Gynecology, Ophthalmology, Orthopedic Surgery, Pediatrics, and Surgery. In 1948, a Section on Microbiology was added. At the time of the Centennial, as noted by Dr. McGuiness, each Section was holding eight scientific meetings each year but, with the decline in attendance during the early 1950s, that number was reduced to five.

## Medical Television

As a means of attracting a larger audience to its medical education programs, the Academy, largely through the efforts of Dr. McGuiness, undertook a significant exploration of the use of television. In 1949, during the 22nd Annual Graduate Fortnight, a demonstration of the radiological examination of the gastrointestinal tract performed at the Presbyterian Hospital was transmitted by closed-circuit television to an audience at the Academy. In the following year, the Graduate Fortnight featured a series of three programs in which surgical procedures being performed at St. Clare's Hospital by surgeons from a number of participating hospitals were telecast to conference rooms in the basement of St. Clare's Hospital.

Following these demonstrations of the feasibility of this type of programming, Dr. Howard Reid Craig sent a letter to the FCC (Federal Communications Commission) on behalf of the Academy urging that agency to allocate 20 percent of its channels to educational television. Dr. Alfred Angrist, a Fellow from Queens, proposed to the Committee that the Academy go further and request the FCC to make specific allocations of TV channels to medical education. In 1952, Dr. Angrist was named Chairman of an Interim Subcommittee on Television, one of whose goals was to persuade New York Governor Thomas E. Dewey to add a person familiar with medical education to his recently established Committee on Educational Television. In January 1953, at a public hearing of the Temporary State Commission on the Use of Television for Educational Purposes, Dr. Angrist suggested that the State support medical television but in its report that Commission opposed the use of State funds for any form of educational television.

Later that year, however, WOR telecast sessions of the Graduate Fortnight on the technique of sternal bone marrow puncture using open-circuit, scrambled-image television, the first time that technique was used for medical television. The programs originated at the station and were shown on special receivers at the Academy.

An attempt in 1957 to procure funding for several medical programs on WPIX failed but, starting in 1962, many medical programs produced by the Academy were telecast by WNYC-TV, the ultrahigh-frequency station of the Municipal Broadcasting System.

Committee on Medical Information

The Committee on Medical Information, the forerunner of the current Committee on Medicine in Society, was founded in 1939 by converting the Bureau of Medical Information into a standing committee. It continued to disseminate information on developments in medicine to the public through print and broadcast media, and to provide a resource for media people reporting on medical news. It also began to concern itself with the social aspects of medicine and, in 1960, its name was changed to the Committee on Special Studies, and finally, in 1964, it assumed its present name, the Committee on Medicine in Society.

Its first Executive Secretary, Dr. Iago Galdston, who achieved worldwide recognition as a medical journalist, was largely responsible for its multidisciplinary orientation. Many years later, in presenting him with the Academy Plaque for 1983, Dr. Duncan W. Clark, then President said, "No one else in its history has told the story of what transpires at the Academy, or so widely, or has done so through the use of so many media, and in so many sophisticated ways."[38]

Lectures to the Laity

Continuation of the Lectures to the Laity, the popular series of meetings for the public, was a major activity of the Committee. Presented monthly except during the summer, each series was assembled into a volume that was published at the end of the year. For example, the thirteenth series presented in 1947–1948 was entitled *Perspectives in Medicine* and was intended to "present in an instructive and perforce in a somewhat optimistic light, current prospects in science. Without attempting to play the prophet, it is our aim, using present knowledge as evidence, to show what the future holds with both the possibility and the promise of reasonable and substantial scientific progress and social improvement. There is good psychological warrant for this approach, for there is far too much gloom about the future and too widespread a feeling that science is a 'menace' in that it places in our hands powers which we seem not wise enough to use constructively."[39]

The quality of the lectures and the eminence of the speakers are demonstrated by the inclusion of *The Atom in Civil Life* by Admiral Lewis L. Strauss, a prominent member of the US Atomic Energy Commission, and *The Inter-relation of Pure and Applied Science in the Field of Medicine* by Dr. James B. Conant, President of Harvard University.

### Other Activities

Another important ongoing activity of the Committee was the annual Eastern States Health Conference, later called the Annual Health Conference. Inaugurated in 1935 and aimed at an audience of health educators and public health officials, these conferences were originally focused on health education, but later their scope was expanded to include social and political issues in health care. The proceedings were first published as separate bound volumes but later they appeared in the *Bulletin*.

An important program on *Ministry and Medicine in Human Relationships* was conducted in 1951, and in 1953, the Committee presented the first of its Institutes on Medical History, a conference on *The Utility and Value of Medical History* that featured as participants such noted medical historians as Owsei Temkin, George Rosen, Edwin H. Ackerknecht and Gregory Zilboorg.

The Committee also arranged symposia to celebrate signal medical anniversaries. These included the 1954 commemoration of the 1,000th anniversary of Avicenna (Ibn Sina), the Baghdad physician whose voluminous medical writings became the fountainhead of medical information during the Middle Ages, the 100th birthday of Paul Ehrlich in 1954, and the 100th birthday of Sigmund Freud in 1956. The proceedings of the Committee's 1951 and 1954 Arden House Conferences on *Panic and Morale,* cosponsored by the Josiah Macy Jr. Foundation became widely read publications.[40]

And, in 1955, in collaboration with the Commonwealth Fund, the Committee undertook a project labeled *"Whither Medicine?"* in which a special committee of sixteen Fellows and invited guests reviewed a broad range of issues ranging from the economics of medical practice to the uses of leisure.

Despite the changes in the name of the Committee and the abandonment of its original role as a source of medical information, the Committee, as reported by Mr. Harry Becker, its Executive Secretary from 1962 to 1967, "successfully met its charge to seek continually an understanding of the new social and economic frontiers of medical care."[41]

## ACADEMY PUBLICATIONS

### The *Bulletin*

The *Bulletin of the New York Academy of Medicine,* launched in 1847 as the *Transactions of the New York Academy of Medicine,* was the 219th medical periodical to be established in the US, but only a few of these have survived through to the 1960s. This makes the *Bulletin* one of the ten oldest medical journals in the country, a list headed by the *New England Journal of Medicine.* Publication of the *Bulletin* was interrupted in 1901 and was resumed in 1925.[42]

In 1937, almost ninety years after it was established, Dr. Mahlon Ashford, who was also Executive Secretary of the Committee on Medical Education, was named the first Editor of the *Bulletin.* He served until 1953, when, as noted earlier, he was succeeded simultaneously in both positions by Dr. Robert L. Craig. During this period, the *Bulletin* was a nonspecialist periodical covering all aspects of medicine. Articles covered a broad range of topics, from medical history, public health and clinical experience to reports of complex laboratory research. Access to the wealth of high quality material presented at the Graduate Fortnights, Stated Meetings, and the Sections' programs as well as the other events at the Academy made the *Bulletin* an impressive journal. It became widely read, not as a repository for original research reports, but because of its reviews of clinical practices and its enlightening discussions of the social aspects of medical care.

The *Bulletin* also published items pertaining to regular Academy business such as the annual Presidential Address, the Anniversary Discourse, the names of newly elected Fellows, and formal statements or position papers approved by the Council. To augment its budget allocations, paid advertising was accepted in 1934; this was discontinued in 1971.

## History of Medicine Series

In the 1950s, the Rare Book Room began to publish a series of historically significant volumes. In addition to the Vesalius anatomical atlas described earlier, these included Bernardino Ramazzini's *Diseases of Workers,* Edgar Milton Bick's *History and Source Book of Orthopaedic Surgery,* Giovanni Maria Lancisi's *De aneurysmatibus, opus posthuman,* and Joseph Janvier Woodward's *Outlines of the Chief Camp Diseases of the United States Armies* (See Appendix for the complete list).

## Other Publications

To inform the medical community about educational opportunities, the Academy published a *Daily Surgical Bulletin,* a *Bulletin of Medical Clinics,* and a *Bulletin of Pathological Clinics, Conferences and Rounds* which listed meetings and activities in local hospitals and medical schools which they might attend. These were all discontinued in 1952. The *Gray Folder,* a semimonthly publication containing announcements of forthcoming Academy meetings was distributed to the Fellows and other interested parties; it became a monthly publication in 1949.

Annual Reports

From 1847 through 1885, the Academy reported to its members and the world through the Presidential Address delivered at the annual Stated Meeting, which contained a review of the accomplishments of the past year and plans for the future. The archives contain unpublished handwritten annual reports for the years 1862 to 1920. From 1893 through 1914, annual *Reports of the Treasurer* and, starting in 1915, more comprehensive annual reports have been published. In addition to a Balance Sheet and Financial Statements, they usually include messages from the Director, the President, and the Chairman of the Board of Trustees, lists of those to whom the Academy awards and fellowships have been presented, and a review of the major activities and the issues that were addressed during the year. In the aggregate, they constitute not only a history of the Academy, but also a panorama of changes in medicine and the society it serves.

## ACADEMY PRESIDENTS

From its inception in 1847 until 1990 (*vide infra*), the President of the Academy was elected for a term of two years and served without pay while continuing his everyday professional activities and responsibilities. He presided over meetings of the Council and the Board of Trustees and the annual Stated Meeting, and was expected to make introductory remarks to open Academy conferences, seminars and meetings. He also was obligated to give the Presidential Address at the annual Stated Meeting in which he reported on the accomplishments of the standing committees and the various sections, and outlined issues that remained to be addressed. While election to the Presidency was seen as recognition of a distinguished career as a physician and a reward for service to the Academy, it was an arduous, time-consuming and sometimes difficult role, especially for individuals with continuing personal responsibilities not readily put aside.

Through the 150 years of the Academy's existence, the Presidents, with very few exceptions, have served with grace and distinction. The Academy and medicine itself have been blessed by their contributions.

## Dr. George Baehr, 1945–1948

Dr. George Baehr, noted for his interest in the organization of the delivery of health care and as the founder of the Health Insurance Plan of Greater New York, presided over the Academy during the centennial year. He became a Fellow in 1918, and served as a member of the Committee on Medical Education from 1924 to 1927 and the Committee on Public Health from 1926 to 1941 acting as its Chairman from 1937 to 1941 and again from 1946 to 1953. He served as a Trustee from 1934–1939 and also from 1941–1945.

In his Presidential Discourse at the March 6, 1947 dinner at the Waldorf-Astoria celebrating the Centennial, Dr. Baehr extolled the Academy as an "indispensable instrument of American medicine."[43] In it, echoing what James Q. Wilson had earlier defined as the critical tasks confronting the Academy, he set forth a three-pronged agenda. First, he said, "(T)he Library must maintain its present position as the most useful and influential depository of medical and related scientific literature in the world." To achieve this, he called for the building of a new Library building and expansion of the Library staff.

Second in importance for the future, he said, is the continuing education of physicians. This would not be a major concern for the medical schools since "they are already heavily burdened with undergraduate medical training and with graduate training in the specialties."[43] On the contrary, in collaboration with them, the Academy would "serve as the centralizing agency and. . . . will assume an even more important role than heretofore in improving the educational curricula of intern and residency training." Thus, the Academy would "weld together the resources of the 65 major hospitals of this great City so as to make it the center of medical education for the physicians of this nation and of the world."

### Dr. Benjamin P. Watson, 1949–1950

Succeeding Dr. Baehr, as the forty-first President, was Dr. Benjamin P. Watson. Born in Scotland, he attended the University of St. Andrews and then the University of Edinburgh where he received his medical degree and later lectured and did research. He migrated to Canada where he became Professor of Obstetrics and Gynecology at the University of Toronto. After serving in the Canadian army during World War I, he returned to Edinburgh for a time and, in 1926 came to New York City to become Chairman of Obstetrics and Gynecology at the Columbia University College of Physicians and Surgeons, a post he held until 1946. He became a Fellow in 1928 and served on the Committees on the Library and on Awards, as Vice President from 1938 to 1940, and as a Trustee for ten years starting in 1951.

### Dr. William Barclay Parsons, 1951–1952

Dr. William Barclay Parsons, a surgeon who achieved eminence for his skill in surgery of the thyroid and parathyroids, was a graduate of Harvard University and the Columbia University College of Physicians and Surgeons. After military service in World War I, he joined the faculty of the Columbia University College of Physicians and Surgeons on which he served for almost forty years, attaining the rank of Professor of Clinical Surgery in 1949. During World War II, he served as Chief Surgical Consultant for the Southwest Pacific area. He became a Fellow in 1922, and was active in the Section on Surgery, serving as Secretary and then Chairman of that section. His term as President was followed by membership on the Board of Trustees from 1953 to 1962. From 1957 to 1959, he chaired the Committee on Academy Survey, which undertook a major effort to review the goals and functions of the Academy.

### Dr. Alexander T. Martin, 1953–1954

Dr. Alexander T. Martin, a pediatrician, was born of American parents in Ireland in 1886, attended Princeton University, and received his MD from the University of Pennsylvania Medical School. He saw military service in World War I, and later became Head of the Pediatrics Service at Roosevelt Hospital where he was elected Chairman of the Medical Board. He also served as State Chairman of the American Academy of Pediatrics. He became a Fellow in 1928, and served as Recording Secretary and as Vice President.

Dr. Martin's Inaugural Address was prominently reported in the *New York Times* for January 9, 1953 under a banner headline reading, *Doctors Warned on Medical Costs, New Head of Academy Tells Them They Must Help Plans for Paying Bills.* Drawing on the thirteen volume report on *Medicine and the Changing Order* which the Academy had published in 1947, he proposed a plan of action opposing the national health insurance plan being considered by the Congress, calling instead for the subsidization of health insurance by state and federal governments.[44]

### Dr. Edward J. Donovan, 1955–1956

Dr. Edward J. Donovan, the forty-fourth President, was born in 1889, and received his education at Hobart College and the Columbia University College of Physicians and Surgeons. He was a founding member of the American Board of Surgery and had been President of the New York Surgical Society. He was Director of Surgery at St. Luke's Hospital Center and Associate Professor of Surgery at the Columbia University College of Physicians and Surgeons. He became a Fellow in 1827 and served as Vice President from 1952 to 1954.

## ACADEMY FINANCES

At the start of the Academy's second hundred years in 1947, it had an endowment fund of $4,536,562 which produced an income of $383,396. Income from dues that year brought in $90,924. The budget for that year anticipated a deficit of $85,000 at the end of the year but that was more than made up by contributions from individuals and corporations. The successful fund-raising was attributable to a Lay Council established in 1940 with Mr. Walter S. Guilford, President of AT&T, as Chairman.

By the end of 1957, the market value of the Academy's endowment portfolio had risen to $11,667,142, but the income it produced had increased only to $424,562. Dues in 1957 brought in $115,678.

Budgeted expenditures, which had been $347,532 in 1947, almost doubled to $709,450 by 1957 but, thanks to the continuing efforts of the Lay Council, the Academy was able to remain "in the black" throughout that decade. Library expenditures accounted for more than one-third of the operating budget, while the allocations for the standing committees ranged from 21 to 23 percent of the budget. To meet these costs, the Academy's reliance on income from investments grew from 42 percent in 1947 to 59 percent in 1957, while income from dues fell from 23 percent to 16 percent. It became quite clear that without maintaining—and increasing—the endowment income and an ongoing fund-raising effort, the Academy would not be able to survive.


## THE END OF THE DECADE

In the address at the January 3, 1957 meeting at which he ended his term as the forty-fourth President of the Academy, Dr. Edward J. Donovan emphasized the need for continuing concern about its perennially tenuous financial status. "While the Academy is enjoying most vigorous health in every department and certainly, from the short term perspective, Academy finances and staffing are very satisfactory," he reported, "it was proving to be easier to identify problems in an environment of turbulent and rapid change than it was to define the critical organizational tasks whose performance would lead would lead to an appropriate organizational response to the environmental challenges to the Academy's survival.[45]

Dr. Donovan took particular—and justifiable—pride in the fact that City and State agencies had presented requests to the Academy for help in solving "difficult medical problems." He described four reports: a study of perinatal mortality whose findings led the City Commissioner of Health to introduce a program to reduce perinatal deaths; a report on the abuse of barbiturates; a study on expert medical testimony jointly sponsored by the Academy, the Association of the Bar of the City of New York, the Medical Society of the County of New York, and the New York County Lawyers Association; and a statement from the Committee on Public Health on drug addiction which urged treatment of the addict as a sick person and not as a criminal.

Dr. Donovan pointed to the improvement in the quality of the *Bulletin,* but expressed concern about the decline in attendance at medical meetings at the Academy. "Until a few years ago, practically all medical meetings in New York were held at the Academy," he noted, "but now the medical colleges, the various hospitals and numerous special medical societies all have their meetings at which compulsory attendance on the part of their members and staffs is required in order for the institutions to maintain their accreditation." This called, he concluded, for a survey to determine the future role of the Academy as a postgraduate teaching institution which would examine whether reducing the number of meetings at the Academy and, as had been suggested by a number of Fellows, increasing the availability of automobile parking spaces near the Academy building would be the answer.

## NOTES

1 Gabriel RA and Metz KS. 1992 *A History of Military Medicine, Vol. II, From the Renaissance through Modern Times.* New York: Greenwood Press, p. 252f.

2 Kelley R. 1975 *The Shaping of the American Past.* Englewood Cliffs, NJ: Prentice-Hall. vol. 2, p. 844.

3 Adams H. 1986 *History of the United States During the Administrations of Thomas Jefferson.* New York: Library of America. p. 78. (This is a reprint of a work originally published in 1889–1891)

4 Sayre WS and Kaufman H. 1960 *Governing New York City: Politics in the Metropolis.* New York: Russell Sage Foundation. p. 30.

5 Wilson JQ. 1989 *Bureaucracy.* New York: Basic Books. p. 25.

6 ibid. p. 26.

7 ibid. p. 26.

8 Van Ingen P. 1949 *The New York Academy of Medicine: Its First Hundred Years.* New York: Columbia University Press. p. 354.

9 Wiebe RH. 1977 Modernizing the republic, In: Bailyn B, Davis DB, Donald DH, Thomas JC, Wiebe RH and Wood GS. Eds. *The Great Republic.* New York: Oxford University Press. p. 908.

10 ibid. p. 1150.

11 Sayre WS and Kaufman H. op. cit. p. 258.

12 Editorial. 1947 The Academy celebrates. *The New York Times.* March 6, 1947. p. 24.

13 Van Ingen P. op. cit. p. 364

14 New York Academy of Medicine. 1940 By-laws Article IX, Section 1.

15 Van Ingen P. op. cit. P. 534

16 Levy RL. 1967 Howard Reid Craig, an appreciation. *Bulletin of the New York Academy of Medicine.* 43:3–8.

17 Craig HR. 1951 The structure and functions of the New York Academy of Medicine. *Bulletin of the New York Academy of Medicine.* 27:598–605.

18 Cresap, McCormick and Paget. 1958 *The New York Academy of Medicine, A Study of Administration.* New York: Cresap, McCormick and Paget. pp. 11–16.

19 Craig HR. 1956 The New York Academy of Medicine: retrospect and prospect. *Bulletin of the New York Academy of Medicine.* 32:701–712.

20 Medical Library Oral History Program. 1977 *Interview with Janet Doe.* Chicago: Medical Library Association.

21 Medical Library Association Oral History Program. 1978 *Interview with Gertrude L. Annan.* Chicago: Medical Library Association.

22 Heaton CE. 1954 Archibald Malloch, MD, 1887–1953. *Bulletin of the New York Academy of Medicine.* 30:400–401.

23 Garrison FH. 1929 *An Introduction to the History of Medicine.* Philadelphia: WB Saunders Company. p. 55.

24 Doe J. 1952 The Library of the New York Academy of Medicine. *Bulletin of the New York Academy of Medicine.* 28:197–203.

25 Doe J. 1950 The Library *Annual Report of the New York Academy of Medicine, 1950.* Cited in: Annan GL. 1967 Our greatest material heritage, the Library. *Bulletin of the New York Academy of Medicine.* 43:21–32.

26 Van Ingen P. op. cit. p. 539.

27 Corwin EHL and Cunningham EV. 1941 *Thirty Years in Community Service, 1911–1941.* New York: New York Academy of Medicine. p. 6.

28 ibid. p. 4.

29 Committee on Public Health. 1961 *Committee on Public Health, New York Academy of Medicine: Pioneering in Public Health, Twenty Year Report of its Activities, 1941–1961.* Mew York: New York Academy of Medicine. p. 92.

30 ibid. p. 98.

31 Kruse HD and Amster LJ. 1967 The Committee on Public Health: 1946 to the present. *Bulletin of the New York Academy of Medicine.* 43:11–16.

32 ibid. p. 18.

33 ibid. p. 18.

34 Baehr G. 1949 Address inaugurating the Institute on Medical Education. In: Ashford M. *The New York Academy's Institute on Medical Education, 1947.* New York: Commonwealth Fund. p. viii.

35 McGuiness AC. 1967 The Committee on Medical Education, 1946-1966. *Bulletin of the New York Academy of Medicine.* 43:49–69. p. 60.

36 Ashford M, Ed. 1949 *Trends in Medical Education.* New York: Commonwealth Fund.

37 McGuiness, AC. op. cit. p. 60.

38 Clark DW. 1983 Presentation of Academy Plaque to Iago Galdston, MD *Bulletin of the New York Academy of Medicine.* 59:620–625.

39 New York Academy of Medicine. 1947 *Announcement Booklet: 1948–48 Lectures to the Laity.* New York: New York Academy of Medicine.

40 Galdston I and Zetterberg, H. Eds. 1958 *Panic and Morale: Conference Transactions.* New York: International Universities Press, Inc.

41 Becker H. 1967 The Committee on Special Studies, 1956–1966. *Bulletin of the New York Academy of Medicine.* 43:70–78.

42 Cranefield P. 1967 The *Bulletin of the New York Academy of Medicine, 1947–1966. Bulletin of the New York Academy of Medicine.* 43:33–48.

43 Baehr G. 1947 The role of the Academy in the City and the nation. *Bulletin of the New York Academy of Medicine* 23:245-259.

44 Martin AT. 1953 Inaugural address. *Bulletin of the New York Academy of Medicine.* 29:261–265.

45 Donovan EJ. 1957 Two years of the Presidency of the New York Academy of Medicine. *Bulletin of the New York Academy of Medicine.* 33:230–236.

# Chapter 3
# 1957–1967
# The Craig Era II

THE HEALTH RESEARCH COUNCIL OF THE CITY OF
NEW YORK
THE NEW YORK REGIONAL MEDICAL PROGRAM FOR
HEART DISEASE, CANCER AND STROKE
ACADEMY PRESIDENTS
Dr. Robert L. Levy, 1957–1960
Dr. Frank Glenn, 1961–1962
Dr. Harold Brown Keyes, 1963–1964
Dr. John L. Madden, 1965–1966
Dr. Preston A. Wade, 1967–1968
THE END OF THE ERA OF DR. HOWARD REID CRAIG
NOTES

P ERIODICALLY during the life of almost every voluntary organization, it becomes advisable to undertake a reexamination of its
purpose, its structure and its operation. This challenges the relevance of the organization both in terms of the needs and desires
of its members and the changes in the environment and the society in which it exists. It is usually undertaken by its leadership,
ideally with broad involvement of its members, and sometimes
with the assistance of outsiders, either volunteers or paid consultants, and it requires the investment of a considerable effort.
Without such reexaminations (except in "secret" societies whose
arcane rituals often have a life of their own), the organization
might stultify and, ultimately, fade from the scene. When successfully accomplished, the organization usually exhibits a renewed
sense of purpose and marches forward with a new vigor, even
though (or, perhaps, because) there may have been some change
in direction.

The Academy has been no exception. In addition to some introspection with the election of each new President and, more recently, the appointment of each new Director, a broad self-
examination has been performed a number of times during its long
history. And, in 1957, President Robert L. Levy, Dr. Howard Reid
Craig, who was starting the second decade of his twenty-year term

as Director, and the other leaders of the Academy decided that it was time for another comprehensive self-examination.

This exercise had been presaged by presentations to the Committees on Public Health and Medical Information a year earlier by Dr. Craig, later published in the *Bulletin,* in which he had pointed out that, "The Academy, in some aspects, . . . is operating to a degree in the framework of twenty-five years ago." He noted that university medical libraries had grown constituting a "great factor in decreasing the reader census" at the Academy. But, he said, despite staff turnover, "[I]t is my conviction that regardless of demand or operational problems or costs or competition, the Library, as our greatest material heritage and treasure, must be maintained at full strength and effectiveness."[1]

The Committee on Public Health, he suggested, had a happy future in terms of opportunities and challenges, especially in consummating a linkage between preventive medicine and public health, on the one hand, and medical practice, on the other, while the Committee on Medical Information, which originally had responsibility for press relations and lay education, was making a transition as documented in its *Whither Medicine?* project to "a closer community of interest between all the professions and disciplines."

The Academy's programs in medical education, he said, had problems of two orders. First, there were internal problems such as "diminished attendance at meetings, the plethora of meetings in general, the difficulty in setting up programs that are not a rehash and whose speakers are not the same authorities speaking again and again." Second, there were external problems in which the Committee was participating such as internship and residency questions, the education and licensure of foreign physicians, and experiments in medical curricula which badly need to be overhauled. "This," he stated, "is one Committee which with the passage of time needs re-orientation and a possible change of direction." Dr. Craig, it appeared, had a fairly clear view of the strengths and weaknesses of the Academy but was somewhat uncertain about the adaptations that needed to be made. His ultimate conclusion, it appeared, was that only relatively marginal changes in programming and structure were needed.

In an internally circulated memorandum, Dr. Iago Galdston, Executive Secretary of the Committee on Medical Information, presented a different and somewhat provocative view, in which he suggested changes that would enhance the roles of the Executive Secretaries of the Academy's Standing Committees.[2] According to Dr. Galdston, while the reputation of the Academy had increased over the past twenty-five years, there was a need for change in its programs. He pointed to the decline in attendance at its meetings and said, "The Academy is no longer, as it was in the former years, the singular and unique place where physicians gather by the hundreds to hear described and discussed the new and the old in medicine. The objectives of graduate medical education which animated many of the operations of the Academy and which structured its internal organization can no longer, with warrant, command and absorb the major interest and labors of the Academy."

"During the past twenty-five years," he continued, "the graduate education functions of the Academy have been 'taken over' by numerous other organizations. Similarly, numerous governmental agencies at all levels—communal, state, and national have intensified their activities in the field of public health."

To remedy these problems, Dr. Galdston suggested a new emphasis on the social science disciplines such as economics, sociology, and cultural anthropology. This would follow along the lines of such activities as the four-year study of *Medicine and the Changing Order,* the Institutes on Social Medicine, on *Panic and Morale,* on *Ministry and Medicine,* and on *Medical History,* the pilot study, *Whither Medicine?,* and the Eastern States Health Conferences, all of which involved the participation of speakers from a variety of disciplines in the social sciences, the humanities and the law.

Dr. Galdston found fault with the current standing committees. Committee members, he said, provide "peripheral vision," and "adjudicate" rather than "initiate" policy, while stronger leadership by the executive secretaries in setting the program agenda of the Academy is necessary.

As an alternative, he proposed transforming the standing committees into the Divisions of Medical Education, Public Health, and Social Medicine with the staff positions of executive secretaries being be replaced by full-time, salaried officers called "Directors" or "Executive Administrators." He further proposed that these Directors and the Division Chairs (replacements for the Committee Chairs) should both participate in discussions of the work of their divisions by the Council. The Council would then have a better understanding of what is going on in the Academy and the Directors would be better apprised of Academy-wide developments.

The Division of Public Health, Dr. Galdston said, should follow the precedents of the Committee on Public Health and continue to undertake such studies as those on barbiturates, drug addiction, and the role of expert testimony in the courts. At the same time, he suggested that the role of the Committee on Medical Information in public relations and providing information to the media, in which he had achieved such prominence and acclaim, should be abandoned.[2]

Finally, Dr. Galdston proposed that the stated meetings of the Academy be replaced by meetings dedicated to specific topics dealing with the sociological, cultural, and anthropological aspects of medicine, and that the Academy strengthen its ties to the local universities and work with them to provide educational opportunities for graduate students.

The exercise of self-examination was heralded by an announcement in the *Bulletin* to inform the Fellows that the Council had appointed a Committee "to survey, in searching fashion, the objectives, functions and activities of the Academy as they exist today."[3] What prompted the study, the announcement said, in addition to the Academy's growth as an organization, its increasing activities and its desire to retain a position of leadership, was the "even stronger motive for self examination afforded by the altered scene in which the Academy operates" and the many changes in the way medicine was being viewed by physicians and the public: ". . . the impact of insurance, of medical care in industry, of labor union participation, of the educational experiments and programs in uni-

versities and hospitals, the increase in the number of societies devoted to medical specialties, the rise of voluntary health agencies
and the growing part played by governmental public health services." Basic research is also important and "the interplay of professional and lay journalism, as well as the wide potential influence
of radio and television cannot be ignored. The Academy, in order
to meet its obligations and render the greatest possible service,
must adapt to a changing environment."[3]

Past President William Barclay Parsons was named to chair the
Survey Committee and a number of Subcommittees were formed:
Administration, chaired by Dr. Marcus D. Kogel; Building and
Plant, chaired by Dr. Condict W. Cutler; *Bulletin,* chaired by Dr.
Louis D. Soffer; Finance, chaired by Dr. Henry N. Pratt; Library,
chaired by Dr. George Rosen; Medical Education, chaired by Dr.
Dickinson W. Richards, Jr.; Medical Information, chaired by Dr.
John H. Garlock; and Public Health, chaired by Dr. Duncan W.
Clark. Each Subcommittee had from five to eight members most of
whom were Fellows. In all, forty-eight individuals were directly
involved, while all Fellows were "earnestly solicited" to send their
views to Dr. Parsons or to one or more of the Subcommittee Chairmen. Early on, the Subcommittees on Finance and the Library decided to seek expert advice and hired the management consulting
firm of Cresap, McCormick and Paget to study the overall management and administration of the Academy, the administration of the
Library, the internal financial arrangements, and the provision of
administrative and building services.

Dr. Parsons presented the report of the Survey Committee to the
June 30, 1958 meeting of the Academy Council—it was subsequently published later that year.[4] Some of its forty-eight individual recommendations were easily resolved. For example, the recommendation of the Subcommittee on Building and Plant that the
cafeteria and catering food service be improved by contracting
with an outside catering organization had already been implemented. The Council quickly approved two other recommendations: one calling for a similar contracting arrangement for the
provision of housekeeping services; and the other suggesting reno-

vations in some of the rooms, notably some of the rooms off the lobby of the building.

Rejection by the Survey Committee of one of the recommendations advanced by Cresap, McCormick and Paget was confirmed by the Council. They had suggested that a single "Board of Directors" replace the current bicameral governance structure in which the Council covered policy matters and the separate Board of Trustees dealt with property and financial management. It was felt that the "business" of these two bodies was "quite different" and, it was agreed that they should remain independent and distinct from each other, despite the overlap in membership.

Recommendations by the consultants for the Library were approved in principle. In addition to changes in staffing and seeking economies by purchasing longer term subscriptions to periodicals, the Council agreed to explore the creation of a depository library and the acquisition of the garage on East 102nd Street, around the corner from the Academy building, to house it.

During the discussion of the Library, Dr. Craig had expressed concern about its rising costs, noting that its staff of 53 employees and current (1958) budget of $283,000 were four or five times those of other medical libraries (except for the National Library of Medicine which had 220 employees and a budget of one million dollars), Dr. William C. White, a member of the Council and Chair of the Library Subcommittee, echoed this concern commenting that, although the volume of use of library materials and interlibrary loans had not changed, there had been a 50 percent drop in the annual number of visitors to the Library, presumably in response to the growth of smaller libraries in the local medical schools and hospitals. It was agreed that the problems of the Library warranted further consideration.

Cresap, McCormick and Paget also recommended the reorganization of the Comptroller's Office and that a "Business Office" be created and a "Business Manager" be employed to take over responsibility for many of the routine matters that occupied the time of the Director. This Office could deal with all of the internal operational and maintenance matters, while the Board of Trustees would retain responsibility for investment policies and transactions. These recommendations were approved and subsequently implemented.

Much of the discussion at this Council meeting centered on the recommendations relating to the Committee on Medical Information and the work of its Executive Secretary, Dr. Iago Galdston, obviously a matter of some contentiousness. The Subcommittee on Medical Information acknowledged that, in undertaking studies on psychiatry and other subjects, it had "gone beyond the original intent of the charge to the Committee." It also noted that its role in public relations and press information was diminishing as the media turned increasingly to the American Medical Association for medical information.[4] Since these functions might be more effectively handled by a layperson rather than a physician, the Subcommittee suggested that the Committee be abolished and replaced by an advisory body of consultants. Meanwhile, Dr. Arthur Master, a member of the Council as Chairman of the Committee on Medical Information, suggested that activities such as *Whither Medicine?* Lectures to the Laity and the Health Education Conference be continued.

As the minutes report with unusual candor, the discussion turned to Dr. Galdston himself: Dr. Harold Keyes, a member of the Council, was torn between his deep irritation and annoyance with Dr. Galdston's behavior as the Committee's Executive Secretary and the man's apparent brilliance. He suggested that "the work of the Committee be divided and that the Executive Secretary then be retired promptly at age 65, two years hence."

The inclusion of such outspoken remarks in the minutes, which were prepared by or under the supervision of Dr. Howard Reid Craig, implies the Director's concurrence with this perception of Dr. Galdston. Indeed, the Academy's files contain a number of memoranda in which Dr. Craig recorded his displeasure with Dr. Galdston's manner of conducting press briefings. In fact, it should be noted that, despite acknowledgment of Dr. Galdston's brilliance, a number of Fellows and, particularly, members of the Council and the Board of Trustees, were made uncomfortable by his self-assurance and his proclivity for seizing the limelight for his pronouncements on historical events and the issues of the day.

This Council meeting adjourned without taking any further action, the matter of Dr. Galdston and the Committee on Medical Information, and the other recommendations of the Survey Committee being deferred until the next meeting, scheduled for October 1958.

In the meantime, at a meeting of the Survey Committee, and in a formal letter to Dr. Craig, another view of Dr. Galdston and his work was presented by Dr. Duncan W. Clark, Professor and Chairman of the Department of Environmental Medicine and Community Health at Downstate Medical Center of the University of the State of New York, who continues to this day to receive attention for his straightforward views of Academy affairs. Dr. Clark, a member of the Committee on Medical Information who had worked closely with Dr. Galdston over the years, took exception to the recommendations for that Committee. He questioned the wisdom of sacrificing "one of the most productive sources of programming for the Academy" as well as the supposition that the news coverage would be enhanced by turning press relations over to a layperson. He said that the "tangents" that the Committee had pursued included some of the "best activities of the Academy, " and suggested that the tendency to overlap could be obviated if the Council were to articulate clear-cut charges to the Committees: the Committee on Medical Information to handle information needs of the media with respect to medical and scientific matters and also develop programs addressed to nonphysicians; while the Committee on Public Health responded to requests for information and assistance from the official public health agencies.[5]

The discussion apparently continued in the October meeting of the Council, but, this time, its content was not recorded in the minutes, which covered only the decisions that were reached. These included: establishment of a new Committee on Public Relations and Financial Development (which, as it turned out, was short-lived); moving the *Bulletin* and other publishing activities from the Committee on Education to a new Committee on Publications and Medical Information with the Editor of the *Bulletin* as its Executive Secretary; and continuing the Academy's involvement with environmental and sociomedical problems under the aegis of the Committee on Medical Information with its name changed to the Committee on Special Studies to reflect its new mission. In all, some forty of the forty-eight recommendations presented by the Survey Committee were implemented, leading to changes that were largely incremental. Over the next decade, as a result, while there remained some uncertainty about the Academy's educational programs as well as concern about the increasing consumption of resources by the Library, the Fellows participating in the self-examination process, as well as the membership at large, seemed to be content with the structure and governance of the Academy, and satisfied that its activities, on the whole, were healthy and appropriately influential.


## THE COMMITTEE ON PUBLIC HEALTH

One of the recommendations of the Survey Committee called for the Committee on Public Health to initiate more inquiries on its own rather than waiting for requests for such studies from outside sources. The Committee replied by noting that, although some of its activities had been responses to outside requests, they had often been triggered by awareness on the part of the outside agencies of the interest of the Committee in studying the particular issue. Nevertheless, in 1959, the Committee undertook a survey of problems for potential study. A number of interesting issues were suggested, including deficiencies in the quality of medical care, gaps in mental illness services, and opportunities in cancer detection. However, when these were found to be under review by other bodies, the Committee finessed them rather than initiating a competing exercise. In a formal statement, the Committee reaffirmed the right to act on its own initiative when an occasion demanded and, "for the time being, it decided not to undertake work on special problems until its counsel was sought, unless impelling circumstances dictated earlier action."[6] It should be noted that this position is directly opposite from the one recommended by the Survey Committee, but apparently there were no repercussions.

Another recommendation of the Survey Committee suggested that the practice of formulating and issuing opinions on all proposed State legislation, which the Committee had initiated in 1911, be reconsidered in light of the lack of any evidence of impact on official actions. The Committee, however, replied that it had decided in 1954 as a matter of policy that, unless there was a specific request from the Governor's Office, it would discontinue "the practice of sending unsolicited opinions to public officials and legislators except when a very important matter warranted such an action." In response to the recommendation, therefore, the Committee said simply that after a review of its experience, it reaffirmed the policy position already taken in 1954.[7]

One such situation arose in 1959, when the Committee reacted against a bill introduced in the State Legislature that would have automatically suspended the right to practice of any physician who had been confined for more than sixty days in a hospital for the treatment of a mental illness. This response was based on an actual case in which the New York City Department of Correction would have been barred from employing a physician who had recovered from a mental illness. If enacted, the Committee said, the bill would have unduly stigmatized physicians and other health professionals. It was not passed.

## The Committee and the New York City Department of Health

During this decade, in addition to its reports and other activities, the Committee on Public Health, with Dr. Harry Kruse as Executive Secretary from 1952 to 1968, had a close and important working relationship with the New York City Department of Health. Its Commissioners, first Dr. Leona Baumgartner and then Dr. George James, called frequently on the Academy for advice and support as they fought to restore the Department to its former level of emi-

nence. Dr. Craig, who had been appointed Chairman of the Medical
Advisory Committee of the New York City Commission on Personal Health Services (which became known as the "Piel Commission" named for Mr. Gerard Piel, the publisher of *Scientific American*, who served as its Co-Chairman), was also actively involved.

In his January 2, 1964 Anniversary Discourse on "*Can We Solve
Our Growing Problem in Public Health?*" Dr. James extolled this
relationship.

To the New York Academy of Medicine, no Health Commissioner of the
City of New York can give ordinary thanks for help, for its role has been
extraordinary. As the record shows, the Academy was a prime mover
even in the establishment of the Department of Health as we know it. The
Academy has worked along with us every step of the way, not always
agreeing, but always progressive, always open-minded and above all,
always bursting with the vigor of first-rate men ready and eager to volunteer first-rate work for the community. Committees of the Academy consult with us on the Health Department budget. The Academy's Committee on Public Health went over the new Health Code with us time and
time again, draft after draft, word by word. The Health Research Council
of the City of New York, under whose auspices research on city problems
is expanding, includes several members of the Academy, and Dr. Craig
was instrumental in recruiting some of the distinguished scientists who
serve on it. The Academy played a significant role in the final wonderful
victory of fluoridation. In this wildly controversial matter the Academy
showed, as it has again and again for over 117 years, that it has a total
lack of fear to stand for something if that something is based on sound
scientific fact and benefits our people.[8]

## Conference on Perinatal Mortality

Typifying the role of the Academy as a convenor was the invitational Conference on Perinatal Mortality presented in conjunction
with District No. II of the American Academy of Pediatrics, the
New York City Departments of Health and Hospitals, the Association for the Aid of Crippled Children, the Maternity Center Association, the Citizens Committee for Children of New York City,

and the Community Council of Greater New York. It was chaired by Commissioner of Health Leona Baumgartner and Dr. Leonard Mayo, Executive Director of the Association for the Aid of Crippled Children, and was attended by a group of over 100 lay and professional participants carefully selected on the basis of their interest and accomplishments in this area.

Working from the Committee's 1955 report on perinatal mortality, a copy of which was furnished to each participant prior to the sessions, the Conference was organized into ten roundtables, each led by a discussion leader who summarized their deliberations at the final plenary session. Each roundtable addressed one of the following questions: What can be done to improve the management of abnormal presentations and operative deliveries? How can the hospital monthly staff conference be made a more potent factor in improving maternity care and preventing perinatal deaths? What can be done to improve the preparation of house staff physicians responsible for women in labor? How can active measures to prevent prematurity be fostered? How can a common standard be established for perinatal mortality studies? How can hospitals, with other agencies, provide an extension service at home for mothers and infants delivered on ward services? How can prenatal care be improved? How can the public be helped to understand the importance of early registration and other health measures in maternity care? What is the relationship between obstetric anesthesia and analgesia and perinatal morbidity and mortality? What can be done to lessen the incidence of perinatal deaths resulting from maternal complications?[9]

In addition to the many important recommendations that were developed, this Conference represented a high-water mark of cooperation among public, professional and voluntary agencies. In addition, its format, together with the skillful preparation of a singularly practical and meaningful agenda and the care with which a mixture of potentially influential lay and professional participants was selected, constitutes a model for conferences on other topics with implications both for medical practice and for public health.

## Drug Addiction

Another issue that featured prominently among the activities of the Committee during this period was the problem of drug addiction. Recognizing that the recommendations put forth by the Committee in 1955[10] had been misinterpreted (the recommendation that physicians be allowed to prescribe narcotics for some addicts as part of their treatment was misconstrued as a plea to allow indiscriminate use of drugs), the subject was revisited and two additional reports were issued, one in 1963 and the other in 1965.[11,12] These reports reiterated the Committee's views of addiction as a vicious circle in which reliance on the punishment of drug users only increases the price of drugs, and the profits from the drug trade, in turn, encourage drug dealers to push their products with greater intensity, thus increasing the number of addicts. Instead, the Committee advised, the addict should be considered as a sick person in need of treatment and not as a criminal and those who sell drugs to maintain their habits should be treated as patients and not as criminals. "Overbearing" limitations on the clinical judgment of physicians should be erased, the Committee recommended, and "the [Federal] Bureau of Narcotics should gracefully bow out of the practice of medicine." In 1965, Dr. Lawrence C. Kolb, a member of the Subcommittee on Addiction, presented the views of the Committee in testimony before the Permanent Subcommittee on Investigation of the US Senate Committee on Government Operations.[13]

## Blood Banks

In 1956, in response to a request from an ad hoc group of twelve organizations involved in the handling of blood, headed by Dr. August H. Groeschel, Associate Administrator of New York Hospital and Chairman of the Committee on Professional Services of the Greater New York Hospital Association, a Subcommittee, chaired by Dr. Milton J. Goodfriend and staffed by Dr. Harry Kruse, was assigned to study the operations of blood banks in the area. Its report, published in 1958, found blood collection and distribution programs in New York City to be chaotic. For example, many hospitals and health agencies maintained their own blood banks and engaged in activities considered to be counterproductive. Also, the Subcommittee suggested, the practice of basing patients' charges for blood on the type of hospital room they occupied should be replaced by uniform billing.[14]

### Salacious Literature, Sexual Behavior and Venereal Disease

In 1963, the Committee on Public Health reviewed problems relating to sexual behavior. It "explored the medical aspects of the marked increase in the number of salacious publications displayed on newsstands and circulated by mail" much of which, the Committee felt, was "purposefully directed toward teenagers."[15] The Committee argued that "the perusal of erotic literature has the potentiality of inciting some young persons into illicit sex relations, thus leading them into promiscuity, illegitimacy and venereal disease." It suggested that these effects can be mitigated only through the active concern of parents, and called for adequate recreational facilities "to provide a wholesome outlet for youthful energy." Finally, the Committee urged the New York State Legislature to enact a bill prohibiting the sale of such materials to minors.

During this period, the Committee repeatedly registered concern over the prevalence of venereal diseases in the community and, on several occasions, examined the major factors contributing to their presence. For example, in 1964, the Committee addressed what it called a "resurgence" of venereal disease.[16] The Committee noted that, while the US Public Health Service had implemented programs of contact tracing through interviews of persons with venereal disease and their sex partners, a key problem was the failure of physicians in private practice to report cases to the public health authorities. The Committee noted that, "Greater promiscuity in young people has its roots in relaxing of moral and cultural values in present-day society. Contributing to promiscuity . . . . is a national preoccupation with sex . . . . encouraged and kept alive and re-inforced by movies and advertisements. But it receives its most in-tensive promulgation and misuse from a highly-organized, nation-wide campaign of salacious literature directed at youth. . . . Much of this salacious literature is aimed at promoting homosexuality, particularly among the young."

Since venereal diseases are curable, the reporting of cases by physicians to public health agencies is indispensable in getting patients into treatment, the Committee said. It also stressed the importance of educating both teenagers and the medical commu-nity about these diseases. The Committee emphasized that there was a "large homosexual element in the present outbreak of vene-real disease," and that failure to recognize this was leading to diagnostic errors. It said that, "Society was once more certain of its attitude about homosexuality: it registered disgust, ridicule, or pity. But changing mores and moral values may have altered atti-tudes, or at least weakened former feelings. Furthermore, the vic-tims have launched an organized and aggressive action to gain at least tolerance, hopefully to achieve acceptance of its respectabil-ity, and most ambitiously to recognize it as a noble way of life."[17] This factor, together with the practitioner's reluctance to report cases to the public health authorities for fear of losing patients, the Committee suggested, impelled physicians to place a higher value on patient confidentiality than on the health of the public. This report received considerable attention in the press and requests for copies were received from every part of the country.

The Committee's report on homosexuality apparently reflects attitudes on sexual issues that were widespread in the medical community at that time. In its 1964 report on homosexuality, the Committee noted that, in contrast with the situation thirty years earlier, the subject of homosexuality was more frequently and openly discussed, citing as an example the highly publicized annual "Fairy Ball" at which its advocates cavorted.[18] Homosexuality, the Committee declared, is an illness, with family neglect a major causal factor and, citing the work of Bieber and his colleagues,[19] it suggested that homosexuality can be treated and prevented. Sex education is needed, it said, "but America's preoccupation with sex reveals a superficial, immature and artificial attitude. . . . . . . . However, when attempts are made to have society become more mature concerning this subject, and capable of placing it in its proper perspective, there arises a surprising resistance. The argument most commonly advanced is that sex education belongs in the home. But, if the home is not providing that education, where will it be given?"[20]

## Health Education

In a fairly lengthy document published in 1964, the Committee contrasted America's "acknowledged mastery of techniques of advertising and selling" with the "sorry record of health education in this country."[21] The Committee called for improvement and expansion of training programs for health educators, increased financial support for health education, improved coordination of school and health department programs of health education, and placing them under the leadership of professional health educators.

## Clearing Reports with the Council

The high standing of the work of the Committee on Public Health and its importance in the life of the Academy was reflected in its empowerment to bypass the Council in presenting policy statements on behalf of the Academy to the public. This was conferred by the By-laws which stated: ". . . [S]tatements may be issued in the name of the Academy only when they have been approved unanimously by the executive Committee of the Committee on Public Health and by the President of the Academy or by three-fourths of the members of the Committee present and voting at any special or regular meeting of the Committee and by the President of the Academy."[22]

In 1966, however, the Council received a protest about a report on the Office of Chief Medical Examiner of the City of New York that had been issued directly by the Committee. After discussion that stretched over two of its meetings, the Council noted that the report in no way reflected on Dr. Milton Helpern, the Chief Medical Examiner "who had served this City with distinction"[23] and voted to return this report to the Committee for further consideration with the suggestion that Dr. Helpern be invited to meet with the subcommittee that had prepared it. The Council also approved a motion requiring that all future reports of the Academy's standing committees must first be approved by the Council before being disseminated. In 1969, the empowerment of the Committee on Public Health to independently issue position papers was formally rescinded.[24]

## COMMITTEE ON MEDICAL EDUCATION

In 1959, in keeping with the changes in the Academy's structure that had been recommended by the Survey Committee and endorsed by the Council, Dr. Robert Craig, who had been Executive Secretary of the Committee since 1952, was replaced in that role by Dr. Aims C. McGuinness. Dr. Craig, who retained his post as Editor of the *Bulletin,* was designated Executive Secretary of the new Committee on Publications and Medical Information. Dr. McGuiness, who had been Special Assistant (Health and Medical) to the Secretary of Health, Education and Welfare, was given the additional responsibilities of coordinating Committee activities with the Sections and working with the medical schools and hospitals in New York City. He served until the end of 1966 when he left to become Deputy Associate Director of the Educational Council for Foreign Medical Graduates in Philadelphia.

Bowing to a drop in attendance, the Committee reduced the number of its meetings. In 1957, the Graduate Fortnight became a one-week program renamed the Postgraduate Week and later, in 1961, it was discontinued altogether. The number of Stated Meetings per year was reduced from eight to three, held in November, December and April. A special subcommittee made up of Drs. Ludwig W. Eichna of Downstate Medical Center, E. Hugh Luckey of the New York Hospital-Cornell Medical Center, and Rustin McIntosh of the Columbia-Presbyterian Medical Center was charged to review the Committee's activities. It observed that medical practitioners in New York were being inundated with the educational programs being offered by the large medical centers as well as the other hospitals, attendance at which was often required to retain their affiliation appointments and admitting privileges. Accordingly, the Subcommittee recommended the following adjustments in the strategy guiding the Academy's graduate medical education programs: general practitioners might best be reached by open circuit television programs; medical specialists could be reached by the programs offered by the Academy Sections; and the research community could be reached by conferences on specialized topics that would address areas of current interest. An initial conference on electrolyte and fluid metabolism to be held outside of the City, was proposed but, because it could not be funded, it was never held.

In 1958, a Subcommittee on General Practitioners, headed by Dr. Louis Soffer, suggested the presentation of courses devoted to special topics that would cover basic concepts, current trends and developments, clinical applications, and therapy. In 1958, Dr. George Reader of the Cornell University Medical College successfully arranged such a program on practical applications of fluid and electrolyte balance. In 1960, a series of weekly sessions designed for general practitioners, called the *Correlated Clinical Science Course,* was initiated. It attracted a substantial audience for two years and, in January 1963, it was transferred to television.

## Medical Television

At the end of 1962, the Academy, represented largely by Dr. Aims McGuiness, joined Channel 31, the municipal ultrahigh frequency station, in a study to gauge the "acceptability and effectiveness of open-circuit television as an additional medium of continuing medical education in a large metropolitan area."[25] In 1963, as a result of this collaboration, the station started telecasting the Academy's Correlated Clinical Science Seminars. Over the next four years, this weekly program, which was open to viewing by the general public, was aired during the prime time hour of 9 to 10 PM in all but seven of the weeks in that period.

With the support of eleven foundations which joined in providing $100,000 to cover production and evaluation costs, Mr. Herbert Menzel of the Department of Sociology at New York University, together with colleagues at the Columbia University Bureau of Applied Social Research and the National Opinion Research Center, surveyed the audience of this open-circuit TV program in 1963, 1964 and again in 1967.[26] The evaluations probed the size and characteristics of the audience and the effectiveness of the programs as perceived by the general practitioners and internists to whom they had been directed.

General satisfaction with the size of the audience was shown by the 1964 survey. Adjusting for the "unusually high or low popularity of one or another of the programs," the average number of general practitioners, board-certified and noncertified internists who watched at least one program in four was estimated at 12.8 percent of these types of physicians in private practice in the New York Metropolitan area. That figure increased to 17.8 percent when those who watched at least one program in five or six months were included. Repetition of this survey in 1967 yielded similar data.[27]

The effectiveness study conducted in 1964 focused on "levels of information" which the researchers defined as including "not only factual knowledge, but also the saliency of certain problems and possibilities and the doctor's awareness of the uncertainty of medical knowledge on certain subjects."[28] Physicians who were more highly specialized, board-certified, more recently trained, or affiliated with a "quality" hospital or a medical school faculty got higher scores than their colleagues not in these categories. The researchers cautioned that the higher scores might reflect a stronger motivation or a greater interest in the subject rather than better training.

In comparing the information levels among watchers and nonwatchers tested an average of six months after exposure to the program, the researchers found only modest differences and so much variation in the pattern of responses from one program to the next that only a few fairly firm conclusions were warranted. For example, the programs on hypertension and cortico-steroids seemed to benefit those who were more highly trained while the program on tuberculosis seems to have been of greater benefit to those with relatively lower levels of training and specialization. High information scores, the researchers reported, were also "uniformly and consistently" related to the reading of specialty journals such as the *Annals of Internal Medicine* and the *American Journal of Medicine* but, they acknowledged, this might simply have indicated that those who read journals may also may take other measures to keep up with new developments in medicine. In general, they concluded, effectiveness in the enhancing viewers' understanding of the subject was related to their initial levels of education and specialization.[29]

## Academy Sections

Of all of the programs of the Academy and, in particular, those of the Committee on Medical Education, those of the Sections succeeded in attracting the largest attendance. New sections added during the second decade of Dr. Craig's tenure as Director included: Anesthesiology and Resuscitation, and Occupational Medicine in 1961; Physical Medicine and Rehabilitation in 1965; and Plastic and Reconstructive Surgery in 1966. This brought the total number of Sections to 15.

By 1966, the Section meetings had been reduced to five each year as a consequence of the growth of competing programs conducted by the medical schools and by local and regional chapters of the specialty societies. The practice of conducting the "Residents' Night," the popular programs of presentations by residents in their specialties, was continued by a number of Sections (e.g., Ophthalmology, Urology, and Pediatrics). In addition, two of the Sections were especially active in their publication programs during this period. Between 1949 and 1965, the Section on Microbiology produced eleven monographs on such topics as infectious diseases, pathology, and the immune response, while the Section on Anesthesiology and Resuscitation, in collaboration with the National Research Council of the National Academy of Sciences, issued two publications on anesthetic agents.

A noteworthy program was the invitational Conference on *The Future of Medicine in Industry* sponsored in 1966 by the Section on Occupational Medicine. Developed by Dr. Leon J. Warshaw, then Medical Director of Paramount Pictures Corporation and Chairman of the Section, and supported by a grant from the Division of Occupational Health of the US Public Health Service, this was a three-day Conference held in Princeton, NJ, to which forty of the most prominent physicians in this field from around the country were invited. Their "ticket of admission" was a written response to a series of far-reaching questions developed by a Planning Committee made up of Fellows who were occupational physicians, with notable input from Dr. Aims McGuiness, Executive Secretary of the Committee. Copies of all of the responses were circulated so that the participants could review them prior to the meeting and, when they got to Princeton, they spent two full days in plenary sessions actively discussing variations in their views. On the third day, a brief summary of points on which consensus had been reached was presented, followed by reactions from Dr. Richard A. Prindle, Assistant Surgeon General of the US Public Health Service, Mr. Allen Burch, Director of Safety and Accident Prevention for the International Union of Operating Engineers, Mr. George H. R. Taylor, the eminent economist affiliated with the American Federation of Labor/ Congress of Industrial Organizations, and Mr. William G. Sharwell, Vice President of the New York Telephone Company. Funds were not adequate to cover the editing and publication of a formal proceedings, but the document containing the questions and responses has been used repeatedly as a guide to long-range planning not only by both the Industrial Medical Association (now the American College of Occupational and Environmental Medicine) and the Academy of Occupational Medicine but also by the Division of Occupational Health (now the National Institute of Occupational Safety and Health) and a number of universities conducting programs in occupational medicine.

### Fellowships of the Committee on Medical Education

One area in which the role of the Academy was not diminished was the provision of fellowships and scholarships for undergraduate and graduate physicians. Funding of these awards has come either from bequests from physicians and their families or from philanthropic individuals and organizations. In some instances, the funds remain in the custody of another nonprofit organization while the Academy selects the recipients and administers the award process. These awards have gained in significance as government and other funding for research and training have diminished.

Among the more important fellowships originating during this period were the Bowen-Brooks scholarships, originally established by Mrs. Elizabeth Cochran Bowen, widow of Harry S. Bowen, in memory of their son, Alexander Cochran Bowen, and named in honor of Dr. Harlow Brooks, their personal physician. These scholarships are intended to help selected graduates of hospital residency programs by financing one year of study or training in another country. Mrs. Bowen originally provided an annual gift of $2,000. She doubled that amount when Dr. Brooks died in 1936 and, on her death in 1941, her estate included a $100,000 bequest to the Academy to continue these scholarships. They were suspended during World War II, but were resumed when it ended, being targeted to assist young physicians whose study had been interrupted by the war. By 1955, inflation and the rising cost of foreign travel, coupled with gradual diminution of the available funds, dictated changing from an annual to a biannual award. In the late 1960s, they were discontinued largely because of the difficulties the young residents were having in making the needed arrangements for short-term independent studies in Europe. (They will be resumed in 1997, thanks to arrangements, negotiated by Senior Vice President Alan R. Fleischman, through which one individual each year, after completing a residency or fellowship, will have the opportunity of six months of study in a clinical specialty in the Program of Evidence-based Medicine at the Green College at Oxford University and the Radcliffe Hospital.)

The Glorney-Raisbeck Fellowship in the Medical Sciences was established in October 1959 by a grant from the Glorney Foundation, created two years earlier by Miss Ethel Glorney. The Fellowship was intended to honor Dr. Milton J. Raisbeck, her personal physician, whom she named President of the Foundation. Dr. Raisbeck had been Vice Chairman of the Committee on Education since 1961, and had also chaired its Subcommittee on Awards. These Fellowships are awarded to physicians in the New York City Metropolitan Area and provide one year's support for research and study in any field of medicine or the allied sciences. Subsequently, the Glorney Foundation also provided support for a Glorney-Raisbeck Fellowship in Cardiovascular Disease, Glorney-Raisbeck Medical Student Grants, a Glorney-Raisbeck Award for Achievement in Cardiovascular Disease, and a Glorney-Raisbeck Memorial Lecture in Cardiology.

### The Ferdinand C. Valentine Awards

The Ferdinand C. Valentine Medal and Award and Fellowships of the Section on Urology have brought unique prominence to the Academy in that specialty. They also have a most interesting history.

Dr. Valentine was born on March 22, 1851 on board a boat in the North Sea, owned by his grandfather. His birth was registered in the town of Leer in East Friesland, Germany. When he was a young child, he and his parents came to the United States where, in 1876, he graduated from the MacDowell Medical School of St. Louis. He moved to Honduras in Central America, where he became Surgeon General of the Honduran Army and developed an interest in urology. He went to Europe to study genitourinary disease and urological surgery and became an early leader in this emerging specialty. One of the founders of the American Urological Association, he practiced in New York and was affiliated with a number of teaching institutions. He was elected a Fellow of the Academy in 1896, and was a resident of Queens when he died on December 13, 1909.

In his will, he named the Academy as the residuary legatee of his estate, which was to be applied to "the establishment of a trust . . . whose net income shall be paid every two years to the physician who shall have made the greatest advance in that period in the field of genitourinary work and research, in the judgment of the Committee which the said Academy may appoint."[30] There was, however, an additional provision which the Academy found especially troubling: the will required that Dr. Valentine's nephew be Chairman of the Fund Committee for the duration of his life and that he receive 10 percent of the income of the fund as compensation for his services.

Since Dr. Valentine's siblings and their children were life beneficiaries under the will, the Academy received only very modest sums after his death. The death of a major beneficiary in July 1929, however, presented the prospect that a substantial amount of money might become available to the Academy and, accordingly the terms of the bequest were reexamined. On December 18, 1929, the Council, in accord with a recommendation of the Committee on Gifts and Bequests, voted to refuse the Valentine bequest because of the conditions set forth in the will. Some time later, however, Dr. Julius Valentine, the nephew, refused the chairmanship of the Fund Committee and, in 1935, the Council, reversing its earlier decision, voted to accept the funds.

Meanwhile, as the various legatees of the Valentine bequests died, the amount of money in the Fund had been growing. In 1934, Mr. Robert Brereton, then Business Manager of the Academy, had estimated that the value of the stock in the Valentine bequest, which had been $37,400 at its inception in 1909, had risen to $850,000. By the early 1960s. the amounts available for the award were even greater and, on the advice of Counsel, an ad hoc Committee was created and charged to develop an alternative, more practical scheme for the disposal of the Valentine Bequest Fund. This Committee, chaired by Dr. Asa L. K. Lincoln, a physician on the staff of the New York Hospital, recommended that, in addition to the awards, the income from the Fund be applied to research fellowships in urology and to support internal Academy activities such as the Committee on Medical Education and the Library.

Davis Polk & Wardwell, Academy Counsel, then filed a petition on behalf of the Academy under the *cy pres* doctrine requesting the court to allow the income to be used in a manner other than that set forth under the will.[31] This doctrine is invoked when the terms of charitable gifts or trusts become impossible or impractical to carry out. On April 27, 1964, Justice Henry Clay Greenberg of the Supreme Court of New York County ruled that the amounts to be spent annually would depend on the income earned by the Fund and, if no award or grant were made in a given year, the amounts available could be used by the Committee on Medical Education to support the Academy's programs in medical education.

The first Ferdinand C. Valentine Medal was awarded in 1962 to Dr. Charles B. Huggins who received the Nobel Prize in Medicine in 1966 for his work on hormonal treatment of cancer of the prostate. As has become the custom, he also gave the Ferdinand C. Valentine Memorial Lecture. Other Valentine medalists have included Drs. Meredith F. Campbell (1963), Harry Goldblatt (1964), Moses Swick (1965) and Theodore McCann Davis (1966). The Ferdinand C. Valentine Fellowships for Laboratory or Clinical Research in Urology were inaugurated in 1964 and have been continued to the present.

## COMMITTEE ON MEDICAL INFORMATION
## (SPECIAL STUDIES)

As noted above, the Committee on Medical Information changed its name in 1960 to the Committee on Special Studies. The press relations functions were transferred to a newly created Committee on Publications and Medical Information.

### The *Whither Medicine?* Project

The *Whither Medicine?* Project, which had been active from 1955 through 1958 was resumed under the guidance of Dr. Iago Galdston, with Dr. Duncan W. Clark serving as recorder. This Project brought together a selected group of approximately sixteen Fellows and invited guests for a discussion of such "cutting edge" topics as *The Economics of Medical Practice; The Rendering of Medical Services; The Increasing Power and Influence of Labor Unions in the Field of Health Services; The Critical Role of the Medicinal Industries; The Role of Technology in the Practice of Medicine; The Changing Demographic Spectrum;* and *The Challenge of Unobstructed Leisure.* Among the distinguished speakers at the dinner meetings that were a prominent feature of the Project were: The Right Honorable Lord Cohen of Birkenhead, Sir George Pickering, and Drs. Stanhope Bayne-Jones, Raymond E. Trussell, Odin W. Anderson, Michael M. Davis, Talcott Parsons, Willard C. Rappleye, James P. Dixon, and Thomas McKeown. Only a few of the individual presentations appeared in print, and a formal report of the Project was never issued by the Academy. However, in 1965, Dr. Iago Galdston published a book in which he used the presentations and discussions of the *Whither Medicine?* Project as take off points for his comments on a whole range of issues including health insurance, the role of government, changing demographic factors, and the consequences of new technology in medicine.[32]

History of Medicine

In May 1958, the Academy joined the Rockefeller Institute for Medical Research in hosting the annual meeting of the American Society for the History of Medicine. Dr. Galdston was Chairman of the Program and Local Arrangements Committee and the participants included Drs. Owsei Temkin of Johns Hopkins and George Rosen who discussed the seminal work of Henry Sigerist, the noted medical historian. The Academy Library supplemented the presentations by displaying outstanding works in its collection and mounting an exhibit on the work of the Medical Department of the US Army during World War II.

In December 1958, the Committee held an Institute on Social and Historical Medicine at Arden House in Harriman, NY. Speakers at this noteworthy event included J. George Harrar, Ph.D., Director of Agriculture at the Rockefeller Institute, Vihljalmur Stefanson, Consultant on Northern Studies at Dartmouth College, Karl A. Wittfogel, Ph.D., Professor of Chinese History at the University of Washington, and Henry A. Wallace, the former Vice-President of the United States.

In 1961, another Institute on Social Medicine held at Arden House dealt with *Medicine and Anthropology* This particular Institute was supported by the grants from the National Institutes of Health, the Wenner-Gren Foundation, and the Ickenheimer Fund, and the speakers included Drs. Marston Bates of the Department of Zoology at the University of Michigan, René Dubos of the Rockefeller Institute, Paul Fejos, President of the Wenner-Gren Foundation for Anthropological Research, Jurgen Ruesch, Professor of Psychiatry at the University of California School of Medicine, and William Caudill of the Laboratory of Socio-environmental Studies of the National Institute of Mental Health.

The Lectures to the Laity during this period continued to take an adventurous and stimulating tack. For example, the 1959–1960 series was entitled, *On the Medical Frontiers,* and featured presentations by such prominent figures as Drs. Paul Dudley White, the world-famous cardiologist from Harvard Medical

School, and Francis J. Braceland, Director of the Institute for Living in Hartford, Connecticut. The 1963–1964 series included a presentation on "*Man's Travel in Outer Space—Physiological and Psychological Adjustments*" by Eugene B. Konecci, Ph.D., of the US National Aeronautics and Space Administration, and another on "*New Frontiers in Cardiovascular Surgery*" by Dr. Frank Glenn of the Cornell University Medical College.

Replacement of Dr. Iago Galdston by Mr. Harry Becker

In 1962, Dr. Iago Galdston retired after having been at the Academy since 1928, and, as noted earlier, having more than left his mark on the Academy and on medical journalism. He was succeeded by Mr. Harry Becker, who had achieved recognition as an expert on health care financing, health insurance and welfare administration. Mr. Becker, a native of Lincoln, Nebraska, had graduated from the University of Nebraska with a Bachelor's degree and a Master's degree in social work. He had been Director of Social Security of United Automobile Workers, Assistant Vice-President for Program Planning and Research at the Blue Cross Association, and Assistant Director of the Commission on Financing of Hospital Care.

Mr. Becker was much more receptive than some of his colleagues at the Academy to a greater government role in health care and to the concept of universal access to health care through a national health insurance program. His tenure with the Committee lasted only three years but, in that brief period, he changed its focus and that of the Annual Health Education Conference to issues relating to health care financing and the role of government in health care delivery. This was quite relevant in the light of the current lively national debate about whether to establish a new health care financing program for the aged under the Social Security System that was being sparked by bills in the Congress which, with support from Presidents Kennedy and Johnson, culminated in the creation of Medicare in 1965. As a result, there was great interest in the work of the Committee and its meetings, in the planning of which Dr. Harold Jacobziner, Assistant Commissioner for Maternal and Child Health in the New York City Department of Health, played a major role.

For example, the two-day conference in April 1965, on *Closing the Gaps in the Availability and Accessibility of Health Services* attracted over 400 participants. The keynote speaker was Dr. E. Richard Weinerman, Professor of Medicine and Public Health at the Yale University School of Medicine, who concluded his presentation by saying, "To my mind, there is only one answer for a democratic and affluent society; that is a judicious combination of social insurance and tax support for basic medical care and for protective health services."[33] Other speakers included: Dr. Julius B. Richmond, Dean of the Medical Faculty and Chairman and Professor of Pediatrics at the State University of New York in Syracuse; Agnes Brewster, the noted health economist at the US Public Health Service; Dr. Michael E. DeBakey, Chairman of the Department of Surgery at the Baylor University College of Medicine and Chairman of the President's Commission on Heart Disease, Cancer and Stroke; Dr. Herman Hilleboe, former Commissioner of Health of the State of New York who was Professor of Public Health at the Columbia University School of Public Health and Administrative Medicine; Dr. Willard C. Rappleye, Dean Emeritus of the Columbia University College of Physicians and Surgeons; Mr. Robert Ball, Commissioner of the Social Security Administration; and Mr. Morton Miller, Vice President and Chief Actuary of the Equitable Life Assurance Society of the United States.

The Conference on *New Directions in Public Policy for Health Care,* held in April of the following year, attracted over 600 participants. It featured Ms. Eveline M. Burns, Professor of Social Work at the Columbia University School of Social Work, as the Keynote Speaker, and the roster of speakers included: Dr. Martin Cherkasky, Director of the Montefiore Hospital and Medical Center; Dr. Edmund Pellegrino, Professor and Chairman of the Department of Medicine, University of Kentucky College of Medicine; Ms. Lisbeth Bamberger, Acting Chief of Health Programs at the Office of Economic Opportunity; Dr. Lester Breslow, Director of Public Health for the California Department of Health; and Mr. Leon Keyserling, former Chairman of the Council of Economic Advisers.

A key factor in the success of these conferences was that, in contrast to the adamant opposition to Medicare on the part of organized medicine and many in Congress, most of the speakers invited by the Committee were advocates of a larger role for government in health affairs and of expanded entitlements to health care. By presenting such views at the time, the Academy broadened the discussion of these matters among both health professionals and laypersons and expedited the discussion of proposed solutions to the problem. The thousands of the brochures announcing the Conferences that were sent throughout the country enhanced the national prominence of the Academy, particularly among administrators of health programs in both the public and private sectors, while the issues of the *Bulletin* containing the proceedings enjoyed a large sale.

## Social Policy in Health Care

Unlike Dr. Galdston, Mr. Becker was very responsive to the concept of Medicare and strongly supported an expanded role for the federal government in assuring adequate access to health care for all persons. As a federal employee and as a union official, he had strongly endorsed legislative proposals for national health insurance. Knowledge of this position was undoubtedly a factor in the procurement in 1963 of a sizable grant from the Ford Foundation to underwrite a comprehensive review of the issue of national health care that was being debated at that time.

This was a major undertaking. Under Mr. Becker's leadership, a new Committee on Social Policy for Health Care was created and Dr. Norton S. Brown, Attending Physician at Roosevelt Hospital, was appointed Chairman. This was a multidisciplinary Committee with forty members, including both Fellows of the Academy and nationally known experts from the outside. A number of background papers were prepared and distributed and, in 1965, a series of monthly seminars on issues in the organization and financing of health services was launched. Speakers at these seminars included Senator Eugene McCarthy of Minnesota, Dr. Seymour E. Harris, Professor of Economics at Harvard University, Dr. Eveline M. Burns, Professor of Social Work at Columbia University, who had been trained as an economist, Dr. Eli Ginzberg who continues to this day to play a significant role in Academy affairs, Mr. Brian Abel-Smith of the London School of Economics, and Dr. John H. Knowles of the Massachusetts General Hospital.

In 1965, this Committee submitted for review by the Council a *Policy Statement on the Role of Government Tax Funds in Problems of Health Care* which was returned to the Committee with a request that it be "clarified, condensed and shortened." After appropriate revision, it was finally endorsed on May 26, 1965 by both the Council and the Board of Trustees.[34] The Statement deplored the gaps in access to health care that confronted sizable segments of the US population and stated that a "major goal of our democratic society must be that all people have the assurance of an equal opportunity to obtain a high quality of comprehensive health care." It said that the involvement of all levels of government in the financing of "high-quality comprehensive health care for all our people is deemed legitimate and essential," and urged that "the availability of health services, as a matter of human right, should be based on health need alone, and not on ability to pay."

There was no great reaction from the Fellowship, although this Statement, which could appropriately be understood as an endorsement of the Medicare proposal, was clearly at odds with the position taken by the Committee on Public Health and most of the medical organizations in the country.

## ACADEMY PUBLICATIONS

In 1963, Dr. Robert L. Craig, who had been named Editor of the *Bulletin* in 1952, was succeeded by Dr. Paul Cranefield. While successfully discharging this responsibility, Dr. Cranefield, who had obtained his Ph.D. in physiology some years previously, also attended the Albert Einstein College of Medicine from which he graduated in 1964. He left the Academy on December 31, 1966 to join the faculty of Rockefeller University where his work later earned him the 1988 Academy Medal for Distinguished Contributions in Biomedical Science, an award that he shared with Dr. Brian Hoffman.

In 1967, Dr. Cranefield was succeeded in turn by Dr. Saul Jarcho, who served on a half time basis as Editor and as Executive Secretary of the Committee on Publications. Dr. Jarcho, a Fellow of the Academy since 1940, was a prominent medical practitioner who had achieved wide recognition for combining his clinical work with a distinguished scholarly career as a medical historian, author, linguist and translator, and as a pioneer in the field of paleopathology.

### Award to Mr. Charles Morchand

In 1958, the Academy Plaque was awarded to Charles C. Morchand, head of the printing firm that had printed the *Bulletin* since 1928. The citation that accompanied it describes how Mr. Morchand's relationship to the Academy began in 1924, when he was a young man just out of college who had set up a small printing business. In the course of his canvassing for business, he stopped at the Academy, then on West 43rd Street and, the story runs, when he told the person at the entrance desk the purpose of his visit, he was told to take a chair in the corridor. After an interminable wait, a tall, dignified, rather impressive gentleman entered the front door and, as he passed by, asked the young man if there was anything he could do for him. The gentleman was Dr. Linsly R.

Williams, the first full-time Director of the Academy and the day was his first on his new job. Mr. Morchand left with a small order for the printing of some cards, beginning a relationship with the Academy which endured for more that three decades. Reflecting a warm and engaging personality that supplemented his knowledge and skill as a printer, the Academy's association with his firm continued without interruption until 1990, some years after Mr. Morchand's retirement, when the firm was acquired by another organization.

During the 1960s, the Academy published some twenty-one volumes in the History of Medicine series. They included works by Philippe Pinel, Benjamin Rush, René Théophile Hyocinthe Laennec, Bernardo Ramazzini, Theodore Kraepelin, and Isaac Ray (see Appendix).


## THE LIBRARY

From its inception the Library has been confronted by the problem of finding space for its ever-growing collection of books, journals, and artifacts. Space added in the 1950s had been expected to solve the problem for the next twenty-five years but, with the flood of new medical literature, the problem recurred in only three years. This problem was shared by almost every medical library in existence at the time and, in 1957, the Library Committee invited representatives of a number of New York City medical libraries to explore the possibility of a joint venture that might solve it. Similar meetings held over the next few years culminated in the establishment in January, 1964 of the Medical Library Center of New York, as a not-for-profit corporation. Dr. Howard Reid Craig was elected Chairman of its Board of Directors. The Board of Trustees approved the investment of $275,000 in a ten-year first mortgage to finance the acquisition of a building just one block away from the Academy and the payment of the $10,000 assessment for operating expenses that was required from each participating library.

The formal dedication of the Medical Library Center took place on June 15, 1964 and, almost immediately, the Library transferred to it some 6,000 bound volumes and 100,000 foreign medical theses culled from its stacks. These materials, which were considered marginal to the main functions of the Library, could be retrieved within twenty-four hours through the Center's delivery service, which made daily stops at the participating libraries. In addition to housing old and infrequently needed materials, the Center maintains a Union Catalogue of all the periodical holdings, not only of all the member libraries but also of other collections in the New York City area, including museums, botanical gardens and scientific establishments, altogether a total of sixty-eight libraries.

## Regional Medical Library

In 1965, the federal government enacted Public Law 89–21, the Medical Library Assistance Act of 1965, intended to promote the establishment of regional medical libraries. This legislation, which had been drafted by the National Library of Medicine, was introduced by Senator Lister Hill (Dem/Alabama) and Representative John Fogarty (Dem/Rhode Island). It was strongly and widely supported by health professionals and librarians, having been one of two federal programs proposed by the President's Commission on Heart Disease, Cancer and Stroke chaired by Dr. Michael E. DeBakey, (the other was the Regional Medical Program for Heart Disease, Cancer and Stroke). The Commission had called attention to the poor condition of the nation's medical libraries and declared that "... unless major attention is directed to improvement of our national medical library base, the continued and accelerated generation of scientific knowledge will become increasingly an exercise in futility."[35]

Under the Act, grants, and later contracts, were to be given to foster cooperation among libraries and to help the dissemination of information from a network of regional medical libraries. Accordingly, on May 25, 1966, the Board of Trustees and Council, meeting jointly, voted to approve a combined application on the part of the Medical Library Center of New York and the New York Academy of Medicine for a grant to cover the planning of the program in the New York area. It was one of the first to be approved.

Ms. Gertrude Annan, the Academy Librarian, had at first been reluctant to participate in this program out of concern that the necessity of handling and copying articles from the Library's holdings would do grave damage to these irreplaceable materials. The leadership of the National Library of Medicine, which had been designated to administer this program, recognized the wealth of the Library's holdings and conveyed great eagerness for the Academy to play a role. Miss Annan allowed herself to be persuaded, thereby initiating an involvement of the Academy in the Regional Medical Library Program which continues to this day. This decision has enabled the Library to extend its services to other parts of the country and to participate very actively in the current revolution in the dissemination of medical information.

## Exhibitions

A major activity of the Library staff through the years, described in the Academy's *1958–1959 Annual Report* as a "time-consuming but rewarding chore," has been the organization and installation of the exhibits continuously on display in the reading rooms and the lobby and halls of the building. On occasion, a more elaborate and comprehensive "exhibition" is presented. Many are prompted by their timeliness: to commemorate the birth of prominent physicians or other figures prominent in medical history, the anniversary of the publication of an important book, or the birth or the founding of an organization. Often they are scheduled at the request of Fellows. Several represent a regular annual feature: books by Fellows and other New York physicians published during the previous year; the Nobel laureates and winners of other signal honors; and collections of recent text books devoted to a particular subject.[36]

## Acquisitions

The Library also makes acquisitions of current and historical materials. The Friends of the Rare Book Room, established in 1946, is an organization of Fellows and others who share an interest in medical history and whose Life Memberships and annual contributions help to make it possible for the Academy to acquire incunabula and artifacts of great rarity and interest. Many of the acquisitions are donated by Fellows and others. For example, in 1959, President Robert L. Levy presented a deed of gift promising to the Library his outstanding and valuable collection of works on cardiology, which includes a very fine copy of the first edition of *De motu Cordis*, published in 1628, in which William Harvey first described the circulation of the blood. It remains a part of the Levy Collection in the Rare Book Room.

Another major acquisition during this period was the Michael M. Davis Collection on the Economic and Social Aspects of Medical Care, presented by Dr. Davis in 1967, four years before his death. Dr. Davis, who was trained as a medical sociologist and became Director of the Boston Dispensary, achieved prominence as a commentator and writer on health care issues. His meticulously organized and beautifully catalogued collection contains materials on every aspect of health care organization and financing, national health insurance and governmental programs

## THE ACADEMY BUILDING

In January 1965, Dr. John L. Madden, President of the Academy, appointed a Committee to explore the potential of expanding the Academy's physical plant in the light of current and future activities. The Committee was chaired by Dr. Robert L. Levy and included Drs. George Baehr, Stuart Craig, Frank Glenn, M. Ralph Kaufman, Shepherd Krech, Samuel Lambert, James E. McCormack, John L. Madden, William Barclay Parsons, and Bronson Ray, and Dr. Howard Reid Craig, the Academy Director, and Mr.

Robert Brereton, the Business Manager. Members of the staff presented their views of the space needs of the various departments
and offices. The advice of Mr. James Felt, former Chairman of the
New York City Housing Authority and a noted real estate expert,
was enlisted, and a firm of architects was consulted. The Committee met frequently and its deliberations, which were meticulously
recorded, have been preserved and make interesting reading.

Several alternatives were considered. These included the purchase and remodeling of the apartment building on Fifth Avenue
adjacent to the Academy; adding additional floors to the present
building; erecting a connecting building on the three sites just
east of the building which were being used for automobile parking; expanding into the building around the corner on 102nd
Street, which had been acquired for the Medical Library Center;
and, although it meant a loss of income, using some of the space
in the building currently being rented to other organizations for
Academy-related activities. In addition to the questionable adequacy of the Academy's financial resources, these possibilities
raised such obstacles as zoning laws, underground water, the
feasibility of providing access between any constructions and the
Academy building, and the need to evict current tenants. The
upshot was a decision to acquire the two adjacent tenements at
16 and 20 East 103rd Street. This was accomplished in 1967,
and, at the present time, these properties still continue to produce rental income for the Academy and provide a "hedge"
against a future need for expansion.


ACADEMY FINANCES


In 1959 Mr. Arthur A. Eberle retired after twenty-eight years as
Comptroller of the Academy, and was succeeded by Mr. Robert
M. Brereton who was given the title of Business Manager. New
budgetary controls and reporting systems were introduced and
department heads began to be provided with monthly reports of
actual vs. budgeted expenses. Despite very modest operating defi-

cits in 1958 and 1959, the Academy's financial status was considered to be quite satisfactory. The value of the endowment had risen from $4.5 million in 1947 to just under $22 million in 1966, and the income it produced was providing an increasing proportion of the operating budget, from 44 percent in 1948 to 70 percent in 1966. While Fellows' dues as a percentage of income continued to slide, this decline was more than offset by grants and contracts from government agencies and other sources. In all, it appeared, the Academy could justifiably enjoy satisfaction with the status of its financial resources.

## THE HEALTH RESEARCH COUNCIL OF THE CITY OF NEW YORK

On November 10, 1966 the Board of Health and the Department of Health of the City of New York—the Academy had played a role in founding both—celebrated their centennial at the New York Academy of Medicine. Dr. Leona Baumgartner, the celebrated former Commissioner of Health, a Fellow of the Academy, gave an address that revealed her vision of how the Department might reinvent itself to meet the current challenges to the health of the City. It portrayed cooperative arrangements to promote research that would guide the Department in dealing with the fundamental health problems confronting the people of the City, in which the Academy could play a pivotal role.[37]

In her remarks Dr. Baumgartner reviewed the involvement of the Department in health research which, she said, had always been regarded as important. She recalled the work of Dr. Hermann M. Biggs, the great pioneer in public health and social medicine who had been the first Commissioner of Health of New York State. He founded the Department's Diagnostic Laboratory in 1893 and stimulated the publication of seminal studies in epidemiology, pediatrics, disease control and statistics—he was also a Fellow of the Academy. She also recalled the establishment in 1941 of the Public Health Research Institute as a "semi–independent unit" connected to the Health Department that focused on research in viral, infectious and metabolic diseases.

In the 1950s, she said, new risks to health were emerging, but the City's "medical care services were scattered, undermanned, and were failing to keep up with the problems of the time. Space for needed facilities was inadequate. Yet there was talent here and an enormous medical establishment that was not being used to find answers to the growing problems. A municipally financed effort that focused on some of the most acute problems seemed appropriate."[38]

Accordingly, in 1954, the Health Research Council of the City of New York was created (but it did not become operational until 1958). The Council was modeled on the British Medical Research Council, with the field of investigation broadened to include social sciences and engineering, disciplines that certainly could make a contribution to solving New York's health problems. Made up of both scientists and laypersons, it provided grants to support research conducted in local universities, colleges, medical schools and City agencies. From the very beginning, it emphasized helping the careers of young research scientists working in the City, and, by the end of 1965, some 172 scientists had been funded, and by 1969 about $10 million had been allocated for Career Scientist Awards. Prominent among the recipients were Drs. Vincent Dole and Marie Nyswander of the Rockefeller University whose seminal work on methadone in the treatment of opiate addiction culminated in the methadone maintenance programs of the 1970s which still provide care for many thousands of addicts in the City and around the world. Another notable recipient of a Career Scientist Award was Dr. Saul J. Farber who was then working on problems in diabetes and relationships between cardiac and renal function. Dr. Farber subsequently went on to become Dean and Chairman of the Department of Medicine at New York University Medical School and Dean and Provost of the New York University Medical Center. He later served as Chairman of the Academy's Board of Trustees (1991 to 1995). Dr. Howard Reid Craig and a number of Fellows made key contributions to the formation and operation of the Council and, in addition to receiving grants for research projects in alcoholism, narcotics addiction and infant mortality, the Academy was awarded a contract to administer the program.

Originally, it had been hoped to finance the work of the Council by an allocation of one dollar per year per citizen of the City. The City's allocations were matched by contributions from the State of New York and, it was estimated, for every dollar of these funds, nearly five dollars in the form of grants from federal and private agencies were received. Unfortunately, inflation, fluctuations in the economy and increasing competition for allocations of tax-levy dollars ultimately led to the demise of the Council in the 1970s.

## THE NEW YORK REGIONAL MEDICAL PROGRAM FOR HEART DISEASE, CANCER AND STROKE

In 1966, on the recommendation of the President's Commission on Heart Disease, Cancer and Stroke, and as part of its ambitious "Great Society" programs, the Johnson Administration enacted legislation creating the Regional Medical Programs. Their purpose was ". . . to make the latest advances in medical knowledge of the diagnosis and treatment of heart disease, cancer, and stroke available to physicians for the treatment of their patients all over the nation."[39] The goal of these programs was to apply support from the federal government to regional arrangements through which the nation's academic medical centers and medical schools would serve as centers of excellence to disseminate to local community hospitals and medical practitioners the knowledge and skills they had acquired in the treatment of heart, disease, cancer and stroke.

The Associated Medical Schools of Greater New York, which had been formed in 1964 and had previously collaborated with the Academy in establishing the Medical Library Center, joined with the Medical Society of the County of New York and others in proposing that the Academy undertake a project to formulate and carry out a plan for the establishment of a Regional Medical Program for Heart Disease, Cancer and Stroke (RMP) in the Metropolitan New York Area. Dr. James E. McCormack, who had been appointed Associate Director just a few months earlier, was designated to lead the Academy effort. In order to obtain the federal grant, the Academy was designated as an "Advisory Council" and, by the fall of 1966, RMP had been organized and was occupying office space in the Academy building. Dr. Vincent DePaul Larkin, Director of Medical Education at the Methodist Hospital in Brooklyn, was appointed Director. The Academy's Office of Medical Education was involved with the program because of the RMP's continuing education component.

The deans of the local medical schools were ambivalent about participating in the RMP because of the concern that the federal grants would require financial commitments that the institutions would have to continue even after the government's program ended. There was also the requirement that the institutions would have to develop projects that reached out to the community physicians, activities that some of the medical schools were reluctant to undertake.

## ACADEMY PRESIDENTS

### Dr. Robert L. Levy, 1957–1960

Dr. Levy, a graduate of Yale College and the Johns Hopkins University School of Medicine served two full terms as President. A highly-regarded cardiologist, he was an Attending Physician at the Presbyterian Hospital and a Professor of Medicine at the Columbia University College of Physicians and Surgeons. He became a Fellow in 1922, and served on the Committee on Public Health, the Committee on the Library, Chairman of the Nominating Committee, and Vice-President. After completing his Presidency, he served on the Board of Trustees.

### Dr. Frank Glenn, 1961–1962

Dr. Glenn , a native of Illinois, was a graduate of the Washington University School of Medicine in St. Louis. He was Chairman of the Department of Surgery and Surgeon-in-Chief at the New York Hospital. He became a Fellow in 1936 and, in addition to serving at the Academy, he was President of the New York Cancer Society, the New York Surgical Society and the American College of Surgeons.

### Dr. Harold Brown Keyes, 1963–1964

Dr. Keyes, a graduate of Yale College and the Columbia University College of Physicians and Surgeons, was the Director of Surgery and President of the Medical Board at the French Hospital. He became a Fellow in 1919 and served for twenty years as a member of the Committee on Medical Information. He was elected Vice-President in 1957.

### Dr. John L. Madden, 1965–1966

Dr. Madden was a graduate of the George Washington University School of Medicine who became Clinical Professor of Surgery at the New York Medical College and an Attending Surgeon on the staffs of the Flower-Fifth Avenue and Metropolitan Hospitals. He became a Fellow in 1948, and served as Secretary and Chairman of the Section on Surgery, Chairman of the Committee on Medical Education (1959-1960), and as a member of the Council and the Board of Trustees from 1959 through 1974.

### Dr. Preston A. Wade, 1967–1968

Dr. Wade, a graduate of the Cornell University College of Medicine, was affiliated with the New York Hospital and the Hospital for Special Surgery, where he headed a unit for the treatment of bone fractures. He was a past President of the American Association for the Surgery of Trauma. He became a Fellow in 1931.

## THE END OF THE ERA OF DR. HOWARD REID CRAIG

Dr. Howard Reid Craig retired on January 1, 1967, after twenty years of service as Director, a longer term than any of those who preceded or followed him in that position. On presenting him with the Academy Plaque at the Annual Meeting of January 5, 1967, George Baehr, Emeritus Director of Medicine at the Mount Sinai Hospital, who was President during the first years of that term, said,

We soon learned that his gentle demeanor was misleading, for behind it lies the strength, the wisdom and the quiet determination of a statesman. Every department of the Academy has felt his ever watchful presence. The business management of the Academy was completely reorganized on a sound managerial basis under his direction, Our Library has developed at a more rapid rate. New ventures in public service have had their roots in the Academy, such as the creation of a Community Blood Bank and the establishment of a Central Deposit Library to serve medical schools and research institutions throughout this part of the country. . . . Behind these and many other developments in public affairs in which the Academy has participated during the last 20 years, we can discern the unobtrusive guidance and the expertise of a skillful and diplomatic leader.[40]

Writing about Dr. Craig's retirement, Past President Robert L. Levy, Chairman of the Board of Trustees at that time, added, "Under Craig's tenure of office, the Academy grew in stature and in influence, both local and national and, indeed, international."[41] Throughout that period, the Academy retained an influence on health policy issues, enjoying especially close working relationships with both the City and State health departments. Dr. Craig even formed a close relationship between the Academy and the Royal Society of Medicine of London, England.

For two years after retiring as the Academy Director, Dr. Craig continued as a consultant, and also, from 1967 to 1971, he served as a member of the Board of Trustees. On September 8, 1980, he died in his home in Sharon, Connecticut, at the age of eighty-six, a notably long life for one who had taken the position at the Academy because illness precluded continuing his medical practice.

Dr. Craig, however, did not solve all of the Academy's problems. For example, there were the perennial concerns over financing the continuing growth and influence of the Library, and the challenge of the increasing importance of teaching hospitals and the specialty societies in graduate medical education, to say nothing of the emerging problems of the organization, delivery and financing of health care. But, he eminently succeeded in positioning the Academy well within the arena where such issues could be studied and confronted.

## NOTES

1 Craig, HR. 1956 The New York Academy of Medicine: retrospect and prospect. *Bulletin of the New York Academy my of Medicine*. 32: 701–712.
2 Galdston I. July 11, 1957 *A Prospectus for the Academy*. Mimeo.
3 A communication to the Fellows of the New York Academy of Medicine. 1957 *Bulletin of the New York Academy of Medicine*. 33:663–664.
4 Council of the New York Academy of Medicine. Minutes of the meeting of June 30, 1958.
5 Clark DW. 1958 Letter to Dr. HR Craig re Dr. Iago Galdston and the Committee on Medical Information.
6 New York Academy of Medicine. 1960 *A Report of Activities, 1958 and 1959*. New York: New York Academy of Medicine. p. 23.
7 ibid. p. 23.
8 James G. 1964 Can we solve our growing problem in public health?. *Bulletin of the New York Academy of Medicine*. 40:241–255.
9 Transcript of Report on Conference on Perinatal Mortality (October 29, 1957) 1958 *Bulletin of the New York Academy of Medicine*. 34:311–352.

10  Committee on Public Health. 1955 Report on drug addiction. *Bulletin of the New York Academy of Medicine.* 31:592–607.
11  Committee on Public Health. 1963 Report on drug addiction II. *Bulletin of the New York Academy of Medicine.* 39:417–473.
12  Committee on Public Health. 1965 Report on drug addiction III. *Bulletin of the New York Academy of Medicine.* 41:825-829.
13  Kolb LC. Drug addiction: a statement before a Committee of the United States Senate. *Bulletin of the New York Academy of Medicine.* 41:306–309.
14  Committee on Public Health. 1958 *Human Blood in New York City: A Study of its Procurement, Distribution and Utilization.* New York: New York Academy of Medicine.
15  Committee on Public Health. 1963 On salacious literature. *Bulletin of the New York Academy of Medicine.* 39:545–546.
16  Committee on Public Health. 1964 Resurgence of venereal disease. *Bulletin of the New York Academy of Medicine.* 40:802–823.
17  ibid. p. 817.
18  Committee on Public Health. 1964 Homosexuality *Bulletin of the New York Academy of Medicine.* 40:576–580.
19  Bieber I, Dain HJ, Dince TR, Drellick MG, et al. 1962 *Homosexuality: A Psychoanalytic Study.* New York: Basic Books.
20  Committee on Public Health. 1964 op. cit. p. 579.
21  Committee on Public Health. 1965 Health education: Its present status. *Bulletin of the New York Academy of Medicine.* 41:1172–1188.
22  New York Academy of Medicine. 1956 *By-laws* Article XIII, Section 5.
23  Council and Board of Trustees, New York Academy of Medicine. 1956 Minutes of the joint meeting of December 28, 1956.
24  New York Academy of Medicine. 1969 *By-laws* Article IX, Section 4.
25  Menzel H, Maurice R and McGuiness AC. 1966 The effectiveness of the televised clinical science seminars of the New York Academy of Medicine. *Bulletin of the New York Academy of Medicine.* 42: 679–714.
26  McGuiness AC, Menzel H, Fleischman E, and Garten J., 1968 The medical television audience of the New York Academy of Medicine after four years. *Bulletin of the New York Academy of Medicine.* 44::332–345.
27  ibid. p. 334.
28  Menzel H, Maurice R and McGuiness AC. op. cit. p. 681.
29  ibid. p. 703.
30  Valentine FC. 1910 *Last Will and Testament.* Submitted to Probate, Surrogate, Queens County, January 18, 1910.

31 Davis, Polk, Wardwell, Sunderland and Kiendl. 1964 *Memorandum for Hon. F. Hodges Combier. Re New York Academy of Medicine vs. Ferdinand C. Valentine.* January 31, 1964
32 Galdston I. 1965 *Medicine in Transition.* Chicago: University of Chicago Press.
33 Weinerman ER. 1965 Anchor points underlying the planning for to-morrow's health care. *Bulletin of the New York Academy of Medicine.* 41:1213–1225.
34 Committee on Social Policy for Health Care. 1965 A policy statement on the role of government tax funds in problems of health care. *Bulletin of the New York Academy of Medicine.* 41:795-796.
35 President's Commission on Heart Disease Cancer and Stroke. 1964–1965 *Report to the President: A National Program to Conquer Heart Disease, Cancer and Stroke.* Washington, DC: US Government Printing Office. 2 vols, p. 25. In: Bunting A. 1987 The nation's health information network: history of the Regional Medical Library Program, 1965–1986. *Bulletin of the Medical Library Association.* 75, Supplement: 1–62.
36 New York Academy of Medicine *1957–1958 Annual Report.*
37 Baumgartner L. 1969 One hundred years of health: New York City 1866–1966. *Bulletin of the New York Academy of Medicine.* 45: 555:586.
38 ibid. p. 580.
39 President's Commission on Heart Disease, Cancer and Stroke op. cit. p. 28.
40 Baehr G. 1967 Citation and presentation of the Academy Plaque to Howard Reid Craig, MD. *Bulletin of the New York Academy of Medicine.* 43:319–321.
41 Levy RL. 1967 Howard Reid Craig, an appreciation. *Bulletin of the New York Academy of Medicine.* 43:3–8.

# Chapter 4
# 1967–1976
# The McCormack Years

ON JANUARY 1, 1967, after having served for six months as Deputy Director, Dr. James E. McCormack became Director of the Academy, a position he was to hold until 1981.

Dr. McCormack was born in Jersey City, NJ, in 1911. He received his bachelor's degree from St. Peters College in Jersey City where he had majored in classics, and his MD from the New York University School of Medicine. This was followed by five years of postgraduate training at Bellevue Hospital. During World War II, he served as an aide to the Committee on Medical Research at the Office of Scientific Research and Development in Washington, DC. In 1946, he became Assistant Dean at the New York University School of Medicine, and in 1948, he returned to Washington, DC, where he spent two years as Deputy Executive Director and then as Executive Director of the Research and Development Board of the Department of Defense. During that period, he earned certification by the American Board of Internal Medicine. In 1951, he returned to New York to become Associate Dean of the Columbia University College of Physicians and Surgeons and, in 1955, Assistant Vice President of the Presbyterian Hospital. In 1960, he moved back to New Jersey to become Dean of the Seton Hall University College of Medicine and, when it was taken over by the State of New Jersey because of financial difficulties, he was named President of the New Jersey College of Medicine and Dentistry, which succeeded it.

Dr. McCormack became a Fellow of the Academy in 1947. He served on the Committee on Medical Education from 1952 through 1964 and as Chairman of that Committee from 1952 to 1956. Coupled with his six-months' experience as Deputy Director, this provided a knowledge of the Academy which, together with his extensive experience in the administration of medical education and research, made him uniquely qualified to lead the Academy through a period of great change in medical education and health care.

AN IDEOLOGICAL CONFLICT

Unfortunately, almost as soon as he took office as Director, the Academy became embroiled in a heated conflict over issues of ideology and personalities. This conflict lasted for over a year and involved many of the Fellows either as adversaries or would-be mediators. The ideological issue was a proposal to create a unified Health Services Administration for the City of New York, and the personalities involved were Dr. McCormack and Mr. Harry Becker, who had joined the Academy staff in 1962 as Executive Secretary of the Committee on Special Studies (formerly the Committee on Medical Information).

Although they rarely reached such proportions, ideological differences have always been a characteristic of Academy activities. From time to time, the Academy structure, and especially the commitees, confront contentious issues and policies and, because the Fellows are knowledgeable, experienced and articulate, they often have strong opinions. Through discussion and persuasion in the traditionally collegial environment of the Academy, a resolution of differences satisfactory to most of those involved is generally reached. Those who still disagree are free to put forward a minority report or to pursue their viewpoints in other organizations to which they also belong where their positions might be more acceptable.

Clashes of personality are also not unheard of in the history of the Academy, witness the conflict between Drs. Howard Reid Craig and Iago Galdston mentioned earlier.

This conflict had its roots in the attempt of Mayor John V. Lindsay, who had been elected in 1965 as the first Republican in twenty years to hold that office, to bring efficiency to the City government by creating a small group of "superagencies" in which existing agencies and departments could be consolidated. In the area of health, he proposed the creation of a giant "Health Services Administration" that would include the Department of Health. the Department of Hospitals, the Community Mental Health Board, the Office of the Chief Medical Examiner and the Bureau of Medical Services in the Department of Welfare. The rationale for this move was the hope that uniting the preventive services provided by the Department of Health with the curative services provided by the Department of Hospitals would eliminate the fragmentation and duplication of services, while centralizing their administration would bring badly needed efficiency and economies of scale to the management of their operations and make for more effective planning. The Lindsay administration also believed that, even if they had no great background in the health area, individuals with well-developed managerial skills were likely to be more effective administrators than physicians or other health professionals. These changes would require revision of the City Charter and, accordingly, in January 1967, a legislative proposal was developed which Dr. Howard J. Brown, the recently appointed Commissioner of Health, forwarded to the Academy for study and comment, an assignment that the Trustees and Council (they often met jointly in this era) formally voted to accept at their April meeting.

The stage for the conflict was set when study of the Lindsay proposal was simultaneously undertaken by two committees: the Committee on Special Studies and the Committee on Public Health. Also important was the fact that, while the proposal presented a concept for reorganizing the City's role in health care, it was quite vague about how that was to be implemented. The result was not only a jurisdictional dispute but also, based on strongly held preconceived notions about the role of government in health care, two sets of widely disparate recommendations.

Both Committees criticized the budgetary restrictions, the cumbersome administrative procedures and practices, and the outmoded personnel management systems that pervaded not only the health agencies but the entire City government. But from that point on, they diverged.

The Committee on Public Health, which was chaired by Dr. Arthur Fischl, took its cues from Dr. Kruse, its Executive Secretary, who was an early advocate of a diminished role of government in the delivery of health care and what has come to be called the "privatization" of government-operated facilities. In considering the legislative proposal, this Committee broadened its scope to include all personal health services provided in the City, including those provided by private and voluntary facilities as well as by the municipal hospitals. Although there would be a personal health services authority, there would be autonomous units including public and private agencies. The Department of Hospitals as well as the Community Board of Mental Health and Hospitals would be abolished. To make the decentralized structure work, the municipal hospitals would have to be freed from the centralized control of the City and greater authority given to the administrators of the individual institutions. A number of the municipal hospitals would be closed with the remainder being converted into voluntary hospitals. With the advent of Medicare and Medicaid, the Committee argued, there would be no need to maintain a public hospital system.

The Committee on Special Studies took its lead from its Executive Secretary, Mr. Harry Becker, an advocate of a greater governmental role in health care who had been a personal friend of Health Commissioner Brown since they had worked together for the United Automobile Workers in Detroit. Mr. Becker ignored the fact that the Committee on Public Health had a record of involvement in health care issues dating back to 1911, and had recently issued a report on the City's municipal hospitals. Flaunting this history, he felt that it was entirely appropriate for the Committee on Special Studies to take up this matter, a view that, as it turned out, was not shared by Dr. McCormack, the newly installed Director.

In contrast to the Committee on Public Health, the Committee on Special Studies favored a stronger public authority in health care. It called for a single agency to have authority over all of the tax-levy funds allocated to health services as well as the traditional public health functions. This agency would be headed by a physician who would have the qualifications then required of the Commissioner of Health, with deputies assigned as administrators for defined geographic areas. The Board of Health would assume the responsibilities then assigned to the Community Board of Mental Health and Hospitals.

The report of the Committee on Public Health was published in the *Bulletin* with a notation that it "does not necessarily reflect the views of the Council."[1] The report of the Committee on Special Studies was never published.

At the January 26, 1967 joint meeting of the Council and Trustees, the first attended by Dr. McCormack in his role as Director, and also the first for Dr. Preston A. Wade as President, there was an initial discussion of the "overlapping of interest" between the Committees on Public Health and on Special Studies. Dr. McCormack suggested that a change in the By-laws, which had last been revised in 1956, would be necessary to minimize the risk of such conflicts in the future.

Following a suggestion made at the February meeting, a special Subcommittee of the Council was created to undertake reconciliation of the opposing views. Dr. John L. Pool, then Vice President of the Academy, was named Chairman; its members included Dr. Byard Williams, Chairman of the Committee on Special Studies, Dr. Arthur Fischl, Chairman of the Committee on Public Health, Dr. M. Ralph Kaufman, Chairman of the Committee on Medical Education, Dr. John L. Madden, the immediate past-President, President Preston Wade and Director James McCormack. The Subcommittee was also charged to assist the Director to decide, when the question of jurisdiction over an issue arose, whether to assign it to a particular committee or make it a joint study by representatives of more than one standing committee

In his report to President Wade of the April 28 meeting of the Subcommittee, Dr. Pool indicated that the Chairs of the embattled Committees and their staffs had agreed to try to reconcile their views. The Subcommittee suggested that, to avoid such conflicts in the future, there was "the great need for guidelines as to the areas of future study by committees or combinations of committees and for the release of reports and information that emanate from the Fellows and staff of the Academy. While such long-range planning is in development, it recommended that no committee institute conferences, investigations, reports or other work without prior clearance with the Director and the President."[2]

In keeping with that directive, the Subcommittee withheld approval of a recommendation emanating from the Committee on Special Studies that called for emergency measures to alleviate the shortage of hospital beds in the City. And, in May, the Council referred for review by the Subcommittee a proposal from the Committee on Special Studies for a "program of studies in areas which overlap those of other Committees."

In the meantime, the quarrel between Dr. McCormack and Mr. Becker was heating up. The minutes of the April Council meeting included an item attributed to Dr. John L. Madden, the immediate Past-President and a close friend of Dr. McCormack, indicating his concern that Mr. Becker "has been quoted in the papers on more than one occasion on controversial matters and identified as being on the staff of the New York Academy of Medicine."[3] In June, Dr. McCormack wrote to Dr. Byard Williams, then Chairman of the Committee on Special Studies, in response to a proposal to have the Academy's annual seminar on health problems cosponsored by the Community Council of Greater New York (an umbrella organization of private charities, welfare and social agencies in New York City), that he "must categorically refuse permission to have such a meeting under the terms in which it was requested by Mr. Becker" on the grounds that it would put the Academy in the position of being used "as a platform to advance the agenda of a subcommittee of the Community Council of which Mr. Becker was a member."[4] And, a week later, in a letter to Dr. Howard Reid Craig, his predecessor as Director, who had been given a five-year contract as a Consultant to the Academy, he reported that he had given Mr. Becker notice of his dismissal from the Academy staff as of October 1, 1967.[5] Mr. Becker was ordered to return to the Ford Foundation all unexpended funds in a grant made to support the Committee on Social Policy for Health Care (which, as noted earlier, had become the Committee on Special Studies). In addition, Dr. McCormack announced that he had refused to sign an application for renewal of the Career Scientist grant awarded in 1964 by the Health Research Council of the City of New York to Marvin Lieberman, who had been working on projects under the aegis of the Committee on Special Studies. Dr. McCormack subsequently changed his mind on this, and the grant was renewed.

The quarrel became public when Martin Tolchin, then a writer on medical features for the *New York Times,* reported that Mr. Becker had resigned after being informed by Dr. McCormack that the "Committee would henceforth concern itself with education rather than social issues."[6] Dr. McCormack was "not available for comment," it was reported, but Dr. Preston A. Wade, President of the Academy, is quoted as saying, "no policy changes had officially been made."

Members of the Committee, presumably reconciled to the departure of Mr. Becker, who had become a Professor in the Department of Community Medicine at the Albert Einstein College of Medicine, rebelled against what they interpreted as the elimination of the Committee. The *New York Times* article quoted Dr. Martin Cherkasky, Director of Montefiore Hospital, as saying, "It seems that this represents a decision on the part of the Academy to give up its research, examination and probing into the critical matters of community medical-care issues. It was a mark of the vision of the Academy that a quarter of a century ago it became involved in these issues. If one were to pick the most unlikely time for this institution to remove itself from the critical issues of the day, this is it."[6]

This view was echoed by Dr. Irving Graef, Attending Physician-in-Charge at Lenox Hill Hospital, when, as one of a delegation of Committee members appearing before a special meeting of the Council, he said, "a revolution is going on about us and the Academy must play its part." At that meeting, the resignation of Dr. Byard Williams from the Chairmanship, which he had submitted earlier in protest over the way Mr. Becker had been dismissed, was accepted (he remained a member of the Committee). Dr. John M. Cotton, Chief of Psychiatry at St. Luke's Hospital and Past-President of the Medical Society of the County of New York, was elected to succeed him as Chairman.

It was decided to take no action on the fate of the Committee until the revision of the By-laws, then under way, would be completed some months later. To carry on with activities already in progress,

Dr. Caldwell B. Esselstyn was appointed as part-time, interim Executive Secretary. Dr. Esselstyn, who had founded the Columbia Medical Group in central New York State, one of the earliest prepaid group practices in the country, and who was a leader in the Group Practice Association of America, was then serving as Assistant Director of the New York Regional Medical Program which had its offices in the Academy building. Dr. Marvin Lieberman was assigned to assist Dr. Esselstyn in both his Committee activities and his work with the Regional Medical Program.

The combined work load proved to be too great and, in January 1968, Dr. Esselstyn was succeeded as Executive Secretary by Dr. Albert Snoke, who had just retired from the position of Administrator of the Yale-New Haven Hospital. Dr. Milton Terris, Chairman of the Department of Community and Preventive Medicine at the New York Medical College, agreed to chair the subcommittee to plan the Annual Health Conference for 1968, which was to be devoted to the pros and cons of group practice. After much discussion, a request from the Lindsay administration to discuss the report of the Piel Commission was rejected by both the Committee on Public Health and the Committee on Special Studies, but the Academy did offer to provide facilities for public hearings on that report. Also, the work of the Committee on Social Policy for Health Care supported by a grant from the Ford Foundation, was continued.

On February 26, 1969 the Council approved the revision of the By-laws which assigned the kinds of activities that had been pursued by the Committee on Special Studies to a new standing Committee on Medicine in Society. Dr. John M. Cotton was named Chairman and Marvin Lieberman Ph.D. was appointed its Executive Secretary, a post he was to retain until 1995. Dr. Lieberman had received his Ph.D. in Political Science from New York University which he had attended from 1965 to 1968 under a US Public Health Service Fellowship. Having worked with the three previous Executive Secretaries, assisted with the Committee on Social Policy in Health Care, and having helped to plan the Annual Health Conferences, he had become well-acquainted with many of the Fellows involved with the Committee.

## COMMITTEE ON MEDICINE IN SOCIETY

One of the first major undertakings of this newly reconstituted Committee was the April 1970 Annual Health Conference. Planned by Dr. John W. V. Cordice, a distinguished surgeon from Queens who later became a member of the Board of Health, with the able assistance of Dr. John L. S. Holloman, former President of the National Medical Association who later became President of the New York City Health and Hospitals Corporation, the Conference attracted over 700 participants who not only included physicians, but also a broad variety of health professionals as well as some laypersons. Entitled *Community Participation for Equity and Excellence in Health Care,* it featured panels and workshops that dealt with the health needs of the poor and underserved. In the second of his Presidential Addresses, delivered on April 29, 1970, Dr. John L. Pool called attention particularly to the active exchange of information and attitudes that took place at the Conference between "physicians who, after all, are the ones actually delivering health care and the leaders of communities, especially of deprived communities, who are the recipients in need of improved health care today."[7] He emphasized the value of the Academy as a neutral venue particularly suitable for such exchanges.

### Subcommittee on Community Participation

A by-product of the Annual Health Conference was the appointment of a Subcommittee on Community Participation which was charged to explore the potential role(s) of the Academy in improving the health of the community. Under the leadership of Dr. John V. Waller, Attending Physician at Lenox Hill Hospital who became its Chairman, it ultimately decided that the best way was to promote the design and delivery of health education programs (*vide infra*).

Prolonging Life in Terminal Illness

In 1972, Dr. McCormack received a letter from Drs. G. Jarvis Coffin and Samuel W. Lambert on behalf of the Euthanasia Educational Fund, questioning the propriety of using aggressive methods of treatment to prolong life in cases of terminal illness. Dr. McCormack referred the letter to the Committee on Medicine in Society, then chaired by Dr. Milton Terris, which discussed a provisional statement on this issue that had been drafted by Dr. Lieberman. The discussion focused on the suffering that might be inflicted on patients and their families by futile or near futile heroic measures to prolong life in the face of the interdiction of measures to end life common to a number of religions, as well as the "do no harm" credo of the Hippocratic Oath.

The statement ultimately approved by the Committee deliberately avoided the use of the term "euthanasia," which connotes positive actions to hasten death, on the grounds that it obscured the legitimate issues raised by the Coffin-Lambert letter. It went on, however, to say that, "Even within traditions that strongly condemn the willful killing of patients who are suffering from prolonged disease, it is recognized that there is no obligation on the part of the physician to use heroic measures to lengthen life in the face of a terminal illness, and that there is no prohibition against the use of medications to ease pain even if these medications may shorten life." It suggested that: "Mere preservation of life must not be the sole objective of treatment; the physician should discuss the situation with the patient or the family and encourage the patient and the family to express their feelings and wishes about this matter; the opinions and recommendations of the family physician should be obtained even if he is not a physician of record in the particular case; and, the views of religious advisers may be helpful." The statement was unanimously approved by the Committee with the recommendation that it be published and circulated among hospital trustees and administrators and members of the medical profession. This was approved by the Council on December 20, 1972, and it was published.[8]

## COMMITTEE ON MEDICAL EDUCATION

In May 1967, Dr. Robert S. Goodhart succeeded Dr. Aims C. McGuiness as Executive Secretary of the Committee on Medical Education. Dr. Goodhart had graduated from the New York University School of Medicine 1934 and subsequently served on the faculty of its Department of Medicine. He served with the US Public Health Service from 1942 through 1946 and later headed the Health Nutrition Clinic of the New York City Department of Health in Washington Heights. A member of several committees of the National Academy of Sciences-National Research Council, he was co-author of a major textbook on clinical nutrition. Dr. Goodhart held this position until he was succeeded in 1978 by Mr. William C. Stubing.

In 1969, reflecting growing interest in the application of the physical sciences to medical practice and research, a Section on Biomedical Engineering was created. In the same vein, the Section on Micro- and Molecular Biology, which had formerly been known as the Section on Microbiology, changed its name to the Section on Basic Medical Sciences.

## COMMITTEE ON PUBLIC HEALTH

In 1969, Dr. Kruse was succeeded as Executive Secretary of the Committee on Public Health by Dr. Arthur J. Lewis, a native of Hoboken whose medical education included an M.D. from the New York University School of Medicine, a residency in medicine at the Jersey City Medical Center and a fellowship in rheumatology at the Goldwater Memorial Hospital. He later served on the faculty and as Assistant Dean of Seton Hall University Medical Schools during the period in which Dr. James McCormack was its Dean. There, he had observed Dr. McCormack's difficulties with politicians, public officials and some of the trustees, whom he had perceived as meddling with matters that properly were within the purview of physician administrators, and he

came to perceive Dr. McCormack as someone who was very loyal
to colleagues, and whom he respected and trusted. Dr. Lewis
served as Executive Secretary of the Committee on Public Health
until 1972, leaving to join the staff of the Central Office of the
Veterans' Administration, where he remained until he retired in
1995.

He was succeeded by Rudolph Friedrich, D.D.S. A native of
Chicago, he had been a Professor at the Columbia University
School of Dental and Oral Surgery, and had become known to
many of the Fellows through his participation in some of the advisory committees of the New York Regional Medical Program. Dr.
Friedrich was particularly interested in the improvement of efficiency and productivity in the delivery of health services, particularly in ambulatory care settings, and, in fact, organized a conference on this problem. The members of the Committee and Dr.
McCormack felt, however, that, while Dr. Friedrich's concerns
were intrinsically of interest, they were diverting the attention of
the Committee from its assigned area of public health issues. Accordingly, his tenure with the Committee was relatively brief; he
retired in 1976.

### The Abortion Issue

For the fourth time since 1943, when the State of New York
made performance of an abortion by a physician a criminal
offense, the Committee revisited this issue. In 1943, the Academy had issued a statement calling for legalization of abortion
when needed to protect the health of a pregnant woman. The
abortion was to be performed by a trained, licensed physician
in a licensed hospital after receipt of written opinions from
two consultants stating that "the continuance of the pregnancy
would jeopardize the life of the woman or so aggravate the
physical or mental disease from which she suffers so seriously as
to impair her health or threaten her life."[9] Another statement in

1953 added to the conditions that would justify a legal abortion: "rape, incest, or where the child would be born with grave physical or mental defects." And in 1965, the Academy recommended adoption of the Model Penal Code of the American Law Institute which contained similar justifications for a "therapeutic" abortion, a position parallel to that of the American Medical Association.

In 1968, a special New York State Commission appointed by Governor Nelson A. Rockefeller endorsed the Model Penal Code's provisions and added two more justifications for a legal abortion: where the pregnancy began when the mother was unmarried and under sixteen years of age and remained unmarried; and where the mother already has four living children. In support of its recommendations, the Commission argued that there was a need to end abuses resulting from the performance of abortions by untrained persons, a practice not eliminated by the law banning abortions, and also to end discrimination against the poor who, unlike the affluent, did not have the means to travel to jurisdictions where abortions were permitted and to pay to have one safely performed by a trained practitioner.

The 1969 statement from the Committee, called for the Academy to act as an *amicus curiae* in the California Supreme Court case of *People v. Belous* in which the Court had stayed the California State Board of Medical Examiners from holding scheduled hearings of charges against a physician who had performed an abortion. The statement cited court challenges in the Federal Court in the Second District of New York on grounds similar to those in the California case, and closed by noting that it supported the "repeal of those sections of the criminal code referable to the performance of abortions by qualified physicians and further supports the legal changes that would place abortion under the general provisions of the medical practices act of the various states."[10] The Committee's request was approved by the Council and, on September 9, 1969, the California Supreme Court declared the California statute outlawing abortions to be unconstitutional.

The Committee vs. Mayor Lindsay

A conflict between the Committee on Public Health and Mayor Lindsay arose in December 1969. It had its origins in the Mayor's creation of "superagencies" to bring efficiency and economy to the functioning of the City's panoply of agencies and departments, as described previously. One such superagency was the Health Services Administration which encompassed the Departments of Hospitals and Health, the Office of the Chief Medical Examiner and the agency dealing with mental health services. Dr. Bernard Bucove, the former Health Director of the State of Washington, was appointed to head it as Health Services Administrator.

Almost immediately after his reelection in 1969, the Mayor announced that he had requested Dr. Bucove's resignation and was replacing him with Gordon Chase, a thirty-seven-year old Harvard graduate who had been serving as the Deputy Human Resources Administrator. Prior to joining the Lindsay administration, Mr. Chase had been an aide to McGeorge Bundy, Special Assistant to the President on national security affairs, and Deputy Assistant Administrator for Programs at the Agency for International Development, and had headed a 500 member staff at the US Equal Employment Opportunity Commission.[11]

When the proposed appointment was brought to the attention of the Committee by Dr. James Haughton, the First Deputy Administrator under Dr. Bucove, a statement in opposition was prepared. This statement was approved unanimously by the Council and communicated to the Mayor in a letter signed by Dr. John L. Pool, then President of the Academy. The letter, which was also released to the press, said that "the Academy was deeply concerned" by the appointment of "a person without any education or experience in the health field to be the responsible head of program planning and development of all health facilities and services in this complex community of 8,000,000 people."[12] The letter went on to suggest that, as an alternative, Mr. Chase's experience "could appropriately qualify him as a deputy to the

Health Services Administrator to assist him in supervising the fiscal affairs and managerial practices of the Health and Hospitals Corporation and of the several City agencies within the jurisdiction of the Health Services Administration."[12]

The Academy's position was supported by the Medical Society of the County of New York, but a number of organizations and individuals took an opposing view and endorsed the Chase appointment. These included the Public Health Association of New York City, the Health Research Council, Drs. Martin Cherkasky of Montefiore Hospital, Ivan Bennett, Dean of the New York University School of Medicine, and Drs. Lewis Thomas, Walsh McDermott and Samuel Z. Levine, who were current or former members of the New York City Board of Health.

No acknowledgment of the Academy letter was made by the Mayor, who proceeded with the appointment he had planned. Mr. Chase took office in January 1970. Some months later, Dr. Mary McLaughlin, the Commissioner of Health, who, according to the *New York Times* article, had seen "no reason why both the Commissioner of Health and the City Health Services Administrator had to be physicians,"[11] told colleagues at the Academy that health professionals in the Health Department had come to regret the appointment and suggested that the Academy urge the Mayor to rescind it. No action was taken, however. Ultimately Mayor Lindsay's superagencies were dismantled by the mayors who succeeded him.

This episode was in marked contrast to a similar situation some twenty years earlier, in which the Committee had communicated opposition to the proposed appointment as Commissioner of Health of a physician who did not have the eight years of experience in public health administration and/or education required under the City Charter. On that occasion, Mayor William O'Dwyer withdrew the nomination and proceeded to appoint another physician who did meet this requirement, a prerequisite that originally had been suggested by the Academy's Committee on Public Health Relations in 1936.[13]

Other Activities

The Committee pursued a number of other activities during this period. In 1969, it approved a resolution endorsing the use of methadone in the management of opioid addiction. In 1970, with support from the United Hospital Fund, it produced the third edition of the *Autopsy Manual* (the first edition was published in 1950 and the second in 1958. Subsequent revisions were to appear in 1979, 1988 and 1994) Committee studies during this period also dealt with the marijuana problem, the control of lead poisoning, and the issues involved in the malpractice problem.


THE ACADEMY BUILDING

In his Presidential Address for 1969, Dr. John L. Pool reviewed the badly needed major renovations in the Academy building that had recently been completed. These included replacement of the roof, waterproofing the east side of the building, some general refurbishing, and a complete overhaul of the meeting rooms on the second and fourth floors, including replacement of the fixed seating and the installation of air conditioning.

Security in the streets around the building became an issue in 1968 when the members of the Council were informed by Dr. Wade that, in response to letters from some of the organizations holding evening meetings in the Academy building that complained of a "hazard to personal safety," off-duty policemen from the 23rd precinct had been hired to patrol the area around the building in plain clothes while evening meetings were in progress.[14]

A year later, Dr. McCormack wrote to Mayor Lindsay recommending that a picket fence be installed to supplement the stone wall separating Central Park from the west side of Fifth Avenue across the street from the Academy building to "deter young rascals who mug passersby and then climb over the wall into the Park."[15] A high official of the Police Department responded by telephone offering advice, but the fence was never erected.

On December 31, 1972, Sebastian Veseli retired after serving on the building maintenance staff for fifty-nine years. Rightfully calling it a "notable event" in an article he wrote for *Newsnotes,* Dr. McCormack said, " 'Shebby,' as he is affectionately known to large numbers of Fellows, came to the Academy when it was still located on 43rd Street, at the present site of the Princeton Club. He was 19 years old when he started work on January 2, 1924. Having projected slides during these many decades, he has won the regard of untold numbers of Fellows, who now extend to him their warmest wishes for a happy and long retirement."[16]

The Parking Problem

A perennial problem for those visiting the Academy building had been the lack of parking spaces for automobiles. The demolition of the two tenements just to the east of the building that had been purchased in 1969 did provide a badly needed off-the-street parking area. In a presentation at the October, 1972, joint meeting of the Council and Board of Trustees, Dr. McCormack spoke of a plan to construct a multilevel revenue-producing parking structure on this property, the upper floors of which would provide new space for the Library but, apparently, it never went any further. The parking problem was somewhat eased by an arrangement through which Academy Fellows and guests received discounted rates in the parking garage on 102nd Street around the corner from the Academy, an arrangement that has been continued since Mt. Sinai Hospital took over the operation of that garage.

THE ACADEMY LIBRARY

On December 31, 1969, Ms. Gertrude Annan, who had been Librarian of the Academy since 1956, officially retired, although she stayed on until her successor arrived on September 1, 1970. During her tenure with the Academy, she was frequently called on for consultation and advice by medical libraries around the country, and she received many honors, including the Presidency of the Medical Library Association from 1961–1962 and, in 1968, the Marcia C. Noyes Award for outstanding achievement in medical librarianship. Her scholarship, her formidable intellect, and her devotion to the Academy and its Library won her the respect and affection of Dr. McCormack, the Academy staff and the Fellows. In a memorial tribute, Ms. Ursula Poland, former Director of the Schaffer Library of Health Sciences at the Albany Medical College, wrote, "the former New York Academy of Medicine Director, Dr. McCormack, considered Gertrude Annan one of his best instructors on a wide range of topics; he missed her keenly after her retirement and found it difficult to relate to her successors."[17]

Miss Annan's successor was Mr. Thomas Basler, the thirty-year-old librarian of the American Museum of Natural History. Unfortunately, it became clear that he had strong substantive and personality differences with Dr. McCormack, and his stay was brief. He was succeeded in 1973 by Mr. Alfred P. Brandon, one of the most highly regarded medical librarians in the country. After organizing the medical library at the new Medical School of the University of Kentucky, he served for six years as librarian of the Welch Medical Library at Johns Hopkins University and then became the librarian at the new Mt. Sinai School of Medicine. Mr. Brandon was active as a consultant and as a writer, and had a special interest in the history of medicine. He was the author of the famous *Brandon Lists,* which provided guidance on the basic books recommended for medical and allied health libraries.

Unfortunately, Mr. Brandon's term at the Library was a rocky one: first, because he had been quite ill just before his arrival; and second, because of the serious budgetary problems the Academy was facing at that time. Dr. McCormack felt that decisions made by Mr. Brandon with respect to salary adjustments for the Library staff had opened the door to the attempt by District 1199 to unionize the Academy staff which, although unsuccessful, was nevertheless disruptive.

Regional Medical Library

Just before Ms. Annan's retirement in 1969, the Academy received
a grant under the National Library Assistance Program which
created the Regional Medical Library Program. Ms. Annan initially opposed this because she saw it only as a massive interlibrary
loan program and feared that the extensive photoduplication that
would be required would tax the resources of the Library and its
staff and threaten the fragile bindings and pages of the Library's
holdings. It was the view of those directing the Program that the
Academy's failure to participate could severely compromise the
success of the program. In a later tribute to the career of Ms.
Annan, a colleague wrote, "Many of us will remember how
fiercely Gertrude resisted overtures from the National Library of
Medicine and, how, literally, she had to be wooed by its Director to
have the New York Academy of Medicine Library become a regional medical library."[16]

The program was launched in 1969 with Ms. Annan as the first
Director of the New York/New Jersey Regional Medical Library.
When she retired, that mantle was passed to her successors as
Academy Librarian: Mr. Thomas G. Basler from 1970 to 1972;
and Mr. Alfred N. Brandon from 1973 to 1978. Major responsibility for the day-to-day operation of the program was borne by the
Associate Directors: from 1969 to 1971 by Ms. Ann Hutchinson,
who came to the Academy from the New York State Library in
Albany; and Mr. Vernon R. Bruette, the former Associate Librarian at the Library of the SUNY (State University of New York)
Downstate Medical Center in Brooklyn. As cooperation among
the participating medical libraries in the region improved, the Regional Medical Library became an increasingly valuable resource
and remains so to this day. Much of its success is attributable to
the Academy Library's staff whose skill and creativity have enabled it to cope with the periodic alterations in the regional con-
figurations and the changes in the technical specifications required
by the National Library of Medicine.

REGIONAL MEDICAL PROGRAMS

The Regional Medical Programs were created under the 1966 Partnership for Health Act (P.L. 89–239) as part of the federal Heart Disease, Cancer, Stroke and Related Disease Program (the "related diseases" included diabetes mellitus, hypertension, chronic pulmonary disease and renal diseases) as recommended to the Johnson administration by the "DeBakey Commission." Originally, in 1964, that Commission had proposed the creation of a network of federally supported Regional Medical Complexes, which opponents suggested was modeled on building and financing a Memorial-Sloan Kettering Hospital in every region of the US. The strong opposition to such an intrusive federal program, however, was successful in changing it to emphasize cooperative relationships among institutions. A primary element in the program was the communication of the latest findings and techniques in the fight against these diseases through cooperative arrangements among "centers of excellence," community health facilities and medical practitioners. Thus, the continuing education of physicians became a major component of the program.

Policy determination in the New York Metropolitan Regional Medical Program (NYMRMP) was vested in the Trustees of the Associated Medical Schools of Greater New York, of which, as part of its involvement in the Regional Medical Library, the Academy had become a charter member. These included deans of the seven medical schools in the City (Albert Einstein, Columbia College of Physicians and Surgeons, Cornell, Downstate, Mount Sinai, New York University, and New York Medical College (which has been relocated to Valhalla in Westchester County), and the Director of the Academy. The powers of the Trustees included "priority setting, feasibility studies, program direction, data surveys and the philosophy of the NYMRMP."[18] An Advisory Committee with broad representation from the community at large was responsible, in conjunction with the staff, for developing proposals for possible funding. These were reviewed by categorical subcommittees and then by the entire Advisory Committee. When approved by the Trustees of the NYMRMP, the recommendations were forwarded, in turn, to the federal Division of Regional Medical Programs which had the authority to provide funding to support feasibility studies, planning grants, and operational programs in each of the fifty-six regions.

Each of the medical schools and the Academy designated an individual to act as a Regional Coordinator whose salary was, at least in part, paid by the Regional Medical Program. This provided incentives for the participating institutions to work together in planning and providing outreach efforts in continuing medical education.

The first Director of the NYMRMP was Dr. Vincent dePaul Larkin, Director of Medical Education at the Methodist Hospital in Brooklyn. He was succeeded by Dr. I. Jay Brightman, a longtime senior official at the New York State Department of Health, who was followed in turn by Dr. Jesse Aronson, a Cornell Medical College graduate who was certified in public health and had extensive experience with the health departments of New York City, New York State and New Jersey. From its beginning until the program was terminated in 1976, the Academy was designated as the grantee to manage the federal funds and the Program was housed in the Academy building.

One of the activities sponsored by the NYMRMP from 1973 through 1977, with which Dr. Marvin Lieberman was actively involved, was a training program conducted at the Academy for board members of federally funded ambulatory health care centers in New York. Conducted in collaboration with the Association of Neighborhood Health Centers, the courses covered such subjects as quality assurance and new methods of reimbursement, and provided guidance to community board members on various aspects of ambulatory health care. With termination of the federal NYMRMP grant in 1976, funding was made available under a Public Health Service grant to the Association of New York Neighborhood Health Centers and the courses were continued at the Academy for an additional three years.

In 1975, when Gerald Ford became President of the United

States, there were some indications from the Department of Health, Education and Welfare that the new administration was considering the drafting of a legislative proposal for a national health insurance program. This stimulated the NYMRMP to establish a Task Force to study the impact of national health insurance on New York City. Dr. Irving Lewis of the Department of Community and Preventive Medicine at the Albert Einstein College of Medicine was named its Executive Director and, with the help of Drs. Herbert Lukashok and Marvin Lieberman, a series of discussions was held at the Academy. The speakers included Dr. George Silver of the Yale University School of Public Health, Dr. Herbert Lukashok of the Albert Einstein College of Medicine, Dr. George A. Silver of the Yale University School of Medicine, Betty J. Bernstein, Ph.D., from the Citizens Committee for Children of New York, Mr. Frederick O'R. Hayes, former Budget Director of the City of New York, Dr. Frank van Dyke of the Columbia University School of Administrative Medicine, and Paul M. Densen, Sc.D., of the Harvard University School of Medicine. A group of papers commissioned to provide the background for the sessions was subsequently published.[19]

## HEALTH AND HOSPITAL PLANNING

During the postwar period, the Academy was represented on the Health and Hospital Planning Council of Southern New York, the voluntary agency authorized since 1938 by the State of New York to review applications for certificates of need for the expansion or creation of health facilities in the State (the final decision was made by the New York State Department of Health). From 1966 through 1975, the authority to review certificates of need was shared with the Comprehensive Health Planning Agency of New York. Physician representatives to the agency were selected by the local county medical societies; and the Academy was not involved. In 1975, when Public Law 93–641 authorized the creation of regional Health Systems Agencies to receive federal funding for health planning—this was the same law that abolished the Regional Medical Programs—the Comprehensive Health Planning Agency entered into competition with an entity formed by the Hospital Planning Council of Southern New York to determine which would be designated by the State of New York as the Health Systems Agency for New York City. The Academy supported the application of the entity created by the Hospital Planning Council but it did not prevail. This Hospital Planning Council of Southern New York was disbanded in 1976 and, in 1985, its archives were presented to the Academy, where they have been preserved in the Library.

## THE NATION'S BIOMEDICAL RESEARCH PROGRAM

The National Cancer Act Amendments (P.L. 93–352), signed by President Gerald R. Ford on July 23, 1974, renewed the authorization for the National Cancer Program and established the President's Biomedical Research Panel, which was given a broad mandate to review all aspects of the biomedical and behavioral research programs of the National Institutes of Health and the Alcohol, Drug Abuse and Mental Health Administration. When the Academy was asked for its views on these matters, President Dr. Saul B. Gusberg appointed an ad hoc committee of distinguished Fellows to respond to this request.[20]

In the statement it prepared, the Ad Hoc Committee enthusiastically supported the continuation of the National Institutes of Health as an autonomous research center, endorsing both its intramural and extramural programs. Noting that abrupt fluctuations in funding are harmful to the nation's biomedical research effort, the statement urged that these programs receive stable funding with appropriations linked to a percentage of the nation's expenditures for health care. The Biomedical Research Panel, it said, should be a permanent agency to monitor the nation's research program and to suggest changes where necessary.

The Committee supported the peer-review system being used by the National Institutes of Health, stating that, "There is no realistic procedural alternative that provides comparable expertise across the incredibly broad spectrum of biomedical and behavioral sciences."[21] It deplored the growing emphasis on limiting research to particular diseases, arguing that advances made in one disease are frequently transferable to other areas, and it strongly supported the continuation of training grants, emphasizing the inextricable linkage of teaching, research and service in the medical community. Finally, the Committee called attention to the growing unease in the research community created by the growth of contract research.

The Committee's statement was approved by the Council and forwarded to Dr. Charles Lowe, Executive Secretary of the President's Biomedical Research Panel.

## BY-LAWS REVISION

In his Inaugural Address at the 1969 Annual Meeting, Dr. John L. Pool discussed the recommendations developed in two years of work by the By-laws Committee which had been chaired by Dr. John L. Madden.[22] The other members of the Committee were Drs. Dickinson W. Richards, Jr., Jarvis Coffin, Rustin McIntosh, Fred Mettler and James J. Smith. These were the first changes in the Academy's By-laws since the 1956 revision; with Council approval, they became effective in 1969.

The changes specified that the number of stated meetings would be reduced and, although nominations would still be made at a stated meeting to allow for alternate slates, the election would be conducted by mail. The Committee on Special Studies became the Committee on Medicine in Society and was charged to concern itself with the social and economic aspects of medicine.

The contentious issue of the publication of committee reports was resolved. Previously, the Committee on Public Health had been allowed to issue statements in the name of the Academy if they were unanimously approved by its Executive Committee and the President of the Academy, or by three-fourths of the members of the Committee present and voting at any special or regular meeting of the Committee and by the President of the Academy.[23] In the 1969 revision of the By-laws, this was changed to authorize the Council to "receive and consider all reports of the Committees of the Academy and shall have the power to approve or disapprove them. No report shall be made public or published without the authorization of the Council."[24] In explaining the change, Dr. Pool said,

It must be clear to all thoughtful Fellows that policy statements from the Academy should have Council approval, for how can a person outside our Fellowship differentiate between the opinion of a committee and an opinion representative of our whole Fellowship? On the other hand, there may well be scientific studies that are the result of long deliberation, investigation, and thought that emanate from one committee or another which need not pass in review before the Council prior to publication in the *Bulletin*. There obviously remains a gray area between these two statements which will require collaboration and discussion within the Council. Let me remind you that all committees are represented there by their chairmen. Let us hope that the spirit of good will and the desire for the most careful and objective studies remain the goal of our Fellows.[22]

## ACADEMY FINANCES

In the early 1970s, rapid inflation and a "bear market" created concern about the Academy's financial status. A drop in the value of the endowment portfolio, which had peaked at $32 million at the end of 1970, to $20 million at the end of 1974, was accompanied by a drop in its earnings. This was coupled with a concern that the Academy might lose both its exemption from local real estate taxes and its status as a tax-exempt, not-for-profit organization under the federal income tax code. To meet the potential financial crisis, staff salaries for 1972 were frozen and the Library was ordered to reduce its expenditures by canceling 300 journal subscriptions, a major element in its budget. In 1973, to compensate for the salary freeze, the Board of Trustees authorized a new group life insurance program for all employees and an increase in the Academy's contributions to the employees' pension plan.

At the December 1973 meeting, the Board of Trustees, having learned that both the Countway Library at Harvard and the Li-

brary at the Columbia University College of Physicians and Surgeons had cut their journal subscriptions by 1,000, ordered the
Director to cut at least 300, and preferably 500, additional journal
subscriptions during 1974. At the end of that year, President Albert Santy told the Trustees that, "The Library continues to be the
largest drain, followed by the *Bulletin* and its staff."[25] With that,
the Library was ordered to close one hour earlier each day to
produce savings in electricity and fuel, to cut another 300 to 500
journals from its subscription list and to eliminate, by attrition if
possible, at least five staff positions. There was a warning that, "if
inflation continues, both of these items of retrenchment may be
repeated next year at budget time."[24]

At the April 1975 meeting of the Board of Trustees, Dr. Adrian
W. Zorgniotti, Chairman of the Library Committee, protested that
these cuts "constitute a major policy change. Without due consideration and consultation, and without any systematic study of the
needs of the Library, the Trustees may already have changed the
nature and purpose of the Academy without realizing it and without intending to do so."[26] He went on to point out that Academy's
exemption from City real estate taxes rested "almost solely on the
fact that the Library provides service to the general public, incorpo-
rates what was once the medical collection of the New York Public
Library, and is the place to which the New York Public Library
refers patrons who require the use of a medical collection."[25]

This request from the Library Committee to reverse its earlier
decisions, which had been promoted by Mr. Alfred Brandon, the
Librarian, was rejected by the Board of Trustees, presumably with
support from Dr. McCormack. This contretemps undoubtedly contributed to the strained relations between the Director and the
Librarian, alluded to earlier.

The potential crisis for the Academy was eased in 1975 and
1976 by unexpected rental income from the New York College of
Podiatry, which held its classes in the Academy building while
awaiting construction of its new building on 124th Street. By the
end of 1976, the nominal value of the endowment fund had returned to approximately $30 million. Although a number of indi-

viduals voiced criticism of the Academy's reliance on income from governmental grants and contracts, dependent as they are on the fickle attitudes and political fortunes of elected officials, and from cooperative relationships that were not always stable, it was quite clear that grants like those from the Regional Medical Program and the Regional Medical Library had made substantial contributions to the financial viability of the Academy and, as long as they remained available, would continue to do so.

## ACADEMY PRESIDENTS

### Dr. John L. Pool, 1968–1970

Dr. John L. Pool, a surgeon, was graduated from the Columbia University College of Physicians and Surgeons in 1934, and was on the staff of both the Presbyterian Hospital and the faculty of the medical school. He became a Fellow in 1947 and served as Vice President of the Academy from 1965 to 1966.

### Dr. John E. Deitrick, 1971–1972

Dr. John E. Deitrick, a native of Pennsylvania, was a graduate of Princeton and received his MD from the Johns Hopkins University School of Medicine. He spent most of his career at the New York Hospital-Cornell Medical Center in the Department of Medicine and served as Dean from 1957 to 1969. Later, he became Executive Director of the Associated Medical Schools of Greater New York. He became a Fellow in 1943.

### Dr. Albert C. Santy, 1973–1974

Dr. Santy, an internist, was a graduate of Pennsylvania State University and the Cornell University Medical College. He was active in the arts, especially the theater, in which many of his patients were involved. He became a Fellow in 1950, was active on the Library Committee, and served as Vice-President from 1970 to 1971. He also served as Chairman of the Committee on Art which advised the Director on whether to accept the portraits of Past Presidents of the Academy, many of which are hung in the Presidents' Gallery on the main floor of the Academy building.

## Dr. Saul B. Gusberg, 1975–1976

Dr. Saul B Gusberg, who became a Fellow of the Academy in 1957, received his MD degree from Harvard Medical School in 1937 and a Doctor of Science degree from Columbia University in 1949. In 1985, he was awarded an Honorary Doctor of Science degree by the University Autonomia of Barcelona. He held numerous positions in obstetrics and gynecology, a field in which he achieved world-wide recognition for his discovery of adenomatous hyperplasia as a precursor of uterine cancer and the relationship of endometrial malignancy to estrogens. He was Obstetrician and Gynecologist-in-Chief at the Mount Sinai Hospital and, from 1980–1984, was Professor and Chair of the Department of Obstetrics and Gynecology at the Mount Sinai School of Medicine of the City University of New York. He has had a long relationship as Special Consultant for Research and Medical Affairs with the American Cancer Society, and from 1967–1970, he served as President of the New York City division. He was also President of the New York Obstetrical Society, the Society of Pelvic Surgeons, the American Federation of Clinical Oncologic Societies, the Society of Gynecologic Oncologists, and the American Association of Obstetricians and Gynecologists.

## Dr. McCORMACK vs. Dr. DEITRICK

As a general rule, relationships between the President and the Director were harmonious and mutually supportive. While choice of the Director was invariably vested in the leadership of the Academy, usually including past and future Presidents, the Director, although not a member of the Nominating Committee, was in a position to influence the selection of nominees for the Presidency. That was not always the case; however, witness the period of tension between Dr. McCormack and Dr. John E. Deitrick during the latter's Presidency.

Dr. Deitrick waited until the end of his term to formally register his concerns about the Academy, an action that clearly did not meet with the approval of Dr. McCormack. After retiring as Dean of the Cornell University Medical College, Dr. Deitrick had assumed the post of Executive Director of the Associated Medical Schools of New York which had its offices in the Academy building, allowing him to be on hand almost constantly for discussions with Dr. McCormack and other members of the staff. His interest in minutiae and his knack of asking pointed questions resulted in a familiarity with the details of Academy affairs greater than that achieved by many if not most of the Presidents who preceded him. Dr. Deitrick did make an attempt to initiate a formal study of the Academy activities early in his term but, apparently, did not pursue it. Finally, at the October 25, 1972 joint meeting of the Council and the Board of Trustees, he expressed "his personal doubts as to what the Academy is accomplishing and where the Academy is going."[27] He recalled that this question had been studied in 1958 but no such studies had been made since. He suggested that, "instead of creating a special committee, the Council itself act as a 'committee as a whole' to consider the future of the Academy of Medicine."[27]

After reviewing a "number of weaknesses of the Academy that were not cited in the minutes," he posed a number of questions: "what new services and opportunities can the Academy offer to the Fellows; what continuing or new services can it offer the medical profession; and, what unique services can it render to the public?" He went on to voice skepticism about the value of federal and state support of medical education, noting that "what is given one year may be withdrawn at another time," and challenged the wisdom of having medical schools change their policies and programs to gain federal dollars that may only be temporary.[27]

Dr. William Eisenmenger, Chairman of the Committee on Public Health, responded by pointing to the reports and statements produced by this Committee as one way of reaching the public and the profession. He said that many new Fellows had told him that they had been prompted to join the Academy by what they had read about the activities of the Committee on Public Health.[27]

Dr. McCormack responded at great length. "Despite some tendency on the part of some persons to denigrate the performance of the Academy," he said,

> the sections have in general become more active; there is a lot more going on besides the activities of the sections (in the last year at least 20,000 people attended meetings at the Academy); the New York Pathological Society and the Roentgen Society meetings are attended by just about every resident in the area training in these disciplines; the Library is not used less, more programs have been added and, while there may not be as many Fellows in person in the Library, it is still used extensively by them; if it were not for the recommendations of the Library Committee, the Medical Library Center would not be in existence [Dr. Craig was instrumental in raising money to finance it]; the Harvey Society still lists on its programs 'in affiliation with the New York Academy of Medicine;' and By-laws have been changed to get better rotation on the standing committees, thus involving more Fellows.[27]

In rebuttal, Dr. Deitrick questioned "the advisability of the Academy remaining in this area" and suggested that consideration be given to having a more accessible building "in a more appealing location, which could house the Academy and all its activities, the Associated Medical Schools, some of the many foundations located in the city, and offer pleasant dining facilities and adequate parking space."[27]

On November 20, 1972, acceding to President Deitrick's suggestion, the Board of Trustees and the Council held a special meeting to continue discussing the problems of the Academy. Dr. McCormack opened the discussion by recalling that, some two years earlier, he had indicated his belief that all institutions should be subject to introspection. "However," he said, the prime problem today is to neutralize the results of incessant unconstructive criticism which would sometimes create the impression that the Academy is moribund. Conversations with many colleagues since the last meeting elicited the view that the Academy is the last bastion of freedom to speak out with a respected voice on medical matters. This is in part reflected by the imitation of our programs by other independent medical organizations.[28]

He pointed to the leadership role of the Library in the initiation and the continuing operation of the Medical Library Center. He emphasized that the Academy Library is not just a local resource but a national one, as evidenced by supplemental federal grants totaling $229,000 between 1967 and 1971 for culling and preserving its collection. Since 1968, he said, the Library has served as a State resource through its participation in the New York State Interlibrary Loan Program. Further, he added, "we were requested by the National Library of Medicine to serve in the national Regional Medical Library Program. We are aware that one medical school librarian has been actively trying to take this latter grant away from us. However, the other librarians in the area wish the grant to remain at the Academy."[28]

"There is no justification in purchasing 5,000 to 6,000 journal subscriptions," Dr. McCormack said, "since, through the Medical Library Center, the medical schools are at last discussing cooperative action in this regard."[28] He noted a suggestion that the Academy subscribe to most of the rare and less-used items, an action that would be a relief for the school libraries. "However," he pointed out, "this view ignores the fact that the Academy Library is the only medical library open to the public and, consequently, it must have the less rare material as well."

He described three initiatives for the Library for which he is seeking outside support: establishment of a History of Medicine Division based in our Rare Book Room to serve those medical schools which desire to cooperate; a formal graduate training program in medical library service; and, improved humidity control and air conditioning in the Rare Book Room.

Dr. McCormack called attention to the activation of the History of Medicine Series of publications and pointed out that the *Bulletin* continues to be sent in exchange for over 300 journals that come to the Library.

Pointing to the stature of the three standing committees, Public Health, Medical Education and Medicine in Society, Dr. McCormack emphasized three reasons for continuing such Academy involvement: "the status of the public health professional has been downgraded and some medical voices must be heard; the assaults upon undergraduate medical education and the unfortunate plight of many medical schools are an appropriate concern of the Academy; and, the continuing growth and evolution of socioeconomic problems which impinge on medicine make an alert ear attuned to these elements desirable."[28]

Despite what was apparently an intense and heated discussion, the meeting ended without any formal action having been taken. It was clear that, while some may have shared his disquiet, Dr. Deitrick had failed to convince his colleagues that further study and deliberation were needed, and that Dr. McCormack remained in control. According to the minutes of the next meeting, both Dr. McCormack and Dr. Deitrick became ill and, by the time they recovered, things had quieted down. Dr. Deitrick was succeeded in the Presidency by Dr. Albert Santy, with whom Dr. McCormack was much more comfortable, and the kinds of dissatisfaction with the operation and status of the Academy that had been voiced by Dr. Deitrick receded to remain under the surface until the late 1980s when they reemerged to stimulate the complete restructuring of the Academy of the 1990s.

## NOTES

1 Committee on Public Health. 1967 Health Services in New York City. *Bulletin of the New York Academy of Medicine*. 43:843–849.

2 Pool JL. 1967 *Letter to Preston L. Wade, May 1, 1967*. Council of the New York Academy of Medicine. 1967 Minutes of the meeting of April 16, 1967.

3 Council of the New York Academy of Medicine. 1967 Minutes of the meeting of April 16, 1967.

4 McCormack JE. 1967 Letter to Byard Williams, June 6, 1967.

5 McCormack JE. 1967 Letter to Howard Reid Craig, June 14, 1967.

6 Tolchin M. 1967 Medical Group Faces Breakup: Dispute Over Role Threatens Committee at Academy. *The New York Times.* September 4, 1967, p. 19.

7 Pool JL. 1970 The responsibility of the New York Academy of Medicine in the community. *Bulletin of the New York Academy of Medicine.* 46:649–656.

8 Committee on Medicine in Society. 1973 Statement on measures to prolong life in terminal illness by heroic measures. *Bulletin of the New York Academy of Medicine.* 49:349–351.

9 Committee on Public Health. 1961 Pioneering in public health for fifty years. *Bulletin of the New York Academy of Medicine.* 37:108–110.

10 Committee on Public Health. 1970 The present status of abortion laws. *Bulletin of the New York Academy of Medicine.* 46:281–286.

11 Sibley J. 1969 New city health administrator named. *New York Times,* November 30, 1969, p. 68.

12 Sibley J. 1969 New health aide is under attack. *New York Times,* December 10, 1969, p. 30.

13 Van Ingen P. 1949 *The New York Academy of Medicine,: Its First Hundred Years.* New York: Columbia University Press. p. 522.

14 Council of the New York Academy of Medicine. 1968 *Minutes of the meeting of January 24, 1968.*

15 McCormack JE. 1969 *Letter to Mayor Lindsay, March 4, 1969.*

16 McCormack JE. 1973 A message from the Director. *Newsnotes.* May, 1973, p. 3.

17 Poland U., 1994 Some reflections on Gertrude Annan. *Bulletin of the Medical Library Association.* 82:460–461.

18 New York Regional Medical Program. 1968 Responsibility in the Regional Medical Program. *MetroNews.* 1:2.

19 Lieberman M, Ed. 1977 *The Impact of National Health Insurance on New York,* New York: Prodist.

20 The Committee included: Drs. Stanley E. Bradley, Bard Professor of Medicine at Columbia University College of Physicians and Surgeons; Thomas C. Chalmers, President and Dean of Mt. Sinai Medical Center; Gordon Douglas, Professor and Chairman, Department of Obstetrics and Gynecology at New York University Medical Center; J. Frederick Eagle, Jr., Assistant Commissioner, Maternal and Child Health Services, New York City Department of Health; Edward Fischel, Di-

rector, Department of Medicine, Bronx-Lebanon Hospital and Professor of Medicine, Albert Einstein College of Medicine; Alfred M. Freedman, Professor and Chairman, Department of Psychiatry, New York Medical College; Solomon G. Hershey, Professor of Anesthesiology, Albert Einstein College of Medicine; Joseph Post, Professor of Clinical Medicine, New York University Medical Center; Keith Reemtsma, Professor and Chairman, Department of Surgery, Columbia University College of Physicians and Surgeons. Dr. Marvin Lieberman served as Executive Secretary of the Committee.

21 Ad hoc Committee of the New York Academy of Medicine for the President's Biomedical Research Panel. 1976 Statement on the nation's biomedical program: September, 1975. *Bulletin of the New York Academy of Medicine.* 52:253–258.

22 Pool JL. 1969 Annual meeting of the New York Academy of Medicine: Inaugural address. *Bulletin of the New York Academy of Medicine.* 45:721–722.

23 New York Academy of Medicine. 1956 *By-laws* Article XIII, Section 5.

24 New York Academy of Medicine. 1969 *By-laws* Article X, Section 4.

25 Board of Trustees of the New York Academy of Medicine. 1974 Minutes of the meeting of December 18, 1974.

26 Zorgniotti AW. 1975 *Memorandum to the Board of Trustees from the Library Committee.* Attachment to: Board of Trustees of the New York Academy of Medicine. Minutes of the meeting of April 23, 1975.

27 Board of Trustees and Council of the New York Academy of Medicine. 1972 Minutes of the meeting of October 25, 1972.

28 Board of Trustees and Council of the New York Academy of Medicine. 1972 Minutes of the meeting of November 20, 1972.

# Chapter 5
## 1977–1981
# CME, School Health Programs and Physician Discipline

DURING THE LAST FIVE YEARS of Dr. McCormack's term as Director, he served with Presidents whom he found to be very congenial and very supportive. However, during this period, his own health problems became increasingly troublesome. The cooperative arrangements that were so important to the Academy programmatically and financially were continuing in good order and new meaningful activities were being launched, most notably a program of health education for school children. There were significant changes in the Academy staff, and a period of staff discontent over salary freezes and inequities was weathered.

## LABOR DIFFICULTIES

In 1978, reacting somewhat belatedly to the wage freeze followed by the relatively small salary increases of the early 1970s and the continuing high level of inflation, a majority of the staff petitioned the National Labor Relations Board (NLRB) for an election to determine whether District 1199 of the National Union of Hospital and Health Care Employees, should represent Academy employees as their agent for collective bargaining.

The staff discontent was fueled by the fact that entry-level employees in the hospital industry represented by District 1199, notably those at Mt. Sinai Hospital just a few blocks south of the Academy, were receiving wages higher than those earned by entry-level Academy staff. There was also unhappiness with perceived inequities in the distribution of the 5 percent salary increase budgeted for the Library.

To the displeasure of Dr. McCormack, Mr. Brandon, the Librarian, had awarded more generous increases to professional librarians than to the lower-paid nonprofessional personnel. Also, when an Associate Librarian retired, she had been replaced by two higher salaried Assistant Librarians, further skewing the payroll.[1]

The Board of Trustees opposed the unionization of the staff. It pointed out that the fringe benefits of health and disability insurance and pension contributions that were entirely employer-paid represented a package that was quite generous and competitive with any not-for-profit health care organization. It was also noted that, in contrast to the Academy, hospital personnel expenses were considered in the State's determination of allowable hospital charges and, accordingly, they could be passed along to third-party payers.

The election was held on May 5, 1978, and ended in a tie which, according to the NLRB rules, was declared a victory for the employer. A year later, the union tried again and, in a second election held on September 12, 1979, lost again, this time by two votes. There was an upgrading of the fringe benefits, but there was a continuing feeling among the employees that salary levels were still too low. Nevertheless, no further attempts to unionize the Academy employees were made.

## COMMITTEE ON PUBLIC HEALTH

In February 1977, Dr. Maurice Shils became the Executive Secretary of the Committee on Public Health. A pioneer in the field of parenteral nutrition, he was a co-editor of the standard textbook, *Nutrition in Health and Disease.* He had received his BA and ScD degrees from Johns Hopkins University and his MD from the New York University School of Medicine. He held a series of academic appointments in biochemistry, nutrition, and medicine, and had a long-standing affiliation with the Memorial Hospital-Sloan Kettering. He continued to act as Director of Nutrition at that hospital while serving as Executive Secretary of the Committee on a part-time basis.

Under Dr. Shil's leadership, the Committee and the Academy had good working relations with both the City and the State Commissioners of Health. Both were always willing to speak at the Academy and they often came to the Committee for advice and consultation.

On one occasion, in 1977, a misunderstanding developed with the State Department of Health with respect to an arrangement whereby physicians designated as consultants to conduct medical reviews in hospitals would be compensated directly by the Academy, which would then be reimbursed by the State. When it was learned that these medical reviews were under litigation with the hospital industry in the State, information that had not been disclosed to the Academy by the Department of Health, the Academy elected to cancel the contract. The matter was resolved amicably: the State officials involved apologized and a new relationship was agreed upon whereby the Academy would advertise the need for such consultants to the Fellows while the Department of Health would handle all the arrangements with the physicians involved, including paying them directly.[2]

## Amebiasis

In 1979, the Committee's interest in amebiasis was aroused when Dr. Joseph Post, a gastroenterologist who was then President of the Academy, reported that he had encountered many more patients with amebiasis during the past six months than he had seen in his previous twenty years of practice. Of these 33 patients, 13 were admitted homosexuals, 13 others had traveled abroad, and 7 had not left the country during the past three years. The New York City Department of Health had contended that the spread of the disease among male homosexuals was largely responsible for the increase in its local incidence. Dr. Post, however, believed that inadequate attention was being paid to food-borne transmission as a factor in the increase in the disease. He also raised the question of whether such enteric diseases among the large numbers of "undocumented" (i.e., "illegal") immigrants in the City were being underreported.

The Committee studied the problem and, on December 3, 1979, approved a statement that confirmed the increase in reported cases of amebiasis to a peak of 1,875 in 1978 in contrast to the average of approximately 1,000 cases per year prior to 1965. The statement alluded to the perceived rise in incidence among male homosexuals, but emphasized the number of new immigrants from Central and South America and the Caribbean where this disease is endemic and where no studies had been made as yet. The Committee recommended that more active case finding take place in the homosexual community and that studies of its prevalence among recent immigrants be undertaken.

On December 3, 1979, the Committee convened a conference at the Academy in the planning of which Dr. Pascal J. Imperato, the New York City Commissioner of Health, made a significant contribution. In response to the concern first raised by Dr. Post and reiterated in the Committee's statement, the experts who made presentations at this *Symposium on Amebiasis, A New Look at an Old Disease* seemed to agree that, while unsanitary food handling is a method by which amebiasis is transmitted, it does not appear to be a significant factor in the recent increase in its incidence in New York City.[3]

### Indoor Air Pollution

Another outstanding program conducted under the auspices of the Committee was the 1981 Symposium on *Health Aspects of Indoor Air Pollution.* The program was arranged by Dr. Lawrence E. Hinkle, Jr., who headed the Subcommittee on Environmental Health, while the sessions were chaired by Dr. Norman Simon, then Chairman of the Committee.

In the opening paper, Dr. Hinkle and Ms. Susan Murray of the Division of Human Ecology in the Department of Medicine at Cornell University Medical College, defined indoor air pollution as "particles or gases that occur in the air inside buildings that may adversely affect the health of people," and concluded that such "indoor air pollutants are now a major threat to the health of the people of the United States, and specifically to the people of New York City."[4]

It was pointed out at the Conference that, while combustion products were a major cause of death, volatile products were also significant hazards. Asbestos, radon, formaldehyde, and passive cigarette smoke were also cited as substances causing concern "because of their potential but as yet undetermined effect upon the health of the general population."[4]


## In the Event of a Nuclear Accident

In 1981, the Committee met with a number of experts, including Dr. Rosalind Yalow, a Fellow and a Nobel Laureate, to discuss a suggestion that the City was not adequately prepared for the potential of a major accident at the nuclear energy power plant at Indian Point, NY, just north of the City. The Committee observed that, in the event of such an accident, only small amounts of radioactive iodine were likely to be released into the atmosphere. In addition, most of the soluble fission products released into the atmosphere would be removed by snow, rain water vapor, dust, etc. The Committee concluded that the amount of radioactivity that would reach the City would be very small, and that distribution of potassium iodide, which had been suggested as a prophylaxis against the uptake of radioactive iodine, was unwarranted because it would be impractical and would be an ineffective remedy. This conclusion was embodied in a Resolution that was endorsed by the Council and published in the *Bulletin.*[5]


## COMMITTEE ON MEDICAL EDUCATION

In May 1978, Dr. Robert Goodhart who had served as Executive Secretary of the Committee on Medical Education since 1967, was succeeded by William C. Stubing. A native New Yorker, Mr. Stubing had graduated from the Concordia Seminary in St. Louis, Missouri, with an M.Div. degree in 1965, and later received a Master's degree from New York University. He served for six years on the staff of the Office of the Provost at Queens College of the City University of New York, during the last year of which he was seconded to become Assistant Director of Graduate Medical Education of the American Medical Association. There he worked with the Residency Review Committee and with the Liaison Committee on Graduate Medical Education which is involved with the accreditation of US residency programs.

Mr. Stubing made a point of making close personal relationships with the members of the Committee and became a strong advocate of its programs. In addition to developing interesting symposia on medical education, he worked closely to encourage the reanimation of the activities of several Sections that had become relatively inactive, particularly the Section on Pediatrics. He proved to be quite successful in attracting grants for research and training projects to be conducted under the auspices of the Academy.

The Academic Physician: An Endangered Species

The Eighth Symposium on Medical Education addressed the dearth of career opportunities for full-time clinical investigators in academic medical centers. The program, which was arranged and chaired by Dr. Marianne Legato, Associate Professor of Clinical Medicine at the Columbia University College of Physicians and Surgeons, was attended by over 300 participants and was the subject of an Op-Ed article in the *New York Times*.[6] In her introductory remarks, Dr. Legato pointed out that these physician-scientists, who represent only 3 percent of all US physicians, have a primary commitment to research, but also teach and provide care for patients in a university setting. She differentiated these academic physicians from those who, although they may also have teaching responsibilities, are not committed primarily to research and earn their livelihoods by providing care to patients in their offices or in the hospital setting. The lack of appreciation for the contributions of the academic physicians to finding new knowledge that translates itself into making "American medical art where it currently stands: second to none in the world," she said, has resulted in Congressional efforts to cut funding for support of academic physicians and their research.[7]

In his Presidential Welcome to the Symposium, Dr. Joseph Post, who was Professor of Clinical Medicine at the New York University College of Medicine and who had combined an active practice with an outstanding career in research, presented a somewhat different view. He said that he had "little concern about the disappearance of physicians who will be engaged in research" because the "intellectual excitement generated by biomedical phenomena is sufficiently engaging to attract good minds. Indeed, given a reasonable level of funding, it would be hard to imagine otherwise." A mix of part-time and full-time faculty is a good idea, he suggested. "The clinical experiences and interests of full-time physicians tend to be more limited than those of part-time colleagues. It is important that students be exposed to both groups so that they develop a balanced approach to health care and to the complex interactions involved therein."[8]

Following the Symposium, Dr. Legato asked that the Subcommittee that had planned the symposium be continued with a charge to work toward improvement of the outlook for career medical researchers and the encouragement of public policies that would provide the necessary funding. The Committee on Medical Education had no objection to this and referred it for Council approval. The Council replied that it "did not wish to discourage Dr. Legato but the consensus clearly was that the Academy had made its contribution by conducting the Symposium and will make a further contribution by publishing the proceedings. Future effort in the direction of raising funds for the medical schools in order to support full-time clinical investigators is not the responsibility of the Academy. Such an effort would inevitably consume much of the time of Mr. Stubing and the staff of the Committee on Medical Education, which might more appropriately be devoted to Section activities and other functions of the Office of Medical Education."[9]

## Section on Medicine

During the 1980s an outstanding series of symposia on various aspects of infectious diseases was held over a period of several years under the auspices of the Section on Medicine. These were chaired by Dr. Harold Neu, Chief of the Division of Infectious Diseases at the Columbia University College of Physicians and Surgeons, and were supported by grants from a number of pharmaceutical companies. Most noteworthy was the session on *Infectious Diseases,* held on January 14, 1982, when a large audience braved a major snow storm to attend.[10] Later that year, the topic was *Recent Developments in Oral Antibiotic Therapy: Becampcillin Update,*[11] and in April 1983, the symposium addressed *Current and Future Directions in the Use of Antimicrobial Agents.*[12] Subsequent symposia were held under the auspices of Columbia University, but the proceedings continued to be published in the *Bulletin.*

## COMMITTEE ON MEDICINE IN SOCIETY

The Committee on Medicine in Society continued to be active in organizing conferences. These included the Annual Health Conferences, which had been started in 1940 and addressed such topics as *Health Policy: Realistic Expectations and Reasonable Priorities* in 1977; *The Hospital Reconsidered: A New Perspective* in 1978; *Cost Containment and Resource Allocation in Health Care* in 1979; *The Patient and the Health Care Professional: The Changing Pattern of their Relations* in 1980; and *Struggle for the Assurance of Appropriate Medical Care* in 1981. It also launched a new series of annual programs on issues in long-term care, held in collaboration with the New York City Chapter of the National Association of Social Workers and the New York State Nurses Association. This collaboration was intended to send the message that cooperation among all the professional groups involved in providing long-term care is necessary if the interests of the public in improving these programs are to be advanced. The Committee also collaborated with the New York State Department of Health on developing guidelines for the medical practitioner on the treatment of Alzheimer's disease.

Ethical Issues in Occupational Medicine

Thanks largely to the efforts of Dr. Norbert J. Roberts, the Committee received a grant from the National Institute of Occupational Safety and Health to conduct a Conference on *Ethical Issues in Occupational Medicine*. The meeting was held on June 21–22, 1977, a time when industry was under attack because of media reports of environmental pollution and failures to protect workers against occupational hazards, and when occupational physicians were being accused of sacrificing workers' health and welfare to the monetary interests of the companies that employed them. Dr. Roberts, who chaired the program, was the Vice President and Corporate Medical Director of Exxon Corporation. Prominent in the field of occupational medicine and a leader in the American Occupational Medical Association, he had been an active member of both the Committee on Medicine in Society and the Academy Section on Occupational Medicine.

The highlight of the conference was a presentation by Prof. Robert Ackerman, a member of the faculty at the Harvard Business School, who reported on a study of how more than four dozen corporations were approaching social issues. He emphasized that "Social responsiveness is not easily measured by the financial control system. . . . Some of the costs may be determinable and immediate, while benefits are usually unknown and often occur in the future."[13] He outlined a strategy for making corporations more socially responsible. Although the technical support of specialists in occupational health is necessary, the solution, he said, is the "visible, tangible support of the chief executive." In the final analysis "the firm that can learn to execute these responses more effectively and can manage the challenge of organizational learning is likely to be a more successful competitor in the long run."[13]

In addition to the medical directors of a number of major US corporations, the roster of speakers included Dr. Donald Shriver, President of the Union Theological Seminary. They joined in a lively discussion of the ways in which occupational physicians might maintain their professional integrity and discharge their ethical responsibility for employees' safety and health in the face of pressure from employers to avoid the costs of the necessary protective measures.

## The Doctor-Patient Relationship

The Annual Health Conference held on April 23–24, 1980 addressed *The Patient and the Health Care Professional: the Changing Pattern of their Relations.* The program was chaired by Dr. Stanley Reichman, Chairman of the Department of Medicine at the North General Hospital. Among the many outstanding speakers were Prof. Eli Ginzburg of Columbia University, Dr. Edmund D. Pellegrino of Catholic University, and Dr. Mark Siegler of the Department of Medicine at the Pritzker School of Medicine of the University of Chicago.

Dr. Siegler presented a model for the doctor-patient encounter which had been quite influential in shaping the deliberations of the President's Commission for the Study of Ethical Problems in Medicine, Biomedical and Behavioral Research, created by President Carter and continued during the Reagan administration. This model, which he called "the accommodation model," emphasizes the autonomy of both the physician and the patient. It rejected the old notion of the paternalistic physician who "knows what is best for the patient" as well as newer models of consumerism in which the patient sees the physician as a passive agent. The physician must respect the patient's goals with regard to the outcomes of treatment, he said, but the physician is free not to enter a physician-patient accommodation if this would "violate the conscientious physician's sense of professional and moral responsibility."[14]

## Role of the Resident in Patient Care

In January 1978, the Committee formed a Subcommittee on Hospital Practice that was charged "with the study of the moral dilemmas and organizational conflicts arising out of the increasing authority assigned to residents" in caring for patients. The Subcommittee, chaired by Dr. John K. Guck, Attending Physician at the Lenox Hill Hospital, heard presentations by a number of senior attending physicians and the staff interviewed the chiefs of services at several local hospitals. It heard complaints that there was inadequate supervision of the residents in some of the City's leading hospitals, as well as a lack of candor in informing patients of the role that the residents were playing in their care. Attending physicians complained that, once patients were admitted to some hospitals, their care was taken over by the residents, who wrote orders without consulting or communicating with them. In other hospitals, residents complained that, while continuing to bill the patient as the physician of record, some attending physicians shirked their supervisory and teaching responsibilities. It was found that the practices varied from department to department in almost every academic medical center, and that there were many residency programs in which a proper balance between patient care and training responsibilities was maintained.

The Subcommittee's deliberations were the basis of the 1978 Annual Health Conference on *The Hospital Revisited.* Among the speakers were: Martin Kempner, PhD, the Philosopher-in-Residence at the Academy who was studying ethical issues arising out of hospital practice under a grant from the New York Council for the Humanities; Alisdair MacIntyre, Professor of Philosophy at Boston University; Dr. Joseph Post, Professor of Clinical Medicine at the New York University School of Medicine; and Dr. Stuart Orsher, a Resident in Medicine at the Lenox Hill Hospital who would become President of the Medical Society of the State of New York in 1995.

Dr. Post argued that the role of the attending physician is in danger of becoming superfluous in some hospitals in New York City. He was particularly concerned about how the rules giving residents the authority to write orders for patients were being implemented, and called for their reform "lest others less qualified will lay down simplistic rules which may aggravate the difficulties and create new ones."[15] Professor MacIntyre commented that the "patient is always offering the resident and the medical student and the attending physician an opportunity to learn." He went on to suggest that the key to the relationship between residents and attending physicians is the way the relationship of the patient in the institutional setting to both of them is perceived.

Following the Conference, the Subcommittee issued a Report which contended that "good training and good patient care can and do co-exist under a variety of residency program arrangements. An essential ingredient in these arrangements is the principle of close supervision by a responsible physician or surgeon, with the patient informed about the respective roles of the resident and the attending physician."[16] The Report called for a reaffirmation of the authority of attending physicians to make decisions about the care rendered to their patients and their responsibility for the supervision of potentially hazardous procedures performed by residents. The magnitude of participation in surgical procedures by residents should be at the discretion of the attending surgeon and the chief of service while being consistent with the particular resident's level of competence. Patients should be informed about the extent of residents' participation in their care, and should retain the right to refuse to be examined or treated by residents, medical students or any other member of the hospital staff. "The directors of service should acknowledge the monitoring of the quality of care delivered by their respective services as their primary responsibility."[16] The Subcommittee's Report was approved by the Committee and by the Council and was endorsed by the Medical Society of the State of New York. It was subsequently summarized in the May, 1981 issue of the *Observer*, the newsletter of the American College of Physicians.

As a complement to this Report, the Committee on Medical Education decided in 1979 to conduct a symposium on the *Care of Private Patients in Teaching Hospitals: The Role of Residents*. This was a topic of particular interest to Mr. Stubing, its Executive Secretary, and one that was regarded as part of the jurisdiction of this Committee. The distinguished speakers included a number who had major responsibility for supervising the training of residents: Dr. Jeremiah A. Barondess, then Clinical Professor of Medicine and Attending Physician and Chief of the Private Medical Service at the New York Hospital-Cornell University Medical Center who is now President of the Academy; and Dr. Saul J. Farber, Chairman and Professor of the Department of Medicine at the New York University School of Medicine and Director of the Medical Service at Bellevue and University Hospitals who later became Chairman of the Academy Board of Trustees

Dr. David Lehr, Professor of Pharmacology and Associate Professor of Medicine at the New York Medical College, who chaired the Symposium Planning Committee, opened by noting

a number of situations and practices (or shall I say 'malpractices') in the case of hospitalized patients have the potential of creating serious difficulties and misunderstandings. . . . The most obvious are: 1) neglect clearly to inform patients about the role of the physician-in-training; 2) assignment of tasks to residents which exceed their training, especially in surgery, and inadequate supervision by the attending physician; 3) increasing the authority and responsibility granted residents, such as decisions about treatment and the writing of orders, which may bring residents into conflict with attending physicians.[17]

Dr. Barondess, describing experiences with the residency training programs on his 160 bed service which had been reorganized in 1974, indicated that structuring a teaching and training function on a private service requires a number of elements. These include access to an appropriate patient population in terms of numbers of admissions, spectrum of disease, and a mix of acute and chronic disorders; a commitment to the teaching service by the attending staff; and, as a corollary to such a commitment, staff input into the design of the program. A structured teaching program is vital, he said, as is an appropriate number and distribution of house officers. Also, the system should assure involvement of the house officer in clinical decision-making, and should emphasize full and free communication with the attending staff as an integral part of the training. Finally, he concluded, in institutions with a full-time faculty, including these individuals in teaching activities along with the panel of admitting physicians not only emphasizes the teaching commitment of the service, but also demonstrates the importance of a single standard of patient care.[18]

The presentations at this meeting described the progress being made in resolving issues arising in medical residency training and, most important, the arrangements being introduced in major teaching institutions to achieve the proper balance of patient care and teaching.

The School Health Curriculum Project—*Growing Healthy*

The origins of the School Health Curriculum Project can be traced to the 1970 Annual Health Conference on *Community Participation for Equity and Excellence in Health Care* at which a resolution was approved recommending that a committee be established to encourage consumer participation in Academy efforts to improve the quality of health care. In response, Dr. Milton Terris, Chairman of the Committee on Medicine in Society which had sponsored that Conference, appointed a Subcommittee on Consumer Participation. Over the next few years, this Subcommittee, chaired by Dr. John W. V. Cordice, Jr, an attending physician at the Columbus Hospital, attempted to explore the role of the community in health care delivery and, particularly, in the governance of health care institutions, but it made very little headway. There was great difficulty in framing a practical agenda that would engage the interest of the leaders of organizations serving the disadvantaged segments of the community, most of whom indicated they were too occupied by more pressing concerns to be able to attend Subcommittee meetings at the Academy.

In 1976, when Dr. Post became Chairman of the Committee on Medicine in Society, he appointed Dr. John V. Waller, a specialist in vascular disorders on the staff at Lenox Hill Hospital, to succeed Dr. Cordice as Chairman of the Subcommittee, with the specific assignment of identifying some kind of activity through which the Academy might serve to the community. Dr. Waller, acting on the conviction which, he said, he had learned from his father, that children need to learn good health habits at an early age in order to improve their health in later life, became interested in health education in the school system. This interest in school health education, he said later in a 1982 interview, did not come out of anything he saw in his practice. "It came out of an interest in the general welfare. It seemed to me that the problems of family life planted seeds of behavior disruptive to health, and this could be turned around by introducing a health education program in the schools—and the younger the children we reach, the better."[19]

In 1977, representatives of all the voluntary and public health agencies in the city with an interest in health education were invited to attend a meeting at the Academy to discuss what was happening in health education of the public and to develop suggestions for Academy activities in this field or, more important, what could be done collaboratively. The letter of invitation, signed by Dr. Waller on behalf of what had become the Subcommittee on Health Education, stated that the purpose of the meeting was

> to have our organizations work more closely with each other to improve the health of the people of New York City through health education programs. Thus we would like to discuss the development of a new mechanism for cooperation and coordination among organizations concerned with health education. The idea for this conference has been reviewed with and endorsed by representatives of public and private agencies involved in health education during planning meetings over several months.[20]

This was the beginning of the coalition which ultimately began to advance school health education. The expertise of the various agencies and their experience in health education, coupled with the leadership and objectivity of the Academy, endowed the project with the credibility that was essential to its eventual success. The initial steering committee, in addition to Dr. Waller and Mr. Pearson, comprised Ms. Mary Taylor, head of health education activities for Empire Blue Cross and Blue Shield, Mr. Roger Schmidt of the American Lung Association, and Ms. Eleanor Schweppe of the

United Hospital Fund, with Dr. Marvin Lieberman and Mrs. Cynthia Taylor, his administrative assistant, serving as staff.

The first undertaking of the Coalition was visits to programs already providing health education for children: the school district health education program on Long Island being provided by the North Shore Hospital; and the health promotion program of the Canarsie Local School Board in Brooklyn.

Mr. Schmidt told the group about a project funded by the American Lung Association and the US Centers for Disease Control which had already developed a comprehensive health education program for elementary schools. The curricula were being tested in kindergartens through the fourth grade in Seattle, Washington, and from the fifth to eighth grades in Berkeley, California. With the success of these trials, testing of these curricula was being expanded to sites around the country including the school district in North Bellemore on Long Island, just east of the City.

Accordingly Dr. Waller visited Ms. Betty Spectorman, the Health Education Coordinator for the North Bellemore school district, and her assistant, Mrs. Freya Kaufmann, and sat in on classroom demonstrations of the curricula. He was very impressed with what he saw. Both curricula comprised very carefully choreographed approaches with every exercise spelled out in detail. The lessons, conducted by the regular classroom teachers after initial indoctrination, with occasional supervision by experienced health educators, were supplemented by carefully prescribed reading matter, filmstrips, and other materials. After gaining sufficient experience, the classroom teachers were expected to train other teachers, thus spreading the program to other classes and schools.

Dr. Waller and the Steering Committee became quite enthusiastic about adapting these models to the New York City public school system but it was necessary first to obtain the approval of both the Academy and the Board of Education. The project was endorsed by the Committee on Medicine in Society which had been kept informed of its progress and, once they were assured that it would not unduly burden the resources of the Academy, Drs. Ferrer and McCormack were quite supportive.

The leadership of the Division of Curriculum and Instruction of the Board of Education, which was also responsible for health education, was not only willing to allow the demonstration, but also agreed to allocate several thousand dollars to provide initial funding for the project. From the beginning, officials in the Board of Education felt that a cooperative effort with the Academy and the private sector would provide a supportive constituency that could advance such a project in ways that Board officials responsible for health education could not accomplish alone.

Initial funding for the project, supplementing the allocation by the Board of Education, was provided by MetLife, Empire Blue Cross and Blue Shield, the New York Division of the American Cancer Society, Bankers Trust, the New York Telephone Company, the New York Community Trust, and the Morgan Guaranty Trust Company. Once funding commitments were assured, Mrs. Freya Kaufmann was hired to be Project Director. Periodically, the coalition of health agencies was reconvened to keep them informed and to receive helpful advice; the health education staff of the New York City Department of Health was particularly helpful.

In 1979, the program was launched as a five-year demonstration project in five schools, each in a different district. Classroom teachers from kindergarten through the third grade received training from instructors provided by the Academy and, in turn, trained other teachers from their schools. Teaching materials—films, records, tapes and group learning experiences rather than text books—were provided by the Academy for the first year; after that, their cost was shared by the districts. By 1981, more than 3,100 elementary school children in thirteen New York City public schools were participating in the program.

An evaluation of the program at the end of the first year conducted by Dr. Richard L. Andrews, Associate Professor of Educational Administration at the University of Washington, revealed that children participating in the program had greater levels of knowledge and more positive attitudes toward good health habits than those without access to the program. There were also collateral benefits: the teachers participating in the training sessions showed improvement in teaching skills while the children demonstrated improvement in reading, other language skills and social studies.

To verify the quality of the program, arrangements were made for an evaluation by Prof. Dale Mann of Teachers College, Columbia University, in collaboration with the National Center for Health Education. The major finding was that a somewhat more simplified and less ambitious curriculum would be more suitable to the complex environment of the New York City schools. Dr. Mann's recommendations were accepted by a review committee representing the Academy and the Board of Education and, in collaboration with the National Center for Health Education, the curriculum was streamlined, thereby cutting the cost of materials by one-third.

To monitor the progress of the project, a Management Committee was established. It was chaired by Dr. Waller and, in addition to Mr. Pearson and Dr. Lieberman, its original members included Ms. Joyce Bove of the New York Community Trust, Ms. Pauline Miles of Empire Blue Cross and Blue Shield, Ms. Silver Schecter and Mr. Melvin Warren of the New York City Board of Education, Mr. Roger Schmidt of the American Lung Association, and Ms. Eleanor Schweppe of the United Hospital Fund, organizations which had made funding commitments to the Project. Mrs. Leslie Goldman, Adminstrator of Educational Policy at the Central Board of Education who had an M.A. in policy analysis from Teachers College, was hired as the full-time Executive Director. Mrs. Freya Kaufmann stayed on as part-time Project Director, and the firm of Caesar, Lloyd, Brown was retained to provide assistance in preparing progress reports, fund raising, implementation reviews, and encouraging lateral spread to other schools within the selected school districts.

### Improving Physician Discipline

In 1975, in response to a recurrent "malpractice crisis" which had precipitated very large increases in physicians' premiums for malpractice insurance, New York Governor Hugh Carey appointed a Commission headed by William McGill, President of Columbia University, to study the problem. Dr. Irving Lewis, an Academy Fellow affiliated with the Albert Einstein Medical College, was selected to direct this study.

The "McGill Commission" offered a package of malpractice insurance reforms, including moving to a no-fault system, but these were not acted upon. However, its recommendations on changes in the process for physician discipline were adopted. Instead of placing this process entirely within the New York State Department of Education, which was also responsible for physician licensure, an Office of Professional Medical Conduct was created in the Department of Health to be responsible for initial hearings in cases of alleged misconduct. Additional hearings would be held by a Board for Medical Professional Conduct in the Department of Education; and the final decision would be made by the Board of Regents, the governing body for that Department. The Board for Medical Professional Conduct would comprise lay members appointed by the governor and physicians appointed by the Commissioner of Health. The Academy and the Medical Society of the State of New York were empowered to nominate the physician members; the Academy's initial selections were Drs. Joseph Post and Cyril Jones, both members of the Committee on Medicine in Society, and Dr. Frank Iaquinta, a member of the Committee on Medical Education.

A subcommittee comprising Drs. Joseph Post, Cyril Jones, Stanley Gitlow and Jack Harnes, with Drs. McCormack and Lieberman as ex officio members, was appointed to study the effect of these changes. Working with the Committee on Medicine and the Law of the Bar Association of New York City, it made a number of recommendations including increasing the number of lawyers assigned to the process and eliminating the Office of the Attorney General from the proceedings. However, deficiencies continued to exist. They included inordinate delays in hearing cases and writing opinions, inadequate resources for investigators; too many steps in the appeal process; and insufficient delineation of the roles of the lawyers, physicians, lay persons and administrators on the Board. In addition, there was often a conflict between what the Commissioner of Health would recommend and what the Board of Regents would ultimately decide. In many cases, members of that Board would find extenuating circumstances when, in reality, there were none sufficient to justify diminishing the suggested punishments.

## THE LIBRARY

In 1979, Mr. Brett A. Kirkpatrick, who had joined the staff in January 1978 after experience with the Library of the University of Buffalo School of Medicine, succeeded Mr. Brandon as Librarian. In addition to a variety of policy changes affecting reference services, circulation, interlibrary loans, cataloging, and collection development, he supervised the rearrangement of work spaces and the installation of a theft detection system.

In 1980, Ms. Sallie Morganstern was named Curator of the Rare Book/History of Medicine Department and Ms. Miriam Mandelbaum became her assistant. With generous assistance from Mrs. Marietta "Midge" Morchand, the wife of Charles Morchand, the Academy's printer, William Harvey's *De Circulatione Sanguinis* was acquired, bringing the Library's Harvey collection to near completion. In addition, a collection of 148 books on Arabic medicine and pharmacology was purchased from Dr. Sam Hamarneh, former Curator of the Division of Medical Science of the Smithsonian Institution.

The Library continued to serve as the Regional Medical Library for New York and New Jersey under the program of the National Library of Medicine, managing to cope successfully with the repeated changes required by the Regional Medical Library Program.

## FUND-RAISING AND THE "ROGATZ REPORT"

On repeated occasions, when confronted with questions about whether the Academy was fulfilling its potential role in health affairs in the City and State, Dr. McCormack had, in writing and in conversation, indicated his satisfaction with the current state of affairs at the Academy, especially in comparison with similar institutions elsewhere in the country. As noted in the previous chapter, the suggestion from Dr. John Deitrick when he was President of the Academy, that the Academy should undertake a study of its future was not taken up. When Mr. Robert Forrester, who had been engaged as a consultant to develop a fund raising campaign, suggested that it would be advisable to review the Academy's programs, however, a Committee on Fund Raising was established along with a Subcommittee on Planning and Goals. The Subcommittee was challenged by Mr. Forrester's recommendation that the Academy "underwrite special projects which will extend the Academy's statement of mission and, at the same time, enhance its visibility among the community at large."[21]

The members of the Committee on Fund Raising included Drs. Henry Frick, Jack Harnes, Cyril Jones, Frederic Kirkham, Norbert Roberts, Albert Santy, John Waller and Leon Warshaw, Mr. John Humphry, Library Consultant, and Dr. Maurice Saklad, an Associate Fellow. To chair the Subcommittee, President Dr. Joseph Post appointed Dr. Peter Rogatz, with the following as members: Drs. Pascal Imperato, Maurice Saklad, Joseph Post, James McCormack, and Mr. Joseph Terenzio, Mr. Sam Berté and Mr. Robert Forrester. Dr. Rogatz, a Fellow for many years, had earned distinction as the administrator of Long Island Jewish Hospital and Medical Center and of the Stonybrook University Hospital, as a consultant in hospital management, and as Vice-President for Medical Affairs at Empire Blue Cross and Blue Shield.

The Subcommittee's Report, which became known as the "Rogatz Report," was endorsed by the Committee. It stated that, notwithstanding the many successes of the Academy in the past—its Library; the work of its standing Committees; its many authoritative publications (including, of course, the *Bulletin*); its vital contributions to public health, planning and legislation in New York; and its studies, conferences and numerous contributions to the education of the public— are widely known and admired. Nonetheless, recent reflection on the Academy's plans in a rapidly changing world leads to the conclusion that its exceptional resources—both books and people— are not being used to optimum effect.[22]

The Report proposed that the Academy's mission, defined under the current By-laws as "the advancement of science and medicine . . ."[23] be subdivided into four major areas: "promotion of public health; improvement of medical practice; maintenance of a medical library; and education of the public."

Dr. Rogatz explained that the term, "public health," was used as a broad concept and included in it the functions of the Committee on Public Health as well as those of the Committee on Medicine in Society. He suggested the two

committees have carried out activities which, from time to time, have been complementary, supplementary or overlapping. Ultimately, the Council might wish to consider merging these committees into a single larger one, with a number of carefully defined subcommittees; alternatively, the mandate of each of the two existing committees might be sharpened, and additional standing committees might be created. Such a question, is well beyond the purview of this report.

Dr. Rogatz suggested that "the two committees continue as in the past to provide opportunities for physicians to discuss and debate public policy, serve as a catalyst for the development of new ideas, bring people together, and advocate in behalf of the community at large."

Dr. Rogatz urged that medical education programs focus on nonaffiliated physicians and not compete with medical schools and hospitals, stress new technology, and reach out to nurses, social workers and other health professionals. The library should be "maintained and nourished," and given more space for current activities and for the application of new technology. It should expand its preservation and rare book programs, develop a list of materials on health education, and continue its association with the Regional Library Program.

The Report delineated health education of the public as one area that called for major new initiatives on the part of the Academy. It urged an increase in efforts to reach out to other age groups in addition to the children at whom it was originally targeted, and "suggested the possibility of support from foundations for the creation of a 'Health Education Center' which would develop and supply special materials and utilize modern self-instructional techniques."[22]

The Report indicated a need for two additional staff offices: one for the administration of meetings at the Academy and the other for grant management. Obtaining increased operating income, it said, would require a coordinated fund-raising effort guided by a professional fund raising consultant. It suggested steps to improve security around the building such as improved parking, shuttle buses, and security patrols while studying the possibility of relocating the Academy.

Mr. Kirkpatrick, the Librarian, added a comprehensive review of the Library's collection and its future needs, pleading for a "comprehensive inventory of the Library, computerization of its operations, conservation of a deteriorating collection including adequate climate controls, and long-range planning for adequate space." He suggested the development of a for-profit "information brokerage" that could accommodate the demand for information services and also offer medical documentation and bibliographic services, programs for consumer health education, a learning resources center, and expansion of the duplication and data processing services.

The Report was received by Dr. McCormack and discussed by the Council at its November 1980 meeting, but there was obviously no readiness to begin a serious discussion of the future of the Academy. The report was seen simply as a list of possibilities, and no follow-up was planned. In retrospect, it seemed that, with Dr.

McCormack so close to retirement, what he and the Council had really desired was a rationale for embarking on a fund raising program rather than a proposal for restructuring the Academy. Thus, Mr. Forrester's challenge was partially met, and the hope of Dr. Rogatz and the Subcommittee that the Report would trigger a serious discussion of the future of the Academy and its programs was not to be fulfilled at that time.

## DEVELOPMENT AND PUBLIC RELATIONS OFFICE

One decision taken on Mr. Forrester's advice was the creation of a Development and Public Relations Office. On March 25, 1981, Dr. McCormack announced the appointment of Mr. George H. Weiler, Jr. as its full-time Director, a position he had previously held at the National Multiple Sclerosis Society.

In addition, a Resource Development and Public Affairs Committee was created with President Norbert J. Roberts assuming the responsibility of the chair. The first meeting, which took place on May 26, 1981, was not very encouraging: it was not well attended and some of its members expressed skepticism about the need for a major fund raising activity. In addition, it was noted that institutions such as medical schools and hospitals seem to have the first call on contributions from physicians, suggesting that physician membership organizations like the Academy would find it difficult to raise funds from their members.

## DR. McCORMACK'S DEATH

Dr. McCormack had announced his intention to retire at the end of 1981 and steps had been initiated to search for a possible successor. Unfortunately, he became gravely ill during the summer of that year and he died on September 22, 1981 before that search had been completed.

When Mr. McCormack first became ill, the Council and the

Board of Trustees had approved the recommendation from President Roberts that Dr. Marvin Lieberman, be appointed as "Acting Director" pending Dr. McCormack's return or the appointment of a new director." Having joined the Academy staff in 1964 and served as the Executive Secretary of the Committee on Medicine in Society since 1970, Dr. Lieberman was the senior staff member with the longest tenure at the Academy. Although invited to apply for the position of Director after Dr. McCormack's death, he declined because of doubts that the Academy would select a non-physician for that role, and the feeling that the duties of the Director as the Academy as then structured would not be as satisfying as being Executive Secretary of the Committee on Medicine in Society.

After Dr. McCormack's death, the Council voted to name the Council room the "McCormack Room" as a memorial to him. It was dedicated as such on May 26, 1982 in a formal ceremony that was attended by Mrs. McCormack and their six children, as well as many friends and colleagues. She was presented with a hand-lettered manuscript of the Council's memorial resolution which outlined the highlights of Dr. McCormack's professional career: "his distinguished deanships, his participation in the earliest use of penicillin therapy, his selfless commitment to the highest ideals of his profession, his interest in the problems of foreign medical graduates, his work in Washington on problems of military medicine, his wise judgment and stalwart dedication to the improvement of the Academy."[24]

## ACADEMY FINANCES

On July of 1979, Robert Brereton, the long-time Business Manager of the Academy, retired after suffering a period of ill health. He was succeeded on July 1, 1979 by Mr. Samuel C. Berté, a retired colonel, who had handled financial matters during his many years in the Army. Mr. Berté instituted a series of improvements in financial and administrative management, including: a system for property fund and depreciation accounting which provided a more accurate base for property accounting, better costing of operations and a more systematic technique for property replacement; a more refined budget system; and improved control over programs and expenditures. In 1980, to improve staff communication, a *Personnel Policies and Procedures Handbook* was published and distributed to all employees.

## ACADEMY PUBLICATIONS

### The *Bulletin*

First published in 1847, the *Bulletin of the New York Academy of Medicine* suspended publication after 1901. Volume 1 of Series 2 was published in 1925 and the *Bulletin* has been issued regularly ever since.

In February 1977, Dr. William D. Sharpe became its Editor serving on a part-time basis. He had studied at Cornell University, the University of Toronto and the University of Buffalo, receiving Bachelor and Master degrees in the classics. He graduated from the Johns Hopkins University School of Medicine and became a specialist in pathology. At the time of his appointment as Editor, he was Director of Laboratories at the Cabrini Health Care Center in New York City. Dr. Sharpe was an expert on chronic radium intoxication and in radiobiology, as well as a student of the history of the Civil War, with an emphasis on its medical history.

## ACADEMY PRESIDENTS

### Dr. José M. Ferrer, Jr. 1977–1978

A surgeon and medical educator at the Columbia University College of Physician and Surgeons, Dr. Ferrer was Chief of Surgery at the Harlem Hospital Center, affiliated with the Columbia University College of Physicians and Surgeons. He later served as Associate Dean for Graduate Education at the medical school. Dr. Ferrer was elected to Fellowship in 1950 and had served from 1954 to 1961 on the Committee on Public Health and from 1968 to 1982 on the Committee on Medical Education of which he was also Chairman. He was also a Trustee of the Academy from 1969 to 1973, and Vice President from 1975 to 1976.


Dr. Joseph Post 1979–1980

Dr. Post, who was born in New York City, graduated from the University of Chicago School of Medicine and received a Doctor of Medical Sciences degree from the Columbia University College of Physicians and Surgeons. He combined an active practice with research on liver disease and cancer at the New York University School of Medicine where he was Professor of Clinical Medicine. He had published approximately ninety papers on liver disease and on the biology of tumor cells. He became a Fellow of the Academy in 1949 and served as a member of the Committee on Medicine in Society from 1964 until his death in 1995 and from 1975 to 1979 as its Chairman.


Dr. Norbert J. Roberts 1981–1982

Dr. Roberts was a graduate of the Medical School of the University of Buffalo and trained in medicine at the Mayo Clinic. He was certified in occupational medicine by the American Board of Preventive Medicine and, later became Corporate Medical Director of the Exxon Corporation. He was one of the leaders in the field of occupational medicine having been elected President of the American Occupational Medicine Association. He became a Fellow in 1959, was active in the Section on Occupational Medicine, and served on the Committee on Medicine in Society from 1973 to 1980 After his term as President, he served as a Trustee from 1983 to 1987.

## NOTES

1 Board of Trustees, New York Academy of Medicine. 1977 Minutes of the meeting of December 21, 1977.

2 Council, New York Academy of Medicine. 1977 Minutes of the meeting of November 30, 1977.

3 Imperato PJ. 1981 Conclusions about amebiasis. *Bulletin of the New York Academy of Medicine.* 57:240–242.

4 Hinkle LE, Jr. and Murray SH. 1981 The importance of the quality of indoor air. *Bulletin of the New York Academy of Medicine.* 57: 827–844.

5 Committee on Public Health. 1981 Resolution concerning the stockpiling of Potassium Iodide in New York City in the event of a nuclear accident. *Bulletin of the New York Academy of Medicine.* 57:395–402.

6 Legato MJ. 1980 Medicine's threatened. *New York Times,* September 30, 1980. p. A27.

7 Legato MJ. 1981 Symposium on the academic physician: An endangered species: Introductory remarks. *Bulletin of the New York Academy of Medicine.* 57:413–414.

8 Post J. 1981 Symposium on the academic physician: welcome. *Bulletin of the New York Academy of Medicine.* 57:411–412.

9 Council of the New York Academy of Medicine. 1980 Minutes of the meeting of November 26, 1980.

10 Section on Medicine. 1982 Symposium on infectious diseases. *Bulletin of the New York Academy of Medicine.* 58:667–756.

11 Sections on Medicine and Pediatrics. 1983 Symposium on recent developments in oral antibiotic therapy. *Bulletin of the New York Academy of Medicine.* 59:420–525.

12 Sections on Medicine, Pediatrics and Surgery. 1984 Symposium on current and future directions in the use of antimicrobial agents. *Bulletin of the New York Academy of Medicine.* 60:313–440.

13 Ackerman RW. 1978 The organizational environment and ethical conduct in occupational medicine: A perspective. *Bulletin of the New York Academy of Medicine.* 54:707–714.

14 Siegler M. 1981. Searching for moral certainty in medicine: A proposal for a new model of the doctor-patient encounter. *Bulletin of the New York Academy of Medicine.* 57:56–69.

15 Post J. 1979 Changing house staff-attending staff relations. *Bulletin of the New York Academy of Medicine.* 55:46–51.

16 Committee on Medicine in Society. 1980 Report of the Subcommittee on Hospital Practice, January 14, 1980.

17 Lehr D. 1980 Opening statement: Symposium on the care of private

patients in teaching hospitals: the role of residents. *Bulletin of the New York Academy of Medicine.* 56:356–357.

18 Barondess JA. 1980 An academically organized private medical service: Structure, function, problems and lessons. *Bulletin of the New York Academy of Medicine.* 56:358–362.

19 School Health Curriculum Project 1982 Interview with John Waller. *SHCP News,* May 1982.

20 Waller, JV. 1977 Letter of invitation, September 20, 1977.

21 Forrester R. 1980 Report on fund-raising, October 14, 1980.

22 Rogatz P. 1980 *The New York Academy of Medicine: Its Mission in the Decade Ahead. Report of the Subcommittee on Planning and Goals.* November 17, 1980.

23 New York Academy of Medicine. 1979 *By-laws of the New York Academy of Medicine.*

24 Council of the New York Academy of Medicine. 1981 Resolution in Memory of Dr. James E. McCormack, October 29, 1981.

# Chapter 6
# 1982–1986
# Environmental Issues, Ethics, and Information Management

THE JAMES BEARD GALA AND THE BEEF INDUSTRY
COUNCIL
FILMING AT THE ACADEMY
COMMITTEE ON MEDICINE IN SOCIETY
Nuclear Weapons
Growing Healthy in New York City
"Project Stay Well"
Professional Medical Conduct
Care of Patients with Terminal Illness
"Do Not Resuscitate"
Alzheimer's and Related Diseases
National Health Policy Seminars
COMMITTEE ON PUBLIC HEALTH
Alcoholism and Drug Abuse
Nuclear Plant Accidents
Office of the Chief Medical Examiner
Maternity and Family Planning Services
Nutrition
Retirement of Dr. Shils
COMMITTEE ON MEDICAL EDUCATION
Financing Medical Education
The Training of Physicians
Role of Academic Medicine in Patient Education
THE ACADEMY LIBRARY
Regional Medical Library
Preservation Program

## THE JAMES BEARD GALA AND THE BEEF
## INDUSTRY COUNCIL

In January 1983, the Ketcham public relations firm, acting on behalf of the Beef Industry Council of the National Meat and Live-
stock Board, contacted Dr. McNutt and suggested arranging a
fund-raising gala at the Academy that would publicize the Library's
remarkable collection of cookbooks and also honor James Beard,
the noted cooking expert. There was much discussion of this proposal over the ensuing months. It was obvious that it was intended
to promote the nutritional benefits of beef. This led some to question whether this was too commercial a venture, but others said
that, in addition to raising funds for the Academy, it would increase
its visibility in the eyes of the public. Dr. McNutt suggested that it be
postponed until January 1984, when the US Department of Agriculture would release the new edition of the *Agricultural Handbook*
with its updated analysis of the nutrient content of beef. Finally, it
was agreed to schedule a dinner at the Academy preceded by a press
conference at which the publication of a book of reminiscences and
recipes by James Beard would be announced. The Academy would
receive a contribution of $10,000 and a collection of the books
written by Mr. Beard would be presented to add to the Library's

cook book collection. All press releases were to be approved by the Academy.

The Gala, attended by Mr. Beard's friends and colleagues as well as the officers and senior staff of the Academy, was held on March 1, 1984 in the main reading room of the Library. Dr. McNutt later reported to the Council that the event had received excellent press coverage and that a check for $10,000 from the Beef Industry Council had arrived, but the Library was still waiting for the set of Mr. Beard's books. (And, apparently, it is still waiting.) No further Galas were to be held until January 1995.

## FILMING AT THE ACADEMY

At the February 23, 1983 Council meeting, there was discussion about the handling of requests from communications, media and promotional organizations to use the Academy facilities for filming, photographing or broadcasting. It was agreed that such activities could not only bring favorable notice to the Academy, but also would bring additional income. Guidelines were adopted that were flexible and minimized interference with Academy activities, and yet would encourage organizations to use the Academy facilities for such purposes. There has been a good deal of filming at the Academy including: *The Chosen,* the feature film based on the novel by Chaim Potok; *Law and Order,* the dramatic television series; and commercials for such organizations as Merrill Lynch and American Express. However, scheduling has become more difficult as the number of meetings held at the Academy has increased.

## COMMITTEE ON MEDICINE IN SOCIETY

In 1982, Dr. Duncan Clark completed his fourth year as Chairman and became President of the Academy. He was succeeded as Chairman by Dr. Peter Rogatz.

## Nuclear Weapons

In 1982, the Council considered a resolution from the Committee which emphasized that medicine has very little to offer in the event of a nuclear war and called "upon the Governments of the United States and the Soviet Union to impose an immediate freeze on all testing, production and further deployment of all nuclear weapons, missiles, and delivery systems in a way that can be checked and verified by both sides; and thereafter begin a progressive reduction of existing nuclear weapon stockpiles."[1] After considerable discussion, the Council concluded that it was the Academy's right and duty to speak out about the medical aspects of nuclear weaponry and, after some minor modifications, approved the resolution which was then distributed to the Fellows and to the appropriate persons in the Congress and the Reagan administration. Some forty reactions were received from Fellows—all but one were positive—and, in addition to perfunctory acknowledgments from some of the public officials, a letter was received from Mr. B. F. Halloran of the US Arms Control and Disarmament Agency, expressing appreciation for the Academy's "reasoned and constructive approach to the issue of nuclear arms."[2]

## Growing Healthy in New York City

With streamlining of the curricula, the School Health Curriculum Project, known as "Growing Healthy in New York City," continued to flourish and expand. The training arrangements brought selected teachers to the Academy for a five day session in which they worked on the curriculum, created study materials and developed lesson plans for use in their classrooms. When they returned to their schools, they, in turn, trained their colleagues. Periodically, the teachers would reconvene at the Academy to share their experiences and, at the end of the academic year, the Academy would host a reception at which they could meet representatives of the Academy, the Board of Education and the approximately fifty organizations funding the Project. At these receptions, the achievements of individual teachers would be recognized.

In 1983, the Board of Education recognized the Project as the official health education model to be implemented throughout the elementary school system and the schools' Chancellor recommended to the Mayor that the City allocate $1.3 million of tax-levy funds per year for the next five years to cover the cost of materials and stipends for the teacher training. The Academy would continue to seek private funding to cover the management, coordination, quality control and evaluation of the Project.

By the end of the 1985–1986 school year, the Project was in place in 144 schools in twenty community school districts. Fifteen hundred teachers had been trained in the curriculum and 120,000 elementary school children had been exposed to it. In December 1983, Governor Mario M. Cuomo, in recognition of the accomplishments of the program, presented the Academy with an Eleanor Roosevelt Community Service Award Certificate of Merit.

In 1986, the eighth year of the Project, a six-month study funded by the New York Community Trust and the Morgan Guaranty Trust Company was undertaken to explore the feasibility of its further expansion the City's junior high schools.

### "Project Stay Well"

One result of the School Health Curriculum Project was a request from Mrs. Janet Sainer, Commissioner of the New York City Department for the Aging, for assistance in designing and implementing a health promotion program for the elderly attending senior citizen centers operated by the Departments for the Aging and Social Services. Under the direction of Dr. John Waller, Academy staff assisted in developing *Stay well,* a twelve session curriculum that featured classes in exercise and stress management and forums providing education on health problems of the aging: e.g., communicating with health professionals; safety in the home; medication management; diabetes; hypertension; cancer; arthritis; nutrition;

vision; hearing; and sexuality. Over forty community agencies participated in a Voluntary Agencies Committee and provided speakers, discussion leaders, films and other materials for the sessions. At the end of each course, a volunteer training program was offered, in which older adults were trained to lead the health promotion activities in their centers. There were no fees to the participants. In its first year, the program was implemented in four communities—Boro Park in Brooklyn, Flushing in Queens, North Central Bronx, and Central Harlem in Manhattan—and, since then, in one form or another, it has become a fixture in most of the Senior Citizen Centers in the City, with the Academy no longer involved.

## Professional Medical Conduct

The Ad Hoc Committee on Professional Medical Conduct, which included Drs. Joseph Post, Cyril Jones, Frank Iaquinta, David McNutt and Marvin Lieberman, continued to monitor the activities of the newly created Board of Professional Medical Conduct, and remained dissatisfied with its procedures. On November 28, 1984, an invitational seminar to review this process was held at the Academy with cosponsorship by the New York State Department of Health. The group of some thirty multidisciplinary participants included Dr. David Axelrod, the State Commissioner of Health, Assemblyman James R. Tallon, Jr., Chair of the Assembly Health Committee, Mr. Philip Pinsky, Counsel to the New York State Senate Majority Leader, and Mr. Martin Barell, Vice Chancellor of the Board of Regents. Out of this Seminar came a report that recommended simplifying the process of medical discipline in the State and providing greater resources to the program. The report was endorsed by a subcommittee of the Committee on Medicine and the Law of the Bar Association of the City of New York that was chaired by Dr. Marvin Lieberman.

On February 25, 1985, the Committee on Medicine in Society learned of a proposal in the Governor's Executive Budget suggesting an increase in physician licensure fees to be devoted to the work of the Office of Professional Medical Conduct. In a statement that was approved by the Council, the Committee endorsed the fee increase providing that the funds would be earmarked to support the licensure and disciplinary process. Even then, the statement noted, the amounts to be set aside in a Special Revenue Account would not be adequate to support the improvements needed in the Departments of Health and Education. Because of such reservations, which were shared by other organizations, the Legislature did not adopt the proposed increase in the license fees.

The statement also emphasized the importance of expediting the adjudication process in order to reduce the backlog of cases accumulated through the years. That process required a panel to conduct a preliminary investigation to verify that prosecution of the accused physician was warranted. The panel's findings and recommendations were then reviewed by the Commissioner of Health, and then by a Professional Discipline Committee comprising three members of the Board of Regents. Finally, the full Board of Regents, after hearing oral arguments by the respondent and his or her attorney and a lawyer representing the Department of Health, made the final determination. The object of this lengthy and cumbersome process was to allow fairness to the respondent and, at the same time, to protect the public safety and interest. It opened the door, however, to legal maneuvering and procedural delays that allowed a physician ultimately found guilty of egregious incompetence and misconduct to continue to treat patients for many years before such penalties as suspension or revocation of his or her license could be invoked.

The Committee's statement recommended streamlining this process by essentially eliminating the role of the Board of Regents. It proposed that, after an initial investigation by the same kind of panel, there would be only one review, by a committee chaired by the Commissioner of Health and comprising two members of the Board of Regents. The decision would be embodied in a written opinion that would provide guidance to the profession and to future panels on what constitutes professional misconduct. However, opposition from friends in the Legislature who supported objections of the Board of Regents and the Department of Education to the downgrading of their roles proved to be a formidable obstacle to the enactment of the proposed reforms.

In 1986, the hearing panels were reduced in size from four physicians and one layperson to two physicians and one layperson and, in 1991, major reforms eliminating roles for the Board of Regents and the Commissioner of Health were enacted. These reforms, which simplified the process by allowing only one level of appeal, followed the general outline of the Academy recommendations.[3]


### Care of Patients with Terminal Illness

In 1980 the Committee on Medicine in Society and the Committee on Public Health formed a Joint Committee on the Care of Patients with Terminal Illness, chaired by Dr. John T. Flynn, Chief of Medicine at Beekman Downtown Hospital; Drs. Eugene B. Feigelson, Chairman of the Department of Psychiatry at Downstate Medical Center, and Peter Rogatz, then Chairman of the Committee on Medicine in Society, played leading roles in its work.

Recent advances in medical technology and changing attitudes of physicians and the lay public regarding patient autonomy in health care decision making, had brought the ethical issues involved into the limelight. A major effort in transforming the discussion into a consensus that would influence policy, law and regulation was the work of the President's Commission for the Study of Ethical Problems in Medicine and Biomedical and Behavioral Research, created by President Carter and continued during the Reagan administration. This Commission focused on such issues as the definition of death, the patient's role in decision making, and the withholding of life-sustaining treatment, including cardiopulmonary resuscitation. Many of its recommendations became policy in a variety of jurisdictions in the US through legislative acts, regulations and/or court decisions. In New York State, the Task Force on Life and the Law established by Governor Mario Cuomo attempted to clarify and foster a consensus on these ethical issues. It proposed a bill that embodied many of the recommendations of the Commission, and came to the Academy for its opinion.

The proposed definition of death as the irreversible cessation of function of the cardiovascular system or the brain, however, aroused opposition from the Union of Orthodox Jewish Congregations of America and the New York State Catholic Conference. The position of Agudath Israel (an organization generally representing talmudic authorities) and the Union of Orthodox Jewish Congregations contended that, according to Jewish religious law, death can only be defined as the cessation of breathing or the functioning of the heart. These views were opposed by some authorities within the orthodox community, however, who agreed with current biological science which holds that the brain controls respiration and heart function and defines death as the cessation of brain function, even if respiration and the heartbeat can be sustained by external means.

The proposed bill had initially been approved by the New York State Catholic Conference but Monsignor Smith, Cardinal Cook's theological adviser, who, apparently, had linked the definition of death with such perceived evils as euthanasia and abortion, prevailed upon the Cardinal to have this approval rescinded.

In reaching its conclusions, the Joint Committee relied on a comprehensive review of the medical and bioethical literature. It was particularly impressed by the writings of Christopher Pallis, a pathologist, who said "a dead brain in a body whose heart is still beating is one of the more macabre products of modern technology. During the past thirty years techniques have developed that can artificially maintain ventilation, circulation and elimination of waste products of metabolism in a body whose brain has irreversibly ceased to function."[4] In its statement, the Committee cited the views of Germain Grisez and Joseph M. Boyle, Jr., two conservative Catholic theologians, who wrote that a "correct definition of death, if it would eliminate some false classifications of dead individuals [as being] among the living, could eliminate some of the pressure for legalizing euthanasia—in this case, pressure arising from a right attitude toward individuals really dead and only considered alive due to a conceptual confusion."[5]

The Joint Committee's statement, in essence, reaffirmed the recommendations of the President's Commission, which, based on the model statute drafted by the National Conference of Commissioners on Uniform State Laws, focused on brain death as the definitive finding. It proposed that "either the irreversible cessation of cardiopulmonary function or the irreversible cessation of the entire function of the brain, including the brain stem, is an adequate criterion for the definition of death. . . . A determination of death must be made in accordance with accepted medical standards."[6] The New York State Task Force on Life and the Law endorsed this definition of death (with a dissent by Rabbi J. David Bleich), but did recommend that hospitals and physicians, where feasible, should accommodate the moral or religious views of families.

The proposed bill was held up in the legislature due to the opposition of the orthodox Jewish community and the New York State Catholic Conference. The matter was resolved, however, by an interesting decision by a criminal court in Brooklyn in case of homicide in which the defendant, relying on the common law definition of death as the cessation of heartbeat or respiration, claimed that he could not be held responsible for the death of the person he had shot because the victim's heart had continued to beat until hospital personnel removed him from the respirator after he had been declared brain dead. The Court of Appeals of the State of New York ruled against the defendant, holding that, in light of current scientific knowledge, death would be defined as the permanent cessation of brain functioning, not the cessation of respiration and heartbeat. In this way, the recommendations of the President's Commission and the New York Task Force on the Life and the Law, which had been supported by the Academy's Joint Committee, overturned the earlier common law definition and imposed a modern definition of death.

## "Do Not Resuscitate"

Included in the Joint Committee's statement, which was approved by the Council on May 22, 1985, was a recommendation for legislation that would empower the State Commissioner of Health to prepare guidelines for "do not resuscitate" (DNR) orders for patients who have suffered an in-hospital cardiopulmonary arrest. As the statement notes, "Technology is currently available that is capable of restoring cardiopulmonary functions after a patient has suffered cardiac or respiratory arrest, thus reversing a condition which would result in death in a short period of time."[7]

This issue arose out of the practice in hospitals to have "informal undocumented decisions reserved to the professional staff," a practice that was criticized because "the patient or family may not be involved in the decision nor is there any possibility of accountability or possibility of review as clinical conditions may change."[7]

The statement suggested that "physicians, patients and family members must recognize that competent patients have a right to refuse treatment as well as a right to request and expect efforts at resuscitation if indicated." It went on to propose public education to promote the use of living wills, which contain the wishes of patients on what is to be done, or not done, if they become incapable of making decisions. The statement proposed the legislation of special provisions that would allow family members and physicians to "withhold DNR orders where appropriate, even in cases where the patient is a child or has never expressed wishes and is now or has always been decisionally incapable."[7] Once again, the Joint Committee had followed the excellent document prepared by the President's Commission.[8] Laws regarding DNR regulations were passed in 1987[9] and, in 1990, a bill recognizing health care proxies was enacted.[10] (No law has yet been passed to deal with the situation in which a decisionally incompetent person had failed to appoint a proxy or make his or her wishes known while still competent.)

Alzheimer's and Related Diseases

In July 1984, in collaboration with New York State Health Planning Commission, the Committee on Medicine in Society convened a two-day, invitational *Institute on Alzheimer's and Related Diseases* at West Point, NY. It was planned by a committee that included such well-recognized experts in gerontology as Msgr. Charles J. Fahey of Fordham University, and Drs. Eugene Y. Berger of Morningside House in the Bronx, Robert N. Butler of Mt. Sinai Medical Center, Carl Eisdorfer of Montefiore Medical Center, Robert Katzman of Albert Einstein College of Medicine, Barry Gurland of Columbia University, and representing the Committee, Drs. Duncan Clark, John K. Guck, Peter Rogatz and James J. McCormack. The objective of the Institute was to develop policy recommendations for differentiating the 15 percent of persons aged sixty-four or older who have some form of dementia amenable to treatment from the smaller number diagnosed as having Alzheimer's disease.

The Institute recommended a broad range of initiatives in research and training coupled with innovations in coverage of these conditions by private health insurance as well as by Medicare and Medicaid. It also suggested that the State and the Academy collaborate in convening experts from medical schools to develop "simple low cost diagnostic protocols for diagnosing suspected Alzheimer's disease."[11] As a follow-up, the Academy and the New York State Planning Commission convened a group of experts to develop guidelines that would assist general internists in identifying forms of dementia that could be treated. The product was delivered to the Commissioner of Health, who, for reasons that are not clear, decided not to distribute it throughout the state. The significance of this effort is that it represented a close working relationship between the Academy and the State government; the conference and publication of the report having received financial support from the State.

## National Health Policy Seminars

In 1985, the Committee inaugurated a year-long series of seminars on national health policy that harked back to a similar series of discussions sponsored by the Committee in the 1960s. Major funding was provided by the Ford Foundation, which had supported the work of the Committee on Social Policy for Health Care in the 1960s; supplemental funding came from the United Hospital Fund. These seminars were constituted as a part of a Ford Foundation project to examine *Social Welfare and the American Future* relating to health care issues. To inaugurate this activity, the Committee was asked to hold a weekend "retreat" at which the whole range of policy alternatives could be considered.

To prepare for that meeting, Prof. Lawrence D. Brown, then at the University of Michigan, was commissioned to prepare a background paper outlining various options for broadening health insurance coverage while improving the quality of care and controlling its costs in the United States.[12] This paper was republished by the Ford Foundation and circulated widely.[13] The meeting, which was held at conference center on Long Island was chaired by Dr. Peter Rogatz, Chairman of the Committee.

A series of nine seminars was conducted between October 1986 and March 1988, featuring presentations by Ms. Dorothy P. Rice of the Institute for Health and Aging of the University of California at San Francisco, Dr. David Blumenthal of the Kennedy School of Government at Harvard University, Bruce Vladeck, Ph.D., of the United Hospital Fund of New York, Bradford Gray, Ph.D., of the Institute of Medicine of the National Academy of Sciences, Robert Evans, Ph.D., of the University of British Columbia, Rashi Fein, Ph.D. of the Harvard Medical School, Lawrence D. Brown, Ph.D., now at Columbia University, Louise B. Russell, Ph.D. from Rutgers University, and James A. Morone, Ph.D., from Brown University. They culminated in the publication by the Committee on Medicine in Society of a position statement entitled *Toward a Health Care Financing Strategy for the Nation.*[14]

COMMITTEE ON PUBLIC HEALTH

The Committee on Public Health, chaired by Dr. Norman Simon with Dr. John T. Flynn as Vice Chairman, succeeded in 1984 by Drs. Lawrence E. Hinkle, Jr. and Anita S . Curran, with Dr. Maurice E. Shils as Executive Secretary, pursued a broad range of activities through its subcommittees and working groups.

Alcoholism and Drug Abuse

In March 1982, the Subcommittee on Alcohol and Drug Abuse, chaired by Dr. Robert B. Millman, studied the use of methadone in opioid addiction pioneered by Drs. Marie Nyswander and Vincent Dole of Rockefeller University. The Subcommittee's *Statement and Resolution Regarding Methadone Maintenance Treatment,* which updated an earlier report issued by the Committee on Public Health more than a decade earlier,[15] reaffirmed the importance of medical participation in the treatment of drug addictions and supported the use of methadone for maintenance, but noted that "the regulatory requirements governing its distribution by clinics have led to long waiting lists and a lack of access to needed services." These services should be made available to all who need them, the Subcommittee contended, and thus it "endorses and encourages the implementation of efforts designed to test more effective ways of delivering services, including a pilot project of 'medical maintenance' in which appropriately trained and interested physicians would provide methadone maintenance treatment, pursuant to a protocol which ensures adequate control, monitoring, and evaluation, to a limited number of addicts who have been rehabilitated successfully, who are considered to need on-going chemotherapy, and who wish to do so."[16]

Later in 1982, the Subcommittee presented a two-session course, entitled *The Difficult Patient: Dependency on Prescription Drugs and/or Alcohol,* cosponsored by the New York State Division of Substance Abuse Services. As part of the course, which was given at the Academy, Dr. Anne Geller of St. Luke's-Roosevelt Medical Center, Dr. Robert Millman of New York Hospital, and Dr. Edward Rabinowitz of St. Vincent's Hospital and Medical Center hosted visits to their hospital-based treatment centers. On May 26, 1982, the Subcommittee convened a *Conference on Alcoholism and the General Hospital,* cosponsored by Blue Cross-Blue Shield of Northeastern New York, the Greater New York Hospital Association, the Hospital Association of New York State, the New York State Department of Health and the Office of Alcoholism and Alcohol Abuse Services. In the opening presentation, Dr. Stanley E. Gitlow, noting that "many accidents are alcohol-related but are not labeled as such," made an eloquent and impassioned plea for recognizing alcoholism as the biggest killer of young adults."[17]

In October 1985, assisted by grants from a number of pharmaceutical companies, the Subcommittee revisited the problem of iatrogenic addiction. Prompted by concern that fear of addiction was leading to undertreatment of patients needing narcotic analgesics, it convened a conference on *Iatrogenic Addiction—Developing Guidelines for the Use of Sedatives and Analgesics in the Hospital.*[18] At this conference, Dr. David Musto of the Yale University School of Medicine, a prominent historian of American social policies toward drug abuse and alcoholism, noting the high level of such addictions among health workers and the prevailing attitudes toward iatrogenic addiction through the years, emphasized that it is not really a new problem. Drs. Domenic A. Ciraulo of the Department of Psychiatry at Tufts University Schools of Medicine, Samuel W. Perry of the Cornell University Medical College, and Barry Stimmel of the Mount Sinai School of Medicine emphasized the abuse potential of the benzodiazepines.[19,20] Dr. William A. Frost of the Department of Psychiatry at Cornell University Medical College, who had chaired the conference planning committee, said that the withholding of narcotics from hospital patients reflects the fact that, while pharmacologists and physicians particularly involved in the treatment of pain know better, "there has been relatively little change in the behavior of hospital staff physicians, who do most of the prescribing, and nurses who do most of the dispensing."

Nuclear Plant Accidents

In April 1983, in response to concerns about potential nuclear plant accidents and exposure of their employees to radiation, the Subcommittee on Environmental Health convened a two-day conference that focused on the operation of nuclear power plants, the risks of life-threatening accidents, and the health consequences of both accidents and the responses to them. The Conference, which was attended by over 200 physicians, health physicists, government officials, media representatives and others, was supported by funding from the New York State Department of Health, Long Island Lighting Company, Niagara Mohawk Power Company and the Power Authority of New York State. Dr. Norman Simon, the Chair, noted in his introductory remarks that the Subcommittee had attempted to present a balanced program but the "strongest opponents of nuclear power did not accept our invitations to speak."[21] Commissioner of Health Dr. David Axelrod opened the program by noting that there is much that we do not know about nuclear plant operation and the risks of low-level ionizing radiation. Our ignorance, he said, reflects in part "the limits of modern epidemiology and epidemiologic techniques. We do not know what the radiation health effect is at the very low doses, as low as a few millirems per year, to which we all are exposed. No unequivocal data exist on dose-response relationships for various radiation-induced cancers among exposed human populations. And we do not know the role of competing. . . . biological, chemical, or other physical factors existing at the time of the exposure, or following exposure, which may affect or influence the carcinogenic, the teratogenic, or genetic health effects of the low-level radiation."[22]

Later that year, as Chairman of the Working Group on the Health Aspects of Radioactive Materials, Dr. Norman Simon presented oral and written testimony on the Academy position on the disposal of very low-level radioactive wastes to a hearing of the City Council Committee on the Environment.

Office of the Chief Medical Examiner

During the 1980s, the Subcommittee on Governmental Health Agencies, chaired by Dr. John T. Flynn, studied the operation of the Office of the Chief Medical Examiner (OCME) in the New York City Department of Health. The Committee on Public Health had been a leader in efforts to assure competent review of violent, accidental or suspicious deaths since 1912 when it took a position on reform of the then prevailing coroner system. That effort succeeded, with the creation in 1918 of the OCME as an independent agency headed by a physician selected on the basis of competence appointed by the Mayor from a civil service list, and who could be removed only by the Mayor. The Committee continued to oppose legislative efforts that would curtail the authority of the Chief Medical Examiner and subject the OCME to political control.

In 1965 the Committee took a position in opposition to a proposal by Deputy Mayor John Connorton that the work of the OCME be further centralized in its office in Manhattan. Largely because of the Academy position, this proposal was never implemented.

The OCME lost its independence during the administration of Mayor John V. Lindsay when it was made part of the Health Services Administration, a newly created "superagency." When Mayor Abraham Beame came into office and did away with the superagencies, he appointed a committee headed by Mr. Joseph V. Terenzio, President of the United Hospital Fund and a Fellow of the Academy, to review the operation of the OCME. The "Terenzio Report," submitted in 1977, found the OCME to be in serious disarray, suffering from "poor financial reporting mechanisms, inadequate administration, a minimal role in education and research, and difficulties with personnel and recruitment caused by competitive civil service procedures."[23] The report recommended maintaining the independence of the OCME and the creation of an advisory board to monitor its operation, and asserted that "putting the OCME in the Department of Health would do nothing to solve the administrative constraints and might hamper the recruitment of top flight persons." Notwithstanding this recommendation, the mayoral bill enacted by the City Council in 1977 did place the OCME in the Department of Health and gave its Commissioner the "power to supervise the management of all programs, activities and expenditures."

In 1979, when it became obvious that the OCME continued to have problems, the Committee appointed a working group to review its operations. At that time, it was also being studied by Dr. Leon J. Warshaw, a Fellow who had been seconded from his role as Vice President and Corporate Medical Director of the Equitable Life Assurance Society to serve as Deputy Director for Health Affairs of the Mayor's Office of Operations, an office staffed by experts in various disciplines of management loaned to the City by organizations in the private sector to improve its administration and help Mayor Edward I. Koch to rescue it from the brink of bankruptcy. Dr. Warshaw found the Terenzio report and guidance of the members of the working group to be quite helpful in framing appropriate recommendations for changes in the OCME. Most of them, however, were not implemented, owing to concurrent disarray in the Department of Health and the pressure of other problems, including the Health and Hospitals Corporation, which the Mayor perceived to be more urgent.

In 1984 the Committee launched another study of the OCME that included interviews with Dr. Elliot M. Gross, the incumbent Chief Medical Examiner who came under fire in January, 1985 when local newspapers featured allegations of his incompetence and misconduct, and also featured a survey of the opinions of local hospital pathologists in which the OCME did not get good scores. The report of this study, which was approved by the Council in May 1985, offered detailed recommendations for the organization and operation of the OCME which were extremely helpful to Dr. Martin Cherkasky, a Fellow of the Academy who was acting as an ad hoc advisor on medical affairs to Mayor Koch. With the implementation of many of these and the appointment of Dr. Charles S. Hirsch, the highly regarded Chief Medical Examiner for Suffolk County on Long Island, the OCME was able to regain much of the luster it had lost. (Dr. Hirsch became a Fellow of the Academy in 1989 and is currently a member of the Board of Trustees.)

## Maternity and Family Planning Services

In February 1982 the Subcommittee on Maternity and Family Planning, chaired by Dr. Hugh R. K. Barber, adopted a statement and resolution entitled *The Setting of Obstetrical Delivery* that was critical of delivery in the home. There was some byplay between the Council, which attempted some editorial revisions, and the Committee, whose request to issue the report without Council approval was rejected by President Dr. Duncan Clark on the grounds that this was prohibited by the By-laws. Dr. Peter Rogatz noted that the report did not mention the Maternity Center Association, which did not do home deliveries but did provide non-hospital maternity care. The statement in the report that "a hospital is the recommended place for planned obstetrical delivery," with no reference to birthing centers, was rightfully interpreted by their supporters as a rebuff. The Council voted to approve the statement with one dissent.[24]

In 1983 the Subcommittee reviewed data indicating that ectopic pregnancies are a major cause of maternal death. Since deaths from this cause are preventable through early diagnosis and treatment, the Subcommittee urged the Commissioner of Health to organize a campaign to raise the awareness of both physicians and women of child-bearing age to the signs and symptoms of ectopic pregnancy and the importance of early treatment.

In 1984 the Subcommittee issued a statement that endorsed the regionalization of perinatal services and called for cooperation among hospitals and medical centers in the provision of optimal care of pregnant women, their unborn babies and critically ill or high risk newborns.[25]

## Nutrition

The Subcommittee on Nutrition sponsored the Registry of Patients on Home Total Parenteral Nutrition, which conducted annual surveys of home-based patients on intravenous alimentation. The Registry, funded by the Dana Foundation and the Oley Foundation for Home Parenteral and Enteral Nutrition, made data summaries available to physicians and other health care professionals, governmental agencies, insurance companies and other interested parties.

Executive Secretary Dr. Maurice Shils served as Principal Investigator of The New York-New Jersey Regional Center for Clinical Nutrition Education, funded by the American Cancer Foundation to promote nutrition education programs in medical, dental and osteopathic schools in the New York-New Jersey area. Under the direction of Dr. Shils and Mrs. Barbara C. Lowell, MS, RD, the Center had inaugurated interhospital teaching rounds and had undertaken the development of model curricula for nutrition education. In March 1983, it sponsored a *Conference on Nutrition Education in Medical Schools* with speakers from the area and from schools in six other states, that was attended by physicians, students and residents.

## Retirement of Dr. Shils

Having reached retirement age, Dr. Maurice Shils, Executive Secretary of the Committee stepped down from that position after more than eight years with the Academy. While serving the Committee, he was also Professor of Medicine at Cornell University Medical College and Director of Clinical Nutrition at Memorial Hospital. In 1983 he received the Joseph P. Goldberger Award in Clinical Nutrition from the American Medical Association. Upon his retirement he continued at the Academy as its first Visiting Scholar, and continued to work with the New York-New Jersey Regional Center for Clinical Nutrition.

Dr. Shils was succeeded in May 1985 by Dr. Susan Hadley, Professor of Medicine at Cornell University Medical College. To take this position, she took a one year leave as Assistant to the Chairman of the Department of Medicine, New York Hospital-Cornell University Medical College.

## COMMITTEE ON MEDICAL EDUCATION

Under the aegis of Chairman Dr. William H. Becker, Vice-Chairman Dr. Marianne J. Legato and Executive Secretary William C. Stubing, the Committee and the nineteen Sections continued to hold about ninety meetings, conferences and workshops attracting a total of approximately 10,000 attendees each year. In 1982, for example, the Section on Otolaryngology offered a year-long basic science course featuring seventeen sessions that attracted almost 400 graduate and postgraduate students. During the same year, Sections sponsored important full-day symposia: *New Concepts in the Treatment of Infectious Diseases* sponsored by the Section on Medicine; *Selected Updates on Gynecology and Obstetrics,* and *The Computer and Obstetrics and Gynecology,* both sponsored by the Section on Obstetrics and Gynecology. In October 1983, as part of a symposium on *The Visual Process* sponsored by the Section on Ophthalmology, two Nobel laureates, Drs. George Wald and Torsten N. Wiesel, delivered the first Sylvia and Herbert Berger Lecture at the Academy, a lectureship created by a gift from Dr. Herbert Berger, Vice Chairman of the Committee on Education from 1978 to 1981. It was a two-part presentation: Dr. Wald spoke on *Human Vision* and Dr. Wiesel spoke on *Development of the Visual Cortex and the Influence of the Environment.* In addition to the Ferdinand C. Valentine Lecture, sponsored by the Section on Urology, as many as eight other memorial lectures were sponsored each year by various sections. (See Appendix.)

Financing Medical Education

In October 1982, the Committee's Ninth Symposium on Medical Education: *Financing Medical Education: The Costs for Students and the Implications for Medical Practice* attracted over 200 participants, more than half of whom were administrators, faculty or students from thirty-three medical schools in fourteen states. The Symposium was cosponsored by the Associated Medical Schools of New York with which the Committee had established a working relationship, and was funded by the Corlette Glorney and Josiah Macy, Jr. Foundations. Dr. Eli Ginzburg, the eminent medical economist from Columbia University, was the featured speaker and the program, planned by a committee headed by Dr. Mary Ann Payne of Cornell University Medical College, included presentations by prominent figures from the Association of American Medical Colleges, the American Medical Association, the Senate Committee for Higher Education, the US Department of Health and Human Services and a number of medical schools. The proceedings were published in the *Bulletin*.[26]

The Training of Physicians

The Tenth Symposium on Medical Education in 1983 was devoted to *The Training of Tomorrow's Physicians: How Well Are We Meeting Society's Expectations?* Once again, demonstrating the appeal of Academy meetings to people outside the New York City area, half the audience of over 300 came from twenty-nine medical schools in eleven states, while national organizations, such as the American Medical Association, the Association of American Medical Colleges and the Education Commission for Foreign Medical Graduates, and twenty-three major corporations were also represented. The Symposium was supported in part by grants from Burson-Marsteller, Inc., Chemical Bank, Citibank, N.A., Mr. Laurance S. Rockefeller, and the Charles E. Culpepper, Corlette Glorney, Alfred Jurzykowsi, and Helena Rubenstein Foundations.

Role of Academic Medicine in Patient Education

Early in 1983, the Committees on Medical Education and Medicine in Society joined in presenting a two-day invitational meeting on the *Role of Academic Medicine in Patient Education,* at the Tarrytown Conference Center in Tarrytown, NY. The proposal for the meeting, which was accompanied by a grant from Pfizer Pharmaceuticals as part of its program to support leaders in academic medicine, was brought to the Academy by Dr. Rita Wroblewski, Vice-President for Medical Affairs at Pfizer and a member of the Committee on Medicine in Society. Dr. Robert J. Haggerty, also a member of that Committee, chaired the sessions, which involved some seventy distinguished leaders in academic medicine and health education. Dr. Lester Breslow, former Commissioner of Health of the State of California, gave the opening address; other speakers included Drs. R. Brian Haynes of McMaster University in Ontario, Anne R. Somers of Rutgers Medical School, M. Alfred Haynes of the Charles R. Drew Postgraduate Medical School in California, and Stuart Bondurant of the University of North Carolina School of Medicine.

The Conference discussed the responsibility of academic medical centers for patient education and reviewed issues of compliance with medical regimens, self-care, changing health behavior, and the roles of the various health professionals involved. In addition to publishing the proceedings in the *Bulletin,* the Planning Committee prepared a Report which was endorsed by both of the sponsoring Committees and then, in May 1984, by the Council.[27]

The Report accepted the definition of health education proposed by Green and Johnson as: "learning experiences designed to facilitate voluntary adaptations of behaviors conducive to health in individuals, groups and communities. Health education strives to help people control their own health by predisposing, enabling and reinforcing decisions and actions consistent with their own goals and values." It went on to define patient education as health education dealing with a "narrower segment of the population, people entering or already under medical care or treatment," which involves "guidance in the selection of clinical services, help to patients and families in asking questions and relating to caregivers, coping with the stress of illness, participating in realistic goal setting, and changing health behaviors in a purposeful way."[28]

Dr. Cecil Sheps defined the academic medical center as "a complex administrative organization consisting of a medical school, hospitals, and other educational institutions and patient care facilities," and emphasized that these centers were not doing enough to fulfill their potential for good because a role in patient education has not been assigned to them.[29] Dr. R. Brian Haynes of McMaster University added that outpatient settings in academic medical centers were particularly suitable for providing instruction in patient compliance.

The report recommended that physicians should serve as teachers and counselors and, perhaps even more important, should work toward promoting and contributing to the planning of institutional programs. The important role of nurses in patient education was also detailed. The opportunities health care professionals have to motivate patients and the benefits that it can bring to patients imposes an ethical obligation for patient education. To preserve the integrity of the physician-patient relation, and to maintain the patient's confidence in the information and instructions given to him or her, telling the truth to the patients becomes very important and, for the same reasons, coercion or undue influence on patients are to be strenuously avoided.[30]

The Report emphasized the importance of patient education and its evaluation and suggested that these are ethical obligations of academic medical centers. Its practitioners, the Report said, merit academic recognition and support by foundations, government and the public. Health education of the public through the media "assists and reinforces patient education programs" and consequently merits support by the media, other industry groups and professional organizations.

## THE ACADEMY LIBRARY

On June 16, 1981, the Academy joined ten other cultural institutions on Fifth Avenue, including the Metropolitan Museum of Art, the Frick and the Guggenheim Museums, in the Third Annual Museum Mile Festival. For this occasion the Library mounted an exhibit on *The Red Cross: Its Origins and the American Centennial*. Visitors who came to the Academy at the north end of the "museum mile" were greeted by Mr. Brett A. Kirkpatrick, the Librarian, and Ms. Anne Pascarelli, the Associate Librarian.

### Regional Medical Library

In 1982 the Academy was awarded a $1.6 million, three-year contract by the National Library of Medicine to serve as headquarters for Region 1 of the reconfigured Regional Medical Library Program (RML). Acquisition of the award was a competitive process in which the Academy had to compete with the American College of Physicians in Philadelphia and the Countway Library in Boston which had submitted a joint application in concert with the University of Connecticut Health Sciences Center.

Now one of seven instead of the prior eleven regions, the Library's area of responsibility was expanded from New York and New Jersey to include medical libraries in Maine, New Hampshire, Vermont, Massachusetts, Connecticut, Rhode Island, Pennsylvania, Delaware and the Commonwealth of Puerto Rico. The RML, coordinated by the National Library of Medicine, would now "provide health science practitioners, investigators, educators, and administrators in the United States with timely, convenient access to health care and biomedical information resources."[31] It would enable libraries to share expertise and physical resources, improve efficiency and performance for meeting medical information needs, and test, evaluate and implement improved methods for the exchange of biomedical information.

In 1985 the grant was renewed for five years in a $2,235 million contract, and an additional $1.238 million contract was awarded to the Academy to provide on-line training and services for medical librarians and health professionals in the Eastern On-line Region which included twenty-two states.


### Preservation Program


On December 8, 1983 Librarian Brett A. Kirkpatrick attended a special ceremony at the White House at which President Reagan and William J. Bennett, Chairman of the National Endowment for the Humanities, awarded incentive grants to thirteen independent institutions from around the country selected from among the many more who had applied. The $100,000 grant to the Academy, which had to be matched by $300,000 in other contributions collected over a three year period, was to be used to create a special endowment to support the full-time staff position of Preservation Administrator for the Rare Book and History of Medicine Collections. The award was applauded when it was announced at the Council meeting of December 12, 1982, although a concern was voiced that the necessity of procuring the matching grants might complicate the Academy's general fund-raising campaign. However, by 1985, the end of the three-year period, the required amount was raised through contributions from more than twenty-five foundations and corporations and 800 Fellows of the Academy. This endowment was supplemented in 1985 by a challenge grant of $200,000 from the Andrew W. Mellon Foundation, which was also successfully matched well within the required time.

In 1985 the Preservation Program was formally established with the appointment of Ms. Vanessa J. Piale as Preservation Administrator. Two years later, she was succeeded by Ms. Elaine Reidy Schlefer, who has continued in that role to the present. Since then, in addition to holding classes on the art of book preservation, the department has been restoring and preserving rare books and manuscripts, and constructing customized acid-free boxes and envelopes to hold them. In 1993, the Preservation Department moved into its specially designed laboratory on the fifth floor of the Academy building which Fellows and guests are invited to visit.

## The Book Adoption Program

In 1983, the Book Adoption Program was launched. Materials in the Rare Book Room's collection in need of preservation are posted in a list from which individuals interested in making donations may select one or more items. In return, they receive a "condition" report and an account of the treatment, together with before and after photographs, a copy of the specially inscribed book plate placed on the package to acknowledge their contribution, and the Academy bookmark.

## Books and the Physician

In March 1984, the Committee on Library, chaired by Dr. William D. Sharpe, held its first major meeting, a *Conference on Books and the Physician*. Supported by funding from Sands, Inc. and chaired by Dr. Ralph Engle, a member of the Committee, it featured discussions by prominent librarians from around the country on the creation, development, collection and use of medical literature and information.[32]

## Computerizaton

Since 1984, the Library staff has been presenting *The Basics of Searching MEDLINE, a Seminar for the Health Professional,* a course that is based on the syllabus created by the National Library of Medicine and designed to familiarize health professionals and researchers with the use of its MEDLINE computerized database.

In 1985, after much discussion and objections from a few members of the Library Committee, but with the active support of President Clark which proved decisive, the Trustees approved the purchase of LS/2000, a minicomputer-based local Integrated Library System. The system was purchased from the Ohio College Library Center, a consortium of fifty-four Ohio college and university libraries formed in 1967 to create a cooperative computerized regional library network. In essence, this was an on-line catalog that would greatly facilitate access to the Library's collections of books and monographs by staff, collaborating libraries and the public. For this system and also for on-line circulation control, the Library purchased a state-of-the-art computer that could serve forty-four terminals as well as a printer. During the installation, which was completed in 1986, the computer was informally named "Duncan" by the Library staff and its accompanying printer was called "Ida" in honor of Dr. Clark and his wife, Ida.

## ACADEMY PRESIDENTS

### Dr. Duncan W. Clark 1983–1984

Dr. Clark, a native of New York City, attended Fordham University and received his M.D. from the Long Island College of Medicine. He later served as Dean of that school, and subsequently became Chairman of the Department of Environmental Medicine and Community Health at the Downstate Medical Center in Brooklyn. He served as President of the Kings County Medical Society from 1983 to 1984. He became a Fellow in 1947 and chaired the Committee on Medicine in Society. He also served as Vice President from 1977 to 1988 and as a member of the Board of Trustees from 1985 to 1989.

### Dr. Bernard J. Pisani 1985–1986

Dr. Pisani, a graduate of the New York University School of Medicine, had a distinguished career as an obstetrician-gynecologist, serving for many years as Chief of that department and service at St. Vincent's Hospital. He was elected President of both the Medical Society of the County of New York and the New York State Society of Medicine, and served on the Board of Trustees of the American Medical Association. He became a Fellow in 1941, and served on the Committee on Public Health from 1957 to 1979, on the Committee on Medical Education from 1979 to 1991, as Secretary of the Section on Obstetrics and Gynecology from 1966 to 1968, and as a Trustee from 1979 to 1984 and again from 1988 through 1990.

## ACADEMY FINANCES

It was announced on November 21, 1983 that Mr. Samuel C. Berté would retire after six years as the Academy's Business Manager. Mr. Daniel J. Ehrlich was appointed to succeed him. At that time it was also decided to merge the Business Office and the Office of the Comptroller.

In 1984, on the advice of the Academy Counsel, the methods of accounting for the earnings of the restricted endowment funds was examined and found to be improper. It became apparent that the endowments were not being credited with the capital gains realized when investments were sold while, at the same time, the projects to which the endowment funds were allocated were not being charged their fair share of the Academy overhead. The result was a change to a new accounting firm and installation of an appropriate system retroactive to January 1, 1983

### Fund-raising

Fund-raising remained a continuing challenge for the leadership of the Academy. For example, in explaining "why the Academy needs additional funds over and above its dues, admission fees, and the return on its endowment," the Spring 1984 issue of *Newsnotes* said,

There are four primary reasons: deferred maintenance on its 58 year old building, including rewiring and upgrading the electrical systems in Hosack Hall and the Lobby area, the required provision of emergency lighting in all meeting rooms, rebuilding the smokestack, replacement of the roof and a boiler and other capital items; inflation of 17–20% per year in the cost of books and periodicals; deterioration of over half of the one million items in the Library and museum collections; and the need for new systems and programs. For example, the Academy added two trained security officers and a new security system for the building and parking lot in 1983, and manual bookkeeping for the business and Fellowship offices is being computerized.[33]

Other needs detailed included support of the conservation laboratory, automation of the Library's circulation, reference, and cataloging programs, upgrading of conference rooms, extension of environmental control systems to the Rare Book and History of Medicine Collection, remodeling of book stacks to allow for more space, cataloging and restoring the museum collection, and improving the information and communication capacities of the Academy in relation to the public and government agencies and community organizations. It was pointed out that Fellows' dues were significant but represented only a small proportion—6 percent—of the Academy's revenues and that a record of additional contributions from the membership was an essential justification when seeking funds from other sources.

In 1984, with the departure of Mr. George H. Weiler, Jr., who had been employed in 1981 as its full-time Director, the Development and Public Relations Office was discontinued. The publication of *Newsnotes* was given over to the Office of the *Bulletin*, while primary responsibility for fund-raising reverted to the Director, with the President acting as Chairman of the Resource Development Committee.

The City Real Estate Tax Problem

In 1971 the provisions of the New York State Real Property Tax law dealing with exemption from local government real property taxation were changed. The new law set up two classifications: an "unqualified" exemption was given to organizations "organized or conducted exclusively for religious, charitable, hospital, educational, moral or mental improvement of men, women or children. . . . ;" and a "qualified" exemption was given to entities not found in the first category that were organized for some fourteen public benefit purposes such as bar associations, libraries, and medical societies.[34] The new law gave municipalities the discretion to legislate the cancellation of the qualified exemption, thereby requiring such nonprofit organizations to pay the tax, and later that year, because of its financial crisis, New York City enacted a law to do just that.

The City moved very slowly in implementing the law. It did remove the exemptions of the Association of the Bar of the City of New York, and the Swedenborg Foundation, and also requested all nonprofit organizations to pay amounts equivalent to what would have been their water and sewage taxes, something that the Academy, on the advice of Counsel, began to do in 1979.

In 1982, the City declared that the Academy building and the adjacent parking lots were subject to the real estate tax. The Academy responded by beginning a Proceeding against the City claiming that it was a charitable and educational organization and not a medical society, and pointing to its many educational and civic activities.

Some nonprofit organizations whose exemption had been revoked took a similar action. Others, however, notably the Asia Society, pursued remedies in the state courts, claiming that they were, by their very nature, charitable or educational organizations and thus within the mandatory "unqualified" classification. The Appellate Division in Manhattan upheld the City's ruling against the Asia Society. Relying on a very narrow definition of an educational organization, it declared that although the Asia Society provides lectures, conferences and seminars, it does so without a charter from the Board of Regents and because it did not "accomplish these broad ends by 'teaching, instruction, or schooling,' " the City could levy real estate taxes against it.[35,36] This ruling was subsequently overturned by the Court of Appeals.

In March 1982 Mayor Koch appointed a Task Force, chaired by the City's Corporation Counsel, Frederick A. O. Schwarz, Jr., "to undertake a review of the state and local laws and policies governing real estate tax exemptions for non-profit organizations in New York City." In announcing this appointment, the Mayor said "we did not want our tax policy to sap the vitality of non-profit organizations that are performing useful public functions."[37] Completed in October of that year, but not released until the following April, the report noted that the cost of exemption for civic organizations and museums is "inconsequential" and labeled their taxation as "contrary to the City's long term interest." Accordingly, it recommended that they not be taxed. However, the report suggested, some nonprofit organizations, such as social clubs whose purpose is to serve "their members private social interests" should not be tax exempt. The City should return to a broad interpretation of educational or benevolent organizations, it suggested. Further, it argued, while organizations such as "bar associations" and "medical societies" do perform many worthy services, some of which are beneficial to the public at large, they are associations of professionals who have joined together principally to serve their own interests and, therefore, should be taxed.[38]

When the Mayor released the Task Force Report, he announced the scheduling of two days of hearings in City Hall in June 1983. President Duncan Clark, testifying on behalf of the Academy, emphasized the distinctions between an academy of medicine and a medical society and made many references to the work of the Academy. Two weeks later, the Mayor announced a change in the City's policy, separating the Academy from medical societies which continued to be taxed and, after filing the necessary papers to ensure appropriate entries in the City's records and making sure that all of the relevant City departments concurred, a letter confirming the Academy's tax exemption was received along with notification of the correction of the delinquency notices that had threatened to foreclose on the Academy's property unless the tax was paid. During this lengthy process, Edith Spivack, Esq., the Assistant Corporation Counsel of the City of New York, to whom this matter had been referred, commended Dr. Clark for his testimony and confided that, on numerous occasions in the course of her long career in the Corporation Counsel's office, she had received helpful advice and assistance from the Academy. Such attitudes undoubtedly facilitated the ultimate favorable outcome.

### Real Estate Development as a Long-Term Strategy

In 1985, Dr. McNutt proposed for consideration by the Trustees a very ambitious real estate undertaking involving the transfer of the air rights over the Academy building to a real estate corporation so that it might build a high-rise apartment building on the current parking lot. That building would include a parking garage and a conference center for the Academy to be connected to the current building. Dr. McNutt's enthusiasm for this venture reflected his feeling that the proposed venture would enable the Academy to satisfy its needs for space and resources, and enable it to renew its prominence as a focal point in a neighborhood that was being upgraded and transformed.

President Pisani appointed a Building Committee chaired by Dr. John K. Lattimer to review the proposal which had come from the General Atlantic Corporation, a firm prominent in urban development in the City and the State, which was then developing property at Fifth Avenue and 107th Street, a few blocks north of the Academy.

The plan involved the construction of a thirty-story building with mixed residential and commercial uses, including condominium or cooperative apartments, a 150-space parking garage, of which 125 spaces would be reserved for Academy use, and 40,000 sq. ft. of space that the Academy could use for a conference center, library stacks or other purposes. The zoning restrictions would require transfer of the unused air rights over the Academy building.

The development would be financed solely by the developer

with the Academy contributing the title to the current parking lot in addition to the air rights. The Academy would not be responsible for any losses, but would receive half of any profits in cash, in the form of condominium apartments, or in rental values for commercial space. Instead of sharing in the profits, the Academy could opt for accepting a fixed sum either in cash or property.

When it was first presented, the reaction of most of the Trustees was positive. Drs. Duncan Clark and Lawrence E. Hinkle, Jr. opposed it, and filed a number of memoranda explaining their position. Nevertheless, the Trustees approved a letter of intent that initiated detailed negotiations which were to continue over the better part of the next year. They also voted funds to appraise the Academy properties and to obtain the advice of an attorney, Mr. Joseph Sperber from Davis Polk and Wardwell, the Academy Counsel and two real estate consultants, Mr. Abram Barkan and Ms. Debra Fechter from James Felt Realty Services, who were familiar with developments in the area. The Academy also engaged the firm of Beyer, Blinder, Belle for advice on its architectural needs, and the firm of Jones Lang Wooton to explore the possibility of purchasing the remaining two tenements east of the Academy property, a prospect that never materialized.

Dr. McNutt's enthusiasm for the project remained high and he worked with great diligence to prepare materials, consult with the outside advisors, and meet with Dr. Lattimer and the Building Committee and the developers of the project. At one point, hints had been received that Mount Sinai Hospital might be interested in joining the Academy in such a real estate venture but, it became clear, they had no interest in property to the north of the buildings they already owned. They did describe having had difficulties with the Local Community Planning Board, which would have to approve the Academy's joint venture, because of its opposition to private "luxury" housing in the area. This raised some qualms but, nevertheless, in October 1985, the Trustees voted, with dissents by Drs. Duncan Clark and Marianne Legato, to approve the project "in principle." Dr. Pisani would need to sign a Memorandum of Understanding with the developer on October 30. Dr. McNutt would prepare a briefing book for review by the Council before its next meeting. Plans and specifications were to be made final before February 26, 1986 and the basic agreement ratified by the Trustees on April 30, 1986. The Council and Fellowship would then have an additional thirty and sixty days respectively to ratify the agreement and, finally, if the New York State Supreme Court and other necessary regulatory approvals were obtained, construction could begin in two years, with occupancy in late 1989 or 1990.

The minutes of the November 27 Council meeting indicate that, despite the initial agreement about the construction, reservations on the part of influential members of the Council were materializing. Some reflected a general anxiety but others were more specific. Concerns were expressed about the real estate tax implications, the possible crowding of the Academy's agenda by involvement in real estate, the problem of the underground streams flowing through the Academy property, and the need to consider the future mission and goals of the Academy before undertaking the construction of a new building. It was also suggested that the Academy should seek funds to construct its own parking garage and not surrender its land to the condominium.

As such reservations were mounting, he revealed in a recent interview, Dr. McNutt visited the members of the Council individually and, when it became apparent that the project was not going to go forward, he decided to resign. Another factor in this decision, he acknowledged, had been the reactions to his attempts to take control of the Academy's budget process. However, in his letter of resignation, which Dr. Pisani revealed to the Council on November 11, 1985, he referred to "personal matters, one of which was the offer of an outstanding position to my wife by a major international corporation in the Chicago area." (Dr. McNutt, who took additional training and then served as the head of a unit in Chicago's Cook County Hospital, is currently County Health Officer in DuPage County, a suburb of that city.)

Mr. William C. Stubing, who had been Executive Secretary of the Committee on Medical Education, was appointed Director when Dr. McNutt left that office on December 31, 1985, It was evident that Mr. Stubing had little enthusiasm for this real estate proposal. He believed that it was more important for the Academy to make decisions about its mission before embarking on such a major construction project and felt that it would be an unnecessary distraction for him and for the Academy.

The project was discussed in great detail on December 12, 1985 at a special dinner meeting of the Council and Trustees during which Dr. McNutt reported that the architects had uncovered a problem in the current building that would hamper the flow of people from Hosack Hall to the proposed banquet facilities in the new building. Additional concerns were voiced and alternative suggestions were offered. Finally, although Dr. McNutt noted that a formal response from the Academy was not required until May 31, 1986, it was voted to terminate the project.

## NOTES

1 Council of the New York Academy of Medicine. 1982 Minutes of the meeting of April 28, 1982.
2 Halloran BF. 1982 Letter to the New York Academy of Medicine, September 22, 1982.
3 New York State Public Health Law: Title IIA—Professional Medical Conduct, Section 280. In: *McKinney's Consolidated Laws of New York, Annotated.* St. Paul, Minn: West Publishing Company. 1990 and 1996 Pocket Parts.
4 Pallis C. 1982 ABC of brain stem death: Reappraising death. *British Medical Journal* 285:1409–1412.
5 Grisez G and Boyles, JM, Jr. 1979 *Life and Death with Liberty and Justice: A Contribution to the Euthanasia Debate.* South Bend, IN: University of Notre Dame Press. p. 61.
6 Joint Committee on the Care of Patients with Terminal Illness. 1984 Statement and resolution on the definition of death. *Bulletin of the New York Academy of Medicine.* 60:955–958.
7 Joint Committee on the Care of the Terminally Ill. 1985 Statement and resolution on resuscitation for patients who have suffered in-hospital cardiac arrest. *Bulletin of the New York Academy of Medicine.* 61:599–603.

8  President's Commission for the Study of Ethical Problems in Medicine
   and Biomedical and Behavioral Research. 1983 *Decisions to Forego
   Life-Sustaining Treatment.* Washington, DC: US Government Printing Office.
9  New York State Public Health Law. Article 29B Orders Not to Resuscitate. In: *McKinney's Consolidated Laws of New York Annotated.*
   St. Paul, Minn: West Publishing Company. 1990 and 1996 Pocket
   Parts.
10 New York State Public Health Law. Article 29C Health Care Agents
   and Proxies. In: *McKinney's Consolidated Laws of New York Annotated.* St. Paul, Minn: West Publishing Company. 1990 and 1996
   Pocket Parts.
11 *Alzheimer's Disease: Implications for Public Policy in New York
   State, an Institute Convened by the New York Academy of Medicine
   in Cooperation with the New York State Health Planning Commission,* West Point, NY, May 31–June 1, 1984.
12 Brown LD. 1987 Health policy in the United States: Issues and options. *Bulletin of the New York Academy of Medicine.* 63:417–429.
13 Brown LD. 1988 *Occasional Paper Number Four, Ford Foundation
   Project on Social Welfare and the American Future.* New York: Ford
   Foundation.
14 Committee on Medicine in Society: 1988 *Toward a Health Care Financing Strategy for the Nation: A Position Paper of the National
   Health Policy Seminar.* New York: New York Academy of Medicine.
15 Committee on Public Health. 1970 Methadone management of heroin addiction. *Bulletin of the New York Academy of Medicine.*
   46:391–395.
16 Subcommittee on Drug Abuse, Committee on Public Health. 1982
   Statement and resolution regarding methadone maintenance treatment. *Bulletin of the New York Academy of Medicine.* 58:579–
   584.
17 Lewis DC and Gordon AS. 1983 Alcoholism and the general hospital:
   The Roger Williams intervention program. *Bulletin of the New York
   Academy of Medicine.* 59:181–197.
18 Subcommittee on Alcoholism and Drug Abuse, Committee on Public
   Health. 1985 Iatrogenic addiction: Developing guidelines for use of
   sedatives and analgesics in the hospital. *Bulletin of the New York
   Academy of Medicine.* 61:691–768.
19 Perry SW. 1985 Irrational attitudes toward addicts and narcotics.
   *Bulletin of the New York Academy of Medicine.* 61:706–727.
20 Stimmel B. 1985 Under-prescription /over-prescription: narcotics as

a metaphor. *Bulletin of the New York Academy of Medicine.* 61: 742–752.

21  Simon N. 1983 Chairman's introductory remarks. *Bulletin of the New York Academy of Medicine.* 59:863–864.

22  Axelrod D. 1983 Introduction. *Bulletin of the New York Academy of Medicine.* 59:865–868.

23  Terenzio JV, Chairman. 1977 *Report to the Mayor on the Office of the Chief Medical Examiner.* New York: Advisory Committee on the Office of the Chief Medical Examiner. p. 35.

24  Committee on Public Health. 1983 Statement and resolution on the setting of obstetrical delivery. *Bulletin of the New York Academy of Medicine.* 59:401–402.

25  Committee on Public Health, Subcommittee on Maternity and Family Planning Services. 1984 Statement and resolution on the regional perinatal network. *Bulletin of the New York Academy of Medicine.* 60:851–854.

26  Committee on Medical Education. 1983 Financing medical education: The cost for students and the implications for medical practice. *Bulletin of the New York Academy of Medicine.* 59:533–608.

27  Committees on Medical Education and Medicine in Society. 1985 The role of academic medicine in patient education. *Bulletin of the New York Academy of Medicine.* 61:115–224.

28  Green LW and Johnson KW. 1983 Health education and health promotion. In: Mechanic D, Ed. *Handbook of Health Care and the Health Professions.* New York: Free Press. p. 744.

29  Sheps CG. 1985 Implementing changes within the academic medical center. *Bulletin of the New York Academy of Medicine.* 61:175–183.

30  Committee on Medicine in Society and Committee on Medical Education. 1985 The role of academic medicine in patient education: Report of findings and recommendations. *Bulletin of the New York Academy of Medicine.* 61:218–224.

31  Bunting A. 1987 The nation's health information network: History of the Regional Medical Library Program. 1965–1985. *Bulletin of the Medical Library Association.* 75 supplement:36.

32  Committee on Library. 1985 Conference on books and the physician *Bulletin of the New York Academy of Medicine.* 61:227–298.

33  [Anonymous]. 1984 1983 Annual support results and 1984 needs, and beyond. *Newsnotes,* Spring 1984 p. 5–6.

34  New York State Real Property Tax Law Section 421, Subdivision 1.

35  *The Asia Society, Inc. v. The Tax Commission of the State of New York,* March 3, 1983, (Appellate Division. 1st Dept) 92 AD 2d 781, 459 NYS 2d, 620.

36 Swords P. 1981 *Charitable Real Property Tax Exemption in New York State.* New York: Columbia University Press.
37 Schwarz FAO, Jr, Chairman. 1982 *Report of City Task Force on the Exemption of Non-Profit Organizations from Real Property Tax* October 4, 1982.
38 Goodwin M. 1983 A Court Approves City's Right to Tax Non-Profit Groups. *New York Times,* March 5, 1983, p. 1.

# Chapter 7
# 1986–1990
# Reorganization

THE AIDS PROBLEM
  An AIDS Coalition?
  AIDS Centers
HONORARY FELLOWSHIP FOR DR. ANATOLY
  KORYAGIN
THE MEDICAL PROFESSION AS A MORAL COMMUNITY
COMMITTEE ON MEDICINE IN SOCIETY
  Alternative Health Care Delivery Systems
  Comprehensive School Health Education Program
  The Tenth Anniversary of Growing Healthy in New York
    City
  Lobbying by Organizations Receiving Federal Grants
  Next Steps in Health Care Financing
  Changing Agenda for Health Care in America
  Socio-economic Changes and the Practicing Physician
THE COMMITTEE ON PUBLIC HEALTH
  Tobacco and Health
  Low Birthweight Babies
  Information Systems and the Medical Sciences
  Health Claims and the Food and Drug Administration
  Motor Vehicle Injuries
  Drug Testing in the Workplace
  Symposium Dedicated to Dr. Norman Simon
  Nutrition and Children
  Quality of New York City's Drinking Water
COMMITTEE ON MEDICAL EDUCATION
  Corporate Influences on Patient Relations
  Gifts to the Academy

IN APRIL 1986, William C. Stubing, became Director of the Academy. He had joined the staff as Executive Secretary of the Committee on Medical Education in 1978 and, following the resignation of Dr. David McNutt on December 31, 1985, had been appointed Acting Director. In an item in *Newsnotes,* the newly redesigned Academy newsletter, he pointed out that he was "the first 'lay' person to hold this position, a curious designation for a seminary graduate." *NewsNotes* went on to report: "The new Director views the next few years as especially critical for the Academy. Economic pressures on physicians, changing practice patterns, and increased competition between and within specialties leave physicians little time and less inclination to engage in the voluntarism without which the Academy cannot fulfill its purpose. Yet the public's need for physician leaders to look beyond the profession's interests has never been greater."[1]

While Mr. Stubing acknowledged the many problems facing the Academy, he commented that its strengths: "the experience and commitment of the Council and staff, the resources in the Fellowship, and the endowment inherited from the past—all represent significant assets which give the Academy a fighting chance in tackling the problems."[2] He then outlined areas which would receive his attention in the months ahead; they included such general items as management and administration, staff development, long-term planning, public relations, fundraising, membership development, facility improvement, revenue enhancement, program development, and self-improvement.

His immediate plans included the recruiting of Executive Secretaries for the Committees on Medical Education and Public Health. He reported progress in matching the Mellon Foundation grant for the Preservation/Conservation Laboratory, and announced a meeting of the Council with Mr. Harold Burson of Burson-Marsteller to discuss the Academy's public relations efforts. He said he was planning the distribution of a Newsletter to the Fellows shortly, which would immediately be followed by the Annual Support Campaign.

At the stated meeting on April 10, 1986, the Academy Plaque was awarded to Past-President Duncan W. Clark. The citation, read by Dr. Mary Ann Payne, Treasurer of the Academy, noted that Dr. Clark had served as Chairman of the Committee on Medicine in Society and as Vice President and President of the Academy, and was currently serving as a Trustee and as Chairman of the Portfolio Committee of the Trustees. He was described as "someone who, in striving for the public good, had never avoided controversy. He had no hesitation in taking a minority position, but often was able because of his outstanding intellectual ability, tenacity and integrity to change the views of the majority of colleagues. Dr. Clark has been a Fellow of the Academy for close to 50 years, making that long subway trip from Brooklyn to 103rd Street on a regular basis."[3] The citation also cited the accomplishments that took place under Dr. Clark's leadership as President, which included the restoration of Hosack Hall and the introduction of a

computer-based integrated library system with an on-line catalogue of the Academy's collections that allowed greater public
access to the Library's holdings.

At the same meeting, Dr. Irving S. Wright, the distinguished
cardiologist, received the Academy Medal for outstanding contributions to science and medicine. Dr. Wright, a respected clinician
and teacher, had earned world-wide recognition as a pioneer in the
research and treatment of vascular disease and thromboembolism,
and particularly in the use of anticoagulants.

Dr. Pisani was succeeded as President of the Academy in 1987
by Dr. Mary Ann Payne, a native of Frederick, Maryland. Dr.
Payne, the first woman President, was Clinical Professor of Medicine at Cornell University Medical College. She had received an
M.A. and a Ph.D. in endocrinology from the University of Wisconsin, and an M.D. from Cornell University Medical College. She
had served as a Trustee and as Treasurer of the Academy, and had
been active on the Committee on Medical Education.

## THE AIDS PROBLEM

Each year, Dr. David Axelrod, the State Commissioner of Health,
addressed a special meeting of the Committee on Public Health at
which he reviewed problems and issues in public health in the State
and shared his concerns with the informed and not unsympathetic
audience. At one such meeting on June 2, 1986, he devoted the
bulk of his presentation to a review of AIDS epidemiological data
and State programs to combat this disease, calling AIDS "one of a
series of tragedies facing our society" which, along with poverty
and violence, are not being adequately addressed by our societal
institutions.

An informative conference on AIDS was held by the Section on
Medicine on December 17, 1986. In a paper jointly authored by
Stephen C. Joseph, Commissioner of Health of the City of New
York, and his colleagues, Drs. Stephen Schulz, Rand Stoneburner,
and Margaret Clark, Dr. Joseph described the spread of the disease

in New York City that made it the "North American epicenter of what the head of the World Health Organization had described as 'a health disaster of pandemic proportions.' "⁴ He associated the issues confronting the City, among which was an ominous upsurge in the incidence of tuberculosis. He pointed to a reduction in risk-taking behaviors by gay men that was being offset by the spread of the disease among intravenous drug users, and reiterated his support for prevention through counseling, health education to promote the use of condoms, and needle exchange programs for intravenous drug users, and called for more funds for research on AIDS.

The Committee on Public Health took up Dr. Joseph's suggestion of a pilot needle exchange program. The rationale for this was that, because it was illegal in New York State to purchase or possess hypodermic needles or syringes without a physician's prescription, addicts using intravenous drugs were sharing and reusing them without proper cleansing raising sharply the risk of thereby transmitting the AIDS virus.

As a result, Dr. Joseph had noted, although gay men still accounted for the greatest proportion of reported cases of AIDS, its incidence among intravenous drug users had risen from 21 percent in 1981 to 36 percent in December 1986. Intravenous drug use had become the primary method of heterosexual transmission of the AIDS virus. To combat such spread, Dr. Joseph was proposing a program to provide needles and syringes to a small group of IV drug users and to compare this group's experience with respect to sero-conversion, needle-sharing practices and other risk behaviors with that of a control group of needle-sharing addicts.

At the March 25, 1987 meeting of the Committee, Don Des Jarlais, Ph.D. of the Beth Israel Medical Center, strongly endorsed the concept and indicated that Beth Israel, which had one of the largest drug abuse treatment programs in the City, was prepared to undertake such a program.⁵

Dr. James Curtis, Chief of Psychiatry at Harlem Hospital and a member of the Committee on Medicine in Society, who had been invited to attend this meeting, opposed the idea. He felt that free needles and syringes would encourage drug abuse. The best way to slow the AIDS epidemic, he said, was to rely on health education, voluntary serotesting and providing counseling on needle-sharing and sexual practices. In 1996, when the Committee on Medicine in Society revisited this issue, Dr. Curtis was to express substantially the same opinion (*vide infra*).

Dr. Robert Millman of Cornell University Medical College supported the needle exchange project. He said that, during his many years of experience in the treatment of drug abuse, he had not encountered anyone who had become a an IV drug user because of the availability of needles. Indeed, he added, making sterile needles freely available would discourage the practice of needle sharing and reduce the incidence of virus transmission. Dr. Lawrence Hinkle, Jr., a former Chairman of the Committee, noted that while he had not seen the details of the proposed study, he believed it should go forward. The Chairman of the Committee, Dr. David Harris, concluded the meeting with a plea that the Academy not stand aloof from this problem. The State and City governments ultimately agreed to allow needle exchange programs to be implemented in New York City. Currently, the New York State AIDS Institute, a unit of the Department of Health, continues to fund a limited needle exchange program in the City.

## An AIDS Coalition?

In December 1987, Vice President Martin Cherkasky, President Emeritus of the Montefiore Medical Center in the Bronx, proposed that the Academy take the lead in forming a coalition to deal with the AIDS in the City. Dr. Cherkasky, serving at that time as an adviser on health issues to Mayor Edward I. Koch and to Commissioner Joseph, had the strong feeling, shared by Dr. Joseph, that there was a need for stronger nongovernmental medical leadership to work with the public health authorities in the struggle against AIDS. Without such leadership, he said, there would be a vacuum in the development of policy which would hamper the implementation of effective programs for the prevention and treatment of the disease.

In response to Dr. Cherkasky's suggestion, President Payne asked each of the Standing Committees of the Academy to designate representatives to serve on an Academy-wide committee to review the issue. The first proposal considered was the creation of a city-wide council which, under the auspices of the Academy, would provide guidance on a wide range of issues arising out of the AIDS epidemic. There was little enthusiasm for this suggestion from the other organizations whose interest in participation was solicited.

Another option considered by the Committee was the resurrection of the Health Research Council of New York City which had been organized in 1958 during the administration of Mayor Robert F. Wagner.[6] It was an agency that provided funding for biomedical research, primarily through the support of career investigators, and for the improvement of research facilities in the City, but it had been discontinued during the City's fiscal crisis of the 1970s. There was little support for this idea in the City government and it was quickly abandoned.

The activities of the Committee apparently petered out, but they were picked up by the Committee on Public Health which held some useful meetings and issued some relevant policy positions (*vide infra*). (With the advent of Drs. David Rogers and Jeremiah Barondess in the 1990s, the Academy became much more involved in the HIV/AIDS problem.)

Dr. Cherkasky was disappointed with the Academy's failure to seize the initiative in mobilizing the medical profession against AIDS at that time. In the meantime, a Commission on AIDS was established and located at the offices of the Fund for the City of New York with Mr. John Zuccotti, the former Commissioner of City Planning, and Mr. John E. Jacob, President of the New York Urban League, as co-Chairs.

## AIDS Centers

The Committee on Public Health conducted a special meeting on various aspects of the AIDS problem on January 4, 1988. It was chaired by Bruce Vladeck, Ph.D., President of the United Hospital Fund. Dr. Nicholas Rango, Director of the New York State AIDS Institute, described its program of designating certain institutions as "AIDS Centers." These Centers provide a comprehensive treatment package that includes in-patient services, out-patient services and case management. He urged that these Centers be supplemented by the establishment of a network of rehabilitative and home care services for AIDS patients. He also urged improved access to health care for persons with AIDS, particularly among the prison populations, and an expansion of AIDS testing and counseling.[7]

Dr. Thomas Killip reported that the Beth Israel Medical Center was one of the hospitals that had been designated as an AIDS Center under the program which provided additional reimbursement to institutions offering specially designed and staffed programs for the treatment of AIDS. He stressed the need for education as a means of preventing the disease and noted that Beth Israel had begun a campaign to prevent hospital personnel from needlestick injuries through which the virus might be transmitted.

Ms. Carol Raphael, Deputy Administrator of the Bureau of Medical Affairs of the Department of Social Services of the City of New York, described the public provider network established by her agency, which offers home health care and home attendant services. She discussed the special case management needs of AIDS patients and the impact of AIDS on Medicaid. She suggested that, in order for AIDS costs to be met, there would have to be greater coverage of AIDS services by private insurers.

## HONORARY FELLOWSHIP FOR DR. ANATOLY KORYAGIN

In July 1987, the Committee on Honorary Fellowship, chaired by Dr. Duncan Clark, with Drs. John K. Lattimer and Fidelio Jiminez as members, received a proposal recommending that Dr. Anatoly Koryagin of the Soviet Union be elected an Honorary Fellow in recognition of his imprisonment for protesting abuse of Soviet psychiatry by the practice of confining political dissenters in psychiatric hospitals where they often received drastic treatments. On January 11, 1988, the Committee decided to reject that proposal. The Committee criticized the Soviet abuse of psychiatry but said, "It is not necessary to award a Fellowship to make this statement. Dr. Koryagin is not the first and has not been the only Soviet physician who has suffered in defense of his profession in the USSR."[8] Further, they recommended against such an action at the moment because new laws put into effect in the Soviet Union may have abolished the practice. "The changing situation will continue to be monitored by a member of the Committee," they said.

During the period of the Soviet abuse of psychiatry and of physicians who protested against it, the Academy considered the problem on several occasions. However, it never really became an active part of the movement to advance human rights throughout the world in which organizations of physicians and scientists like the National Academy of Sciences and the World Congress of Psychiatry played such prominent roles.

## THE MEDICAL PROFESSION AS A MORAL COMMUNITY

Dr. Edmund D. Pellegrino, the John Carroll Professor of Medicine and Medical Humanities and Director of the Center for Advanced Studies of Ethics at Georgetown University and the former President of Catholic University of America, spoke at the Stated Meeting of November 9, 1989 on *The Medical Profession as a Moral Community*. Focusing on what the profession must do as a collective to resolve a major moral dilemma, Dr. Pellegrino pointed out that "Today, our profession faces an unenviable choice between two opposing moral orders, one based in the primacy of our moral obligations to the sick, the other in the primacy of self-interest and the market place. These two orders are not fundamentally reconcilable and, like it or not, the Academy and the profession will be forced to choose between them. In that choice this Academy can play a central role. . . . Without such a clear commitment, the full potential of the Academy's new program will not be fully realizable."⁹

Dr. Pellegrino viewed physicians as a "moral community bound to each other by a set of commonly-held ethical commitments and whose purpose is something other than self-interest." He said, "We should collect the data needed to convince the public and legislators that the free market commercialization and monetarization of medicine is unjust and damaging to the welfare of the sick. . . . . We must demonstrate that our first concern is not our own privilege, prerogative, or income but the welfare of those whose covenant we have to serve. There is enormous power in this position but we have not used it."

"We should resist the uncritical acceptance of the idea that rationing of health care is necessary in America," he continued. "Even a superficial comparison of the magnitude of health expenditures with the ways we spend billions of dollars in discretionary income should convince us that needed medical care need not be withheld." Physicians, he acknowledged, do have an obligation to cut waste, pointing to the target of the "administrative overhead (perhaps 15 to 30% in the opinion of some economists)" imposed on health care expenditures by "managed health care systems with their administrative bureaucracies, advertising, and marketing budgets."

## COMMITTEE ON MEDICINE IN SOCIETY

### Alternative Health Care Delivery Systems

The first Duncan W. Clark Lecture, endowed by a gift from Dr. Iago Galdston in honor of his friend and long-time collaborator, was given by Uwe Reinhardt, Ph.D., James Madison Professor of Political Economy at Princeton University, as part of the 1986 Annual Health Conference of the Academy which dealt with *Alternative Health Care Delivery Systems: Implications for Patients and Providers*. In his lecture, which was entitled, *How to Change the Health Care System,* Prof. Reinhardt paid tribute to Dr. Clark, with whom he had served as a member of the study section of the National Center for Health Services Research.

Dr. Reinhardt, a widely acclaimed health economist, used this opportunity to sound a theme that he has often set forth: "the failure of the US to make health care available to those least able to pay indicates that unlike Britain, Canada, France, Sweden and Germany, the US marches to a different drummer."[10] Because it would impose a new burden on small and medium sized businesses, Prof. Reinhardt opposed the suggestion that mandated employer-paid health insurance should be imposed as the vehicle for establishing universal coverage. Instead, he proposed a national program that would require all Americans to pay a health insurance tax set at a percentage of their adjusted gross income, unless they could provide evidence of a private insurance policy that provided benefits as good or better than those of the federal plan. Most Americans, he said, would opt to purchase a private plan leaving the poor to be covered by the federal program.

"Before judging whether the US is overtaxed," Dr. Reinhardt said, one should consider that, "in comparison with other nations in the industrialized world, the US channels a relatively smaller proportion of its gross domestic product through the public sector." He concluded that the current methods of cost-shifting represent a "sleight of hand" that allows politicians to proceed on the premise that "unless coerced through legislative trickery, the American people would be too miserly to care for their poor and sick fellow Americans."


Comprehensive School Health Education Program

The school health education programs promoted by the Academy, *Growing Healthy in New York City,* continued to flourish under the leadership of Dr. John V. Waller, Chairman of its Management Committee, and Ms. Leslie Goldman, Director of the Department.

By the end of 1986, aided by substantial help from the Division of Student Support Services of the Board of Education in the form of stipends for the teachers attending training sessions and funds for teaching materials, concrete progress had been made in implementing the program in 150 of the City's 625 public elementary schools. After reviewing these results, the Committee on Medicine in Society unanimously approved Dr. Waller's suggestions that the Academy participate in expanding the program to the remaining schools within the next five years and that the curriculum be broadened to include "integrating family life" and sex education; both suggestions were also approved by the Council.

At the same time, after hearing the results of a six-month feasibility study that had been funded by the New York Community Trust and the Morgan Guaranty Trust Company, the Committee and the Council also approved expanding the programs to grades 7 to 9 in the City's junior high schools. Aided by one of the first grants awarded by the newly created Patrolman Edward R. Byrne Substance Abuse Fund and additional funding from the New York Community Trust, the Aaron Diamond and MetLife Foundations, Morgan Guaranty Trust Company and the American Heart Association, *Being Healthy*, as this program was called, was implemented very rapidly. By 1993, it was being used in fifty of the City's sixty junior high schools. Once again, the Board of Education provided stipends for the teachers in training and funds for the classroom materials.

The program has attracted much favorable attention. For example, Marshall Kreuter, Ph.D., Director of the Division of Health Education at the US Centers for Disease Control, noted that "the *Growing Healthy* approach increases knowledge and has some effect on behavior."[11] Mr. Timothy F. Kirn, writing in the *News & Perspectives* section of the *Journal of the American Medical Association,* noted that "by most accounts, *Growing Healthy* is also a prescription for invigorating disillusioned teachers and engaging students, in a City with a dropout rate hovering around 30%."[12] On October 3, 1988, the United Hospital Fund of New York presented its Distinguished Community Service Award to Dr. John V. Waller for "his ability to inspire and coalesce the efforts and resources of public and private agencies and organizations and for his energy in transforming a successful pilot program into a city wide organization." The citation also acknowledged the work of the Committee on Medicine in Society and the Academy in fostering the program.

The Tenth Anniversary of Growing Healthy in New York City

The tenth anniversary of the Comprehensive School Health Education Program was marked on May 30, 1989 by a reception at the Academy that was attended by almost 300 people including Mayor Edward I. Koch whose administration had supported the implementation of the program so strongly. It was reported that, as of that date, some 3,600 teachers had received training and that 188,000 students in 360 schools in 31 community school districts in three boroughs had participated in the program. The program took pride in the announcement that the 1988 evaluation by the Division of Health Education of the US Centers for Disease Control had found higher reading and mathematics scores among students in several grade levels who had participated in the program in comparison with those who did not. There was also some delay in the onset of cigarette smoking.

Lobbying by Organizations Receiving Federal Grants

At its March 16, 1987 meeting, the Committee dealt with a request from the Nonprofit Coordinating Council of New York, of which the Academy is a member, to react to proposed regulations of the Internal Revenue Service that would prohibit lobbying by not-for-profit organizations which, like the Academy, receive grants from the federal government.[13] These regulations should be opposed, the Council suggested, because they included a definition that might be interpreted to consider as lobbying the kinds of educational programs on controversial issues conducted by the Academy. A letter, approved by the Academy Council, was filed; it stated, "It is our view that the proposed regulations include in the definition of lobbying many activities that are not included in the current rules and also introduce the uncertainty that the Tax Reform Act of 1976 was intended to eliminate by making it more difficult to determine whether an activity should be classified as lobbying."[14] According to the Government Relations Department of the Independent Sector in Washington, D.C., the proposed IRS regulations were withdrawn and on August 31, 1990, final regulations were promulgated which were much improved and incorporated the suggestions made by nonprofit organizations. (See 26 Code of Federal Regulations 1, 7, 20, 25, 53, 56. The Independent Sector is an organization which represents the not-for-profit agency world and took a leadership role on this issue.)

### Next Steps in Health Care Financing

The Committee's Annual Health Conference held on May 6–7, 1987 attracted some 230 participants to the Academy to discuss *Next Steps in Health Care Financing*. The second annual Duncan W. Clark Lecture was given by Dr. Karen Davis, Professor and Chairman of the Department of Health Policy and Management at the Johns Hopkins School of Hygiene and Public Health (she was later to become President of the Commonwealth Fund.) Dr. Davis presented a comprehensive review of the factors that are shaping the current health care debate and called for expansion of the entitlements to health care throughout the nation. The goal, she said, should be to see "that no one in the country is denied care because of an inability to pay." She urged expansion of health insurance coverage for acute care, insurance coverage for long-term care, and the implementation of incentives to make the organization of delivery of services more efficient.[15] It should be noted that this presentation was given toward the end of the first Reagan administration, a time when it was still possible to hope and to believe that programs expanding entitlements to health care were politically possible. Other speakers included Prof. Uwe Reinhardt of Princeton University, Constance Horner, Director of the US Office of Personnel Management, Marion Ein Lewin, Director of the Center for Health Policy Research of the American Enterprise Institute for Public Policy Research, and Walter McClure, Ph.D. President of the Center for Policy Studies in Minneapolis.


Changing Agenda for Health Care in America

The topic of the Annual Health Conference held on May 9–10, 1989, was *The Changing Agenda for Health Care in America; Balancing Need and Commitment.* The Duncan W. Clark Lecture which opened the meeting was presented by Prof. Amitai Etzioni of George Washington University, now widely known as the leader of the "communitarian movement" in the United States, a movement which seeks to overcome what it considers to be extreme individualism in American society and replace it with a set of values stressing community solidarity and mutual concern. In his speech, he described the advantages of adding to the variables considered by neoclassical economics, "the range of sociological, psychological and institutional factors included in the analysis of economic behavior." For example, in explaining why there has been a reduction in the consumption of alcohol since 1980, neoclassical economists will focus on what has happened to the price of alcoholic beverages and whether the drinking age has been raised, but they decline to consider the role of social movements such as the new interest in fitness and health and the activities of organizations such as MADD (Mothers Against Drunk Driving). This approach of considering socio-psychological variables has implications for social change in many aspects of health-related behavior, he concluded.[16]

Socio-economic Changes and the Practicing Physician

On June 20, 1988, Dr. John Ball, Executive Vice President of the American College of Physicians addressed the Committee on *Socio-economic Changes and the Practicing Physician*. Dr. Ball, a White House official during the Carter Administration, recalled ironically that "organized medicine," a euphemism for the American Medical Association, had greeted the advent of the Reagan administration with enthusiasm over having gained a "friend" in the White House, but found to its dismay that many of that administration's actions were contrary to the positions it was advocating. These included increased antitrust regulation of physicians, mandatory acceptance of the assignment of Medicare claims, and federal regulation of the treatment of damaged newborns. Dr. Ball called for a reorientation of the values of the medical profession. He saw organized medicine's advancement of the private interests of practicing physicians leading to results that advanced neither the legitimate interests of the profession nor the needs of the public and urged that organized medicine adopt a model of advocacy that better advanced the public interest.[17]

## THE COMMITTEE ON PUBLIC HEALTH

In the fall of 1986, Dr. Jacqueline Messite, a well-known expert in occupational and environmental medicine with many years of experience in occupational health programs at the New York State Department of Labor and the National Institute of Occupational Safety and Health, succeeded Dr. Susan Hadley, as Executive Secretary of the Committee on Public Health. Dr. Messite, a graduate of New York University and of Downstate Medical Center in Brooklyn, was a Regent on Occupational Medicine of the American College of Preventive Medicine. Unlike Dr. McCorkel, whose stay with the Committee was very brief, Dr. Messite was to serve the Committee on a full-time basis until December 31, 1994, when she retired and became a consultant to the Committee and the Academy.

## Tobacco and Health

In October 1986, with the approval of the Council, the Committee issued a *Statement and Resolution on Tobacco and Health* which reviewed the virtually unanimity of the scientific literature on the health hazards produced by the use of tobacco.[18] It went on to cite "a number of epidemiological studies of health risks from passive exposure to tobacco smoke" which suggested that "respiratory symptoms, infections and allergic conditions were exacerbated."

In May 1987, the Committee learned that a regulation issued by the New York State Department of Health that would ban smoking in public places had been nullified by a court in Albany which ruled that the Department lacked the authority to issue such a regulation.[19] The Academy joined the Association of the Bar of the City of New York and a number of voluntary organizations, including the cancer and heart associations, in appealing that decision, first in the Appellate Division, and then in the Court of Appeals. The *amici curiae* brief which was crafted by the Bar Association's Committee on Medicine and the Law, drew heavily on the Academy's Statement. Unfortunately, the appeals were not successful. However, the coalition of voluntary health agencies continued its efforts with the Legislature and, despite the resistance of the tobacco industry and its lobbyists, it was rewarded by the enactment of laws limiting smoking in public places within the State.[20]

There was resistance on the part of some Academy staff members and Fellows to the implementation of a no-smoking policy in the Academy building. To accommodate the smokers, those with offices were allowed to smoke in those "private" spaces and, when the Academy's no-smoking policy was implemented on May 7, 1987, smoking was also permitted in the Hartwell Room of the Library, the "Fellows' " room. It was only later, during the Presidency of Dr. Jeremiah Barondess, that the Academy building became entirely smoke free.

Low Birthweight Babies

On October 28, 1987, with the approval of the Council, the Committee sent a letter to Governor Mario N. Cuomo referring to studies of low birthweight babies and commended him on the enactment of the Prenatal Assistance Act of 1987 and the significant funding of the Prenatal Care Assistance Network it established. The letter urged the Governor to take the further steps of broadening eligibility under this Act to cover women whose incomes are up to 185 percent of the federal poverty level, and promoting the continuity of care by providing more adequate reimbursement to hospitals for prenatal care services to this population. The Governor had previously vetoed a bill on hospital reimbursement,[21] but, subsequently, the Governor and the Legislature came to agreement on this matter.

Information Systems and the Medical Sciences

In 1987, the Committee sponsored a large-scale survey entitled *The Future of Information Systems for the Medical Sciences,* which probed how various segments of the medical community use information and explored their reactions to the potential use of advances in computer technology. The study was funded by grants from the McGraw-Hill Book Company, the *New England Journal of Medicine,* BRS Saunders, University Microfilms International, the Josiah Macy Jr. Foundation, the WK Kellogg Foundation, the Commonwealth Fund, the Rockefeller Foundation, and the Pew Memorial Trust of the Pew Charitable Trusts; and it was conducted by Louis Harris and Associates. Those interviewed included medical school faculty in basic and clinical sciences, medical students, medical residents, physicians active in clinical care, deans of medical schools, and chief librarians in medical school and hospital libraries.[22]

The study found widespread awareness of and some concern about the "information glut." Librarians, for example, highlighted their problems of shortage of shelving space and overcrowding, and emphasized their serious concern about the cost of maintaining their collections. They were most aware of the desirability of sharing library services with other institutions. Office-based physicians, the researchers found, were "sorely out of touch with the advantages of on-line data base technology." Indeed, 50 percent of those responding said they believed card catalogues to be more efficient than computerized data bases. Prophetically (in the light of the rapid advances in computer technology during the decade that followed the study), the study explored the possibility of designing data bases for the retrieval and storage of articles from the medical and scientific literature.

In 1988, the Committee sponsored a conference on *The Future of Information Systems for the Medical Sciences* that was chaired by Dr. Campbell Moses, Chairman of the Committee, and funded by the Josiah Macy, Jr. Foundation. The major presentation by Dr. Edward Huth, Editor of the *Annals of Internal Medicine,* offered a comprehensive review of the consequences of the growing oversupply of medical journals and books, and made a number of suggestions for coping with it.[23] For example, he suggested the storage of marginal journals in CD-ROM format, and improving the speed of searches through better selection of databases and indexing formats that would enable the researcher to determine much more quickly whether the full text of an article was worthy of review. He also suggested that office assistants be trained in accessing Medline and other databases. To enable physicians to use the literature more efficiently, he proposed collaborative efforts to build synoptic (i.e., comprehensive or general) literature databases in which clinical departments trained by medical librarians might create databases for their individual specialties.

## Health Claims and the Food and Drug Administration

On December 3, 1987, Dr. Maurice Shils, former Executive Secretary of the Committee on Medical Education, testified before the

Subcommittee on Human Resources and Intergovernmental Operations of the House Committee on Government Operations regarding a proposal to modify the regulations of the Food and Drug Administration (FDA) to allow the advertising of health claims for the prevention of specific diseases such as cancer, cardiovascular disease or osteoporosis.[24] His testimony was based on a statement, adopted by the Committee, approved by the Council and published in the *Bulletin,* which took the position that, because there are very serious differences of opinion about such health claims in the scientific community and because of the staff limitations and the budgetary constraints under which the FDA must function, it would not be advisable to require the FDA to police them.[25] Accordingly, the Academy recommended that the ban on advertising specific health claims be continued. As a result of different opinions presented in the public debate, the matter was left unresolved by the FDA. However, the Academy position was reflected in the Nutrition Labeling and Education Act of 1990 (Public Law 101–535) which was passed in November 1990 and is in the process of being implemented.[26]

### Motor Vehicle Injuries

On December 7, 1987, the Committee on Public Health held a Symposium on *Motor Vehicle Injuries* which was cosponsored by the New York State Department of Health, the New York State Governor's Traffic Safety Committee, and Traffic Safety Now, Inc. Dr. David Harris, Chairman of the Committee, aptly characterized the Symposium as one that stressed the "multidisciplinary exploration of new ideas and emerging issues in the field of vehicular trauma," and dedicated it to the memory of Dr. William Haddon, Jr., a pioneer researcher and administrator in the field of traffic safety who had served with the New York State Department of Health before becoming the Administrator of the US National Highway Traffic Safety Administration.[27] Dr. Haddon was noted for his promotion of epidemiological investigations of auto accidents and his strategy of focusing on changing automobile design as a key to reducing injuries from accidents.

Senator Daniel Patrick Moynihan, who had worked with Dr. Haddon in 1958 during the Harriman administration in Albany, offered a tribute to Dr. Haddon in which he said that Dr. Haddon regarded the morbidity and mortality associated with road transport as the consequence of crashes that have almost certain discoverable regularities. "Because of Bill Haddon," he said, "New York was the first to propose that design be made a central element in vehicle safety."[28]

In his keynote address at the Symposium, Senator Moynihan emphasized "the interface between medicine and public policy."[29] He recalled that, while serving as Acting Secretary to Governor Harriman, he had many discussions of traffic safety issues with Dr. Haddon and came to the conclusion that, while the very difficult task of modifying drivers' behavior should not be abandoned, a more direct route to greater auto safety would be to modify the consequences of behavior through better automobile design that would protect against crash injuries. He noted that, in his first published paper on this issue, *Epidemic on the Highways,* he had said, "This is a public health problem, which is now being dealt with as a law enforcement problem, and this is accomplishing nothing." Senator Moynihan agreed with Dr. Haddon that "traffic injuries and deaths constitute one of nation's greatest public health problems," and drew an analogy between automobile injuries and getting rid of malaria: "You can't kill all the mosquitoes. Instead, get rid of the water. You can swat mosquitoes forever, but if you empty the stagnant water they don't breed. It works out better to drain the pool rather than swat the mosquitoes. Keep the speed limit down rather tell people not to drive too fast."[30]


Drug Testing in the Workplace

On February 3, 1988, the Committee joined the Section on Occupational Medicine, the New York Business Group on Health and the

National Association on Drug Abuse Problems in cosponsoring a one day Symposium on *Drug Testing in the Workplace*. The drugs discussed included alcohol, prescription drugs and illicit substances. J. Michael Walsh, Ph.D., Director of the Office of Workplace Initiatives at the National Institute of Drug Abuse in Rockville, MD, emphasized the need to balance the employers' "responsibility to provide the best service and product they can to their customers, and protect shareholders from losses to drug abuse" with their responsibilities to "loyal and trustworthy workers who for the most part are not abusing drugs."[31]

Dr. Walsh reviewed the technical and scientific guidelines for federal agencies promulgated by the US Department of Health and Human Services. It is clear, he said, that courts will support testing programs in the workplace in the public sector only when the tests are deemed to be reasonable, that is, when the workers are in positions that are "safety or security-sensitive." Thus, he noted, employers in the public sector apparently have greater leeway than those in the private sector in testing their employees for drug abuse. The guidelines which govern the testing of all federal employees specify that the initial screening should be followed by a confirmatory assay and a review of all positive findings by a physician. He sounded caution by noting that a positive result does not establish illegal drug use since employees may be taking controlled substances like barbiturates, amphetamines or opiates under medical direction. Employee assistance programs and health insurance which covers drug abuse treatment, he suggested, would encourage employees with such problems to become productive members of the workforce.[31]

### Symposium Dedicated to Dr. Norman Simon

Dr. Norman Simon, a distinguished radiologist on the staff of the Mt. Sinai Medical Center for many years, was Vice President of the Academy when he died in 1985. He began his association with the Academy in 1948 when he was awarded the Bowen-Brooks

Fellowship to assist in his training in radiology. He served as Chairman of the Committee from 1981 through 1983, and played a major role in many of the conferences and symposia it sponsored during the 1970s and 1980s. It was, therefore, truly fitting that the Committee should dedicate the September 23, 1988 Symposium on Science in Society: *Low Level Radioactive Waste, Controversy and Resolution* to his memory.[32]

Most of the presentations made the point that the risk to the health of the public from low-level radioactive waste had been greatly exaggerated. For example, Eric J. Hall, Ph.D., of the Radiological Research Laboratory at the Columbia University College of Physicians and Surgeons, said, "By any reasonable assessment, the radiation hazards to human health posed by low level radioactive waste are trivial compared to radiation for medical purposes, which, in turn, is dwarfed by the potential deleterious effects of radon. People who live close to a nuclear power plant or to a burial site for radioactive waste, get far more radiation from radon exposure in their own homes in one day than they get from a whole year of having the power plant or the burial site as a neighbor."[33]

## Nutrition and Children

On March 9, 1989, the Committee conducted a Symposium on *Nutrition and Children* that was cosponsored by the Academy's Section on Pediatrics and the New York State Department of Health. The purpose of the meeting, in the words of Committee Chairman David Harris, Commissioner of the Suffolk County Health Department, was to "identify nutrition-related health problems for which prevention and treatment are possible and, most important of all, to suggest specific changes in medical practice and public policy so that all children (and the adults they will become) may enjoy the full benefit of the vigorous application of medical knowledge."[34]

The Symposium celebrated the one-hundredth anniversary of

the founding of the Academy's Section on Pediatrics by Dr. Abraham Jacobi (1830–1919), a great leader of American medicine and President of the Academy from 1885 to 1888. The program committee was chaired by Dr. Henry L. Barnett, a well-known pediatrician associated with the Children's Aid Society, and the speakers included Matilda Raffa Cuomo, the wife of New York Governor Mario Cuomo, who described the State's initiatives in nutrition education for children. She indicated that she was "particularly proud" of the *Nutrition for Life* program and grateful to the Academy for collaborating in bringing it to the New York City schools.[35]

A major presentation, made by Dr. Myron Winick, a distinguished nutritionist and pediatrician on the faculty of the Columbia University College of Physicians and Surgeons, noted that poverty was a major underlying cause of poor nutrition, and that inadequate nutrition alone is not the cause of the slow development of children. For example, he pointed out, in places like the nation's capital the leading cause of death among teenagers is homicide. Nevertheless, he said, nutritional issues are extremely important. Fundamentally, a major nutritional problem is a diet heavy in fat, saturated fat, and cholesterol which will lead to health problems when the children become adults. Children need to eat more fiber and less beef, Dr. Winick said, while avoiding the problem of being overfed.[36]

Lending additional importance to the conference was the presence of Dr. J. Michael McGinnis, Deputy Assistant Secretary for Health and Director of the US Office of Disease Prevention and Health Promotion, who presented a review of the implications of the *Surgeon General's Report on Nutrition and Health*. He noted that the Report had special policy implications for food service programs in schools. He emphasized the importance of nutrition education and better nutrition for poor children, and expressed particular concern that so many adolescents and young adults get much of their food from fast food restaurants whose servings are heavy in saturated fat and cholesterol.[37]

## Quality of New York City's Drinking Water

In June 1989, following approval by the Council, the Committee issued a *Statement on Preserving the Quality of New York City's Drinking Water*[38] The Statement called for major efforts to preserve the high quality of New York City's water supply because "a broad spectrum of pollution inputs now enter the City's source waters." It recommended "Strict limitations, controls and enforcement for infectious, chemical and nutrient contaminants discharged or otherwise released into the city's watersheds; critical reevaluation of the regulatory requirement of staffing by persons with water quality and public health expertise, and responsible land use controls on developments within the watershed, including prohibitions on development in certain critical areas (especially watershed wetlands and areas adjacent to reservoirs)."[39]

The Statement also recommended the following new approaches to the preservation of water quality:

- Prohibiting new discharges of sewage treatment effluents directly into New York City source waters, a prohibition similar to land use and discharge restrictions in force in the State of Connecticut;
- Purchasing or otherwise legally preserving large tracts of land in ecologically 'sensitive' portions of the watershed and/or obtaining conservation easements from land owners;
- Diverting existing wastewater discharges out of watershed areas; and
- Prohibiting incompatible developments, such as chemical industries in the watershed[40]

As this is being written (March 1996), the City, in conjunction with the assistance of State officials, has successfully completed negotiations with the upstate communities in which the New York City watershed is located to bring about many of the changes recommended in the Committee's Statement.

## COMMITTEE ON MEDICAL EDUCATION

In 1986, James McCorkel, Ph.D., a medical sociologist, became Executive Secretary of the Committee on Medical Education. Dr.

McCorkel had previously been employed at Winthrop University Hospital in Nassau County as Director of Medical Education, and was experienced in the use of computers in medicine and, particularly, in medical education. After three months, however, he resigned and returned to the Winthrop University Hospital. Dr. Campbell Moses, the Chairman of the Committee, assumed responsibility for the Computers in Medicine Project, and Mr. Stubing assumed responsibility for administration of the Sections, Fellowship activities and the balance of the Committee's activities.

In 1987, Dr. Elizabeth Carlsen Gerst, Assistant Dean for Continuing Medical Education at the Columbia University College of Physicians and Surgeons since 1984, became Executive Secretary of the Committee on Medical Education. Trained as physiologist with a Ph.D. from the University of Pennsylvania, she had been Director of Continuing Education in the Health Sciences at P & S since 1978. When Dr. Gerst left in 1989, the role of Executive Secretary was filled by Dr. Marvin Lieberman (who continued in that role with the Committee on Medicine in Society as well) until 1993, when the Committee on Medical Education was eliminated as a standing committee. The Office of Medical Education continued to function as the vehicle to administer the Sections and the other programs in medical education.

Corporate Influences on Patient Relations

The 12th Symposium on Medical Education held on March 6, 1986, was devoted to *Corporate Influences on Patient Relations.* Dr. Marianne J. Legato, Associate Professor of Clinical Medicine at Columbia University College of Physician and Surgeons and Attending Physician at St. Luke's-Roosevelt Hospital Center, who chaired the Meeting, gave the keynote address, *The Doctor, The Patient and the Third Party Payer: Three Begins to Be a Crowd.* In it, she presented a somber forecast of the impact of current trends in the financing of physicians' services. With the enormous acceleration of medical care costs, she noted, corporate America has become concerned about that problem. " 'For-profit,' totally commercially-oriented private groups are springing up as the government backs off from its once enthusiastically espoused notion of providing health care to all over 65." The ultimate outcome, she predicted, will be that "profit will motivate those dispensing care on a scale that has never been seen before."[41]

Gifts to the Academy

Mr. Stubing's efforts to raise endowment support for activities of the Committee on Medical Education came to fruition in 1987–1988. A $300,000 grant was received in 1987 from the Corlette Glorney Foundation to endow the Glorney-Raisbeck Award in Cardiology in honor of Dr. Milton J. Raisbeck, an emeritus member of the Committee. The award, a bronze medal and a $10,000 prize, is given to "recognize scientific achievement and outstanding contributions to basic science or clinical medicine, especially as they relate to cardiology." The first Glorney-Raisbeck Award in Cardiology was presented posthumously to Dr. Raisbeck and was accepted by his widow in a ceremony in the Cathedral House of Grace Cathedral in San Francisco with Mr. Stubing in attendance.

An anonymous gift of $200,000 was received from a Fellow to establish the Paul Klemperer Award, whose purpose was "to recognize contributions to basic science or clinical medicine, as those contributions may relate to connective tissue disease." Dr. Klemperer was a distinguished pathologist-researcher who had served on the faculty at the Albert Einstein College of Medicine, the Columbia University College of Physicians and Surgeons, and the Mount Sinai School of Medicine. He received the Academy Medal in 1962 for his work on the mechanisms of collagen vascular diseases and for his other "contributions to the progress of medicine."[42] After retiring from his career as a pathologist, Dr. Klemperer pursued interests in the history of medicine and wrote introductions to several of the volumes in the Academy's History of Medicine series.

Dr. John Kingsley Lattimer provided a grant of $30,000 to endow the John Kingsley Lattimer Distinguished Lectures in the History of Medicine. Dr. Lattimer, former Chairman and currently Emeritus Professor in the Department of Urology at Columbia University College of Physicians and Surgeons, had served as a Trustee and as Vice President of the Academy. He is a distinguished scholar in American history who has written and lectured widely on the assassinations of Presidents Lincoln and Kennedy.

The New York Community Trust provided a grant of $144,000 to fund the first two years of the David Warfield Fellowship Program in ophthalmology, the first of which was awarded in 1989. And, finally, to celebrate the one-hundredth anniversary of the Section on Pediatrics in 1988, a $50.000 challenge grant from Mr. and Mrs. Richard Brock, parents of a child who required extensive medical interventions, established the Pediatrics Education Endowment Fund, which underwrites inviting physicians interested in issues relating to the health of urban children to lecture at the Academy and to spend a day teaching resident and attending staffs at a local academic medical center. Recent lecturers include: Gwendolyn Scott, M.D. who spoke in 1995 on *Pediatric HIV Infection: Prevention, Therapy, and Future Challenges,* and Stephen Ludwig, M.D., who spoke in 1996 on *Munchausen Syndrome by Proxy: A Common Yet Unrecognized Form of Child Abuse in Pediatric Practice.*

### The National Seminar on Medical Education

In 1988, the Josiah Macy, Jr. Foundation provided a $ 271,400 grant to the Academy to support a *National Seminar on Medical Education.* Director William C. Stubing served as project director. This Seminar, to which twenty-five participants were invited, took place in the Bahamas on June 15–18, 1988 and was chaired by Dr. David E. Rogers, Walsh McDermott Distinguished Professor of Medicine at Cornell University Medical College and former President of the Robert Wood Johnson Foundation. The speakers included: Drs. Victor Neufeld of McMaster University, Marjorie P. Wilson, President of the Educational Commission for Foreign

Medical Graduates, and Jo Ivey Boufford, President of the New York City Health and Hospitals Corporation, and Uwe Reinhardt, Ph.D. of the Woodrow Wilson School at Princeton University.

The Seminar focused on current developments in the structure and financing of medical education at the undergraduate and graduate levels, the relationship of diverse health care settings to the education of physicians, and the policy implications that these generated. Dr. Rogers stated the purpose of the meeting without equivocation: "Our nation needs doctors with a broader and more sensitive view of the place and role of medicine in the larger society. We need doctors who are more skilled in doctor-patient relationships. We must better prepare our new doctors to be dedicated lifetime learners, and medical education must become significantly more self-directed and more personally exciting for medical students."[43]

The conference participants, who included physicians, economists, foundation and governmental officials, recommended six important changes in medical education programs. These included a requirement of community service for all medical graduates; financial incentives to encourage more training in ambulatory care for all medical graduates; and less emphasis on standardized tests for the selection and evaluation of medical students. The proceedings were published in November of 1986 to coincide with the annual meeting of the Association of American Medical Colleges, and the Seminar received excellent press coverage with stories in the *New York Times*, the *Boston Globe*, the *Washington Post*, the *Toronto Globe and Mail* and the *Wall Street Journal*.

### Recredentialling of Physicians

At the February 22, 1989 meeting of the Council, Dr. Campbell Moses, Chairman of the Committee, reported that Dr. Alfred M. Gellhorn, Director of Medical Affairs of the New York State Department of Health, had discussed the issue of physician recredentialling at the February 9 meeting of the Committee. Dr. Gellhorn was also the Co-Chair of the New York State Advisory

Committee on Physician Recredentialling. President Martin Cherkasky, presenting the viewpoint of Chancellor Martin Barell of the New York State Board of Regents, commented that continuing medical education had failed to correct the poor performance of some physicians. The proposal that the State develop a recredentialling program was not, he said, "intended to be punitive but to be supportive of the profession in assuring quality of care."[44] He pointed out that in recent discussions, Dr. Charles Sherman, President of the Medical Society of the State of New York, had suggested that all interested parties might discuss the issue, with the Academy assuming the role of an "honest broker." The discussion that ensued indicated some interest in having the Academy playing such a role but, as it turned out, there really was little support for the idea either in the Medical Society of the State of New York or in the Academy.

## ACADEMY PUBLICATIONS

### Challenge to the *Bulletin*

At the Stated Meeting of April 14, 1987, Dr. Arnold S. Relman, the distinguished Editor-in-Chief of the *New England Journal of Medicine* who had been elected an Honorary Fellow of the Academy, delivered the Anniversary Discourse on *The Purposes and Prospects of the General Medical Journal.*[45] Dr. Relman noted that, in the nineteenth century, most journals had a generalist orientation, reflecting a time when there were few specialists. Among the earliest and most influential were the *New England Journal of Medicine* established by the Massachusetts Medical Society in 1812 as the *New England Journal of Medicine and Surgery and the Collateral Branches of Science,* the *Lancet,* founded independently in England in 1823, and the *British Medical Journal* established by the recently organized British Medical Association in 1840. By 1987, Dr. Relman observed, only about twenty-five to thirty such general journals were being published throughout the world, while all the other periodicals cover a limited scientific or clinical field. Given the recent radical growth of specialization in medical knowledge, the reduction the number of general medical journals is understandable, yet their continuation is indispensable. Medicine, Dr. Relman noted, has a common culture, a common ethic, a common orientation, and a common scientific base that ought to bring all physicians together. He conceded that specialty journals are necessary if a physician is to keep abreast with developments in his or her field but, he said, general journals are really the only periodicals "which say, 'We shall try to present to you those things all doctors ought to be interested in simply because they are doctors, regardless of specialty.' " He pointed out that a collateral benefit of a journal which, like the *New England Journal of Medicine,* uses a highly selective process in accepting articles for publication, is that its content provides a major source of information on medical issues for the popular press.

Despite competition from computerized databases, Dr. Relman remained confident of the continued need for good general publications. The computer needs to be asked a specific question about a particular topic, he said, while readers of a general medical journal can find the unexpected in a form that is more attractive to read and easier to clip. Nonetheless, he continued, the challenge to the general medical journal remains the same as it always has been: "To select a varied menu of the highest quality, interest, and originality that will appeal to physicians of all kinds and will help keep the profession aware of its identity, its traditions, and its social obligations." In these eloquent words, Dr. Relman presented a challenge not only to the *Bulletin* but to the Academy itself.[45]

## THE LIBRARY

In 1986, the Library's integrated library system, the LS/2000, was inaugurated providing an on-line catalog that greatly enhanced access to the collection. The Library also completed the first years of two five-year contracts with the National Library of Medicine:

one, a $2.235 million contract to manage the Greater Northeastern Regional Medical Library Program; and the other, a $1.238 million contract to provide on-line training for librarians and health professionals in the region with a special emphasis on extending network services to physicians in rural areas, in outpatient clinics, and in "store-front" clinics.

Toward the end of 1986, the Library's Publication Committee issued Number 51 of the Academy's History of Medicine Series: *Italian Broadsides Concerning Public Health Documents from Bologna and Brescia in the Mortimer and Anna Neinken Collection at the New York Academy of Medicine,* edited by Dr. Saul Jarcho (see Appendix).

### Rare Book Room and History of Medicine Department

The January 13, 1987 meeting of the Committee on Library was devoted to a wide-ranging discussion of the future of the Rare Book and History of Medicine Department. John Scarborough, Ph.D., Professor of the History of Pharmacy and Medicine at the University of Wisconsin, had been invited to attend as an expert consultant. Dr. Scarborough offered a number of suggestions. First, he suggested a study of what the "competition" is doing. This would avoid duplication of programs and services and help in defining the mission of the Rare Book and History of Medicine Department.

Second, he said, the collection should be inventoried so that it might be better characterized for scholars. Putting the catalogue into a machine-readable format would also be helpful in improving access to the collection.

Third, Dr. Scarborough said, in addition to cooperative ties with other institutions, linkages to academic programs should be explored. The latter might include a "scholars-in-residence" program, affiliation arrangements with medical schools with a focus on promoting study of the history of medicine among their students, and relationships with such general university graduate and undergraduate departments as history, sociology, and demography.

Fourth, Dr. Scarborough thought the Library's collection of medical instruments to be excellent and, since the northeastern section of the United States does not have a truly fine medical museum, transforming the Academy's collection into a museum might serve significant educational functions. Otherwise, further options for the use or disposal of the collection should be considered.

Finally, he pointed out that attention to historical collections is cyclical in nature and currently interest in such collections is on a downturn throughout the world. But this may change, he said, and publicizing the availability of such materials would promote their use.

Dr. Scarborough labeled the current staffing authorization for the Rare Book and History of Medicine Department, which includes a head of the department, a reference librarian, a catalog librarian, and a part-time clerical assistant, as adequate for the present but thought there would soon be a need to develop a curatorial position. Although current funding levels were adequate for current program needs, he warned that additional staff would be needed to follow these suggestions.

## Friends of the Rare Book Room

At the Stated Meeting of the Academy on April 4, 1988, Dr. Fidelio A. Jiminez, Chief of Laboratory Services at the Veterans' Administration Hospital in Brooklyn, presented to President Mary Ann Payne on behalf of the Friends of the Rare Book Room, a copy of the first edition of Thomas Sydenham's first book, *Methodus curandi febres propriis observationabus superstructa,* which was published in 1666. The only other copy in America may be found at the Yale University Library. This, Dr. Jimenez noted, was the Library's 500,000th volume.[46]

As noted earlier, the Friends had been founded in 1946 to assist in obtaining rare medical and historical books and manuscripts for the Library. Up to this point, Dr. Jimenez pointed out, the Friends had purchased some 500 rare volumes for the Rare Book Room's collection.

## Revised Guidelines on Fellows' Library Privileges

In 1987, a revision of the *Guidelines on Fellows Library Privileges*,[47] which had not been updated since 1970, was prepared by the Committee on Library, chaired by Dr. John H. Edgcomb, and approved by the Council at its March meeting. (The latest update was published in 1996.[48]) The *Guidelines* provide an overview of the kinds of services the Library makes available in an age of changing technologies. While the Library is open to the public, only Fellows or Members of the Library (The Library has a subscription plan for corporations and other organizations.) are entitled to borrow books or bound journals. Fellows may use the Rare Book Room without a prior appointment. Fellows are entitled to two free hours per year of "in-depth reference services." On-line bibliographic services are provided to Fellows on a priority basis at one-half the rate for the public. Fellows are entitled to ten free photocopies per year of articles with no more than fifty pages per article. Interlibrary Loans are charged to Fellows on a cost-recovery basis.

Several provisions reflected areas of concern: some limitations were placed on use of the collection by Fellows' family members; and anxiety was expressed over the fact that some Fellows were allowing commercial firms with which they were affiliated to use the Library services at no cost or at the Fellows' rates.

## The Effect of Serials Prices on Collection Development

On November 2, 1988, Ms. Anne Pascarelli, Associate Librarian, addressed the New York/New Jersey Medical Library Association on *The Effect of Serials Prices on Collection Development*. The presentation vividly delineated the serious financial problems medical libraries face in maintaining their collections of journals. Because of its relevance to the problems of the Library, Ms. Pascarelli was asked to summarize it at a meeting of the Council.[49]

She noted that price of domestic medical journals had tripled in the decade between 1978 and 1988, with the average cost of subscriptions increasing from $51.50 to $189. The cost increases of foreign periodical increases were especially sharp in 1988 due to the decline in the value of the American dollar in foreign markets. The price increases could be attributed to many factors: the absence of competition in publishing and the growth of publishing conglomerates; the willingness of Canadian and US markets to pay more than other buyers without regard to exchange rates; the growing importance of for-profit publishers as opposed to not-for-profit entities; a real increase in the cost of production; the proliferation of journal titles; and the "publish or perish" syndrome in academia. Title proliferation was taking the form of what was described as "twigging," a phenomenon of excessive specialization and duplication in titles. The increase in price of monographs (stand-alone publications) was termed a most disturbing trend. Approximately 200 new monographs. she said, are appearing annually at an average yearly subscription price of $60.00. This enormous cost made it impractical for a library to subscribe to all the new publications and , as a result, the Library had, to date, cut seventy-eight titles providing an annual saving of over $33,000.

Ms. Pascarelli's recommendations to the library and academic communities included increased reliance in cooperative ventures among libraries; purchase of single articles rather than whole publications; and more careful analysis of price trends. To the academic community, she urged that faculty not be encouraged to publish "junk," and that institutions police fraud more vigorously. She called for resumption of publishing by not-for-profit entities, and warned the publishing community that there is a limit to library budgets and librarians can no longer purchase every journal that is issued.[50]

Ms. Pascarelli emphasized the implications for the Library. Decisions to reduce the purchase of books and periodicals would have to be made, she acknowledged. But, she warned, there is the danger that, in the future, senior staff discouraged by the impact of Library budget cuts would seek career opportunities in institutions where resources were not under such stress. She reported that the growing trend toward automation and the proliferation of computerized databases was adding significantly to the pressure on libraries, but, she pointed out, these developments also bring hopes of increases in revenue as libraries market additional services to new constituencies.

## Interlibrary Collaboration

The Library has cooperated with the State Education Department and the New York State Library in maintaining linkages between the regional information network and the statewide information network. The Academy has a contract with the New York State, amounting to $460,000 for 1988, to subsidize responding to requests for health information initiated by libraries in the State.

As noted earlier, the Academy was one of the eleven sponsoring institutions that created the Medical Library Center in 1959. In return for the payment of annual dues, the Library receives a variety of services, while the Center also serves as a subcontractor in the Regional Medical Library Program and provides selected services to other regional libraries on behalf of the Library.

In 1972, when legislation was passed providing Federal support for research libraries but excluding those under private auspices, the private libraries formed the Independent Research Libraries Association to advance their mutual interests. This organization, of which the Library was a charter member, provides a vehicle for sharing information and, at the same time, offers greater visibility for the Library.

Another organization with which the Library continued to be associated is the On-Line (formerly Ohio) Computer Library Center, Inc. This is the world's largest electronically linked database, serving 9,400 affiliated libraries.

Not to be overlooked is the relationship with the National Library of Medicine from which the library received five-year grants to operate the Greater Northeastern Medical Library Program and the Eastern Region On-line Training and Information Center. Through these programs, the Library negotiated formal agreements with forty-one of the region's medical school and other specialized health sciences libraries to create a regional medical library network.

## ACADEMY PRESIDENTS

### Dr. Mary Ann Payne 1987–1988

Dr. Mary Ann Payne, Attending Physician at the New York Hospital and Clinical Professor Emerita of Medicine at the Cornell University Medical College, the school from which she had graduated in 1945, was the first woman to serve as President. A native of Frederick, Maryland, she received an M.A. and a Ph.D. in endocrinology. She became a Fellow in 1953 and served as a member of the Committee on Medical Education, and as Vice President and Trustee. It was she who, with Mr. Stubing, took the lead in planning for the restructuring of the Academy. After leaving the Presidency, she continued as a Trustee, as Treasurer, and as Chair of the Committee on Strategic Planning.

### Dr. Joseph Addonizio 1989

Dr. Addonizio, a native of Mt. Vernon, New York, was Professor and Chair of the Department of Urology at the New York Medical College. He became a Fellow in 1979 and served as Chair of the Section on Urology, on the Committee on Medical Education, and as Trustee. He was President during the crucial period when proposals for change in the Academy structure were being developed and adopted. Mr. Stubing credits his spirit of collegiality for facilitating this process.

Dr. Martin Cherkasky (Acting) 1989–1990

Dr. Cherkasky became President upon Dr. Addonizio's untimely death in 1989 and served until 1990 when Dr. Barondess assumed that office under the new structure. At that time, Dr. Cherkasky became Chairman of the Board of Trustees, a post he held until 1991. A native of Philadelphia, he received his M.D. from Temple University Medical School, and became Professor and Chairman of the Department of Community Health at the Albert Einstein College of Medicine. From 1951 through 1981, he was Executive Director of the Montefiore Hospital. As an advisor on medical policy during the three terms of Edward I. Koch as Mayor, he had a great influence on medical affairs in New York City during that period. Dr. Cherkasky became a Fellow in 1952 and, as noted above, has played an important role in a variety of Academy affairs and activities.

## ACADEMY FINANCES

In keeping with the plans he presented on assuming the role of Director in April, 1986, Mr. Stubing visited a number of Foundation executives to discus the potential of the Academy as an institution that could make a positive contribution towards alleviating health problems in the City. He was quite candid in his approach to these individuals, indicating that the Academy had a great potential that was not being achieved primarily because of its financial constraints. These discussions reinforced Mr. Stubing's concern over the way the Academy's investment portfolio was being managed. Accordingly, it was decided to retain an outside consultant and, on the recommendation of Ms. Margaret Mahoney, President of the Commonwealth Fund and a Trustee of the Academy, the Boston-based firm of Cambridge Associates, Inc., was selected from among a number of competitors to evaluate the Academy's financial planning and management. A major factor in the selection of this firm was its considerable experience in dealing with the problems of not-for-profit organizations.


### The Cambridge Associates Report

The consultants made a detailed study of the Academy's finances over the preceding decade as the basis for recommendations for future investment and expenditure strategies which were embodied in a Report presented on May 13, 1987.[51]

In this Report, Cambridge Associates pointed out that "the market value of the Academy's endowment funds had declined slightly over the last ten years, when adjustment is made for the effects of inflation. A major decline took place from 1977 to 1981; since then, with the exception of 1984, there had been increases each year." These unsatisfactory results are "attributable to a combination of poor investment returns, inflation, and a growing rate of endowment spending," the report said. In 1977, the market value of the Academy's portfolio expressed in 1986 dollars was $48,103,400, and in 1986 it stood at $46,356,900.

The Report noted that, since 1983, investment management had been furnished to the Academy largely on a non-discretionary basis by a prominent Wall Street firm. The spending policy had been to "limit spending to the amount of income (dividends and interest) generated by the endowment." Depending on the state of the market, the portfolio would be tilted to produce the revenue needed with the result that "the investment performance of the portfolio has been relatively weak."[51]

The Report recommended that performance should be measured in terms of total return, or the sum of interest, dividends, and capital changes, while the Academy's rate of spending should initially be capped at 8.5% of the market value of the portfolio and then be reduced to a "more sustainable rate thereafter." The Academy, the Report said, must take steps to return to or meet financial equilibrium which, given the history of market performance, means that the rate of "actual spending should not exceed 5–6% of endowment assets."[51]

Comments were made about the diversification of the Academy portfolio. It was suggested that the Academy move to a "multiple manager structure." Further, the Report advised, the Academy's investment strategy should have both a return goal and a time line: the return objectives should have a rolling ten-year time horizon for the overall endowment, and a rolling five-year horizon should be used for evaluating fund components (asset classes and individual mangers).[51]

The recommendations of the Report were approved by the Investment Review Committee, whose members were Drs. Joseph C. Addonizio, Martin Cherkasky, Duncan W. Clark, Bernard J. Pisani and Richard I. Saphir, and accepted by the Board of Trustees at its meeting of October 28, 1987. They proved to be singularly important, for they not only have governed the Academy's investment policies since then, but they also triggered the most fundamental changes in the structure and governance of the Academy since its founding in 1847.

## REORGANIZATION OF THE ACADEMY

At the meeting of the Council on the same day, President Payne announced the acceptance of the report of the Investment Review Committee, and went on to say that, in her judgment, the Academy's existing resources were insufficient to support its present program. She pointed to the impact of the recent sharp decline in the stock market as a stark reminder of this fact, and reported that she and Mr. Stubing had careful reviewed the Academy's situation and concluded that a "hard look" at its structure and programs was necessary. Accordingly, she announced that she would support the creation of a committee to study the Academy's mission and structure.[52]

Mr. Stubing confirmed his view of the urgency of such a review.

He noted that, after being in office for eighteen months, some of the goals he had set for his administration had been realized: growth in the visibility of the Academy; strengthening of the Fellowship by the addition of more leaders from academia; and presentation of more careful work in the standing committees. Financial support for new initiatives is at an all-time high, he reported. But, he said, developments in the financial markets and in the tax laws have caused grave concern. Addressing these financial concerns, he concluded, dictates the proposed study of the Academy's mission and structure and the development of recommendations that would strengthen its overall management.[52]

With the approval of the Council, a Committee on Strategic Planning was created. It was chaired by Dr. Mary Ann Payne and was made up of current members of the Council (Drs. Joseph C. Addonizio, Martin Cherkasky, Paul D. Kligfield, Michael R. McGarvey, Mary C. McLaughlin, and Bernard J Pisani), other members of the Academy (Drs. Carleton B. Chapman, Norbert J. Roberts, and Samuel O. Thier, and Ms. Margaret E. Mahoney, Mr. Christopher York), Mr. Stubing and Mr. Joseph Perl, Assistant Treasurer and Controller of the Commonwealth Fund. It was charged to "examine and redefine the Academy's mission; review existing programs, consider new initiatives and establish new priorities; examine the structure and function of the standing committees; and address the space and financial needs of the institution."[53]

One of the Committee's first actions was to seek the help of Cambridge Associates, the consulting firm that had become quite familiar with the Academy, its people and its activities during the course of its study of the Academy's financial management and planning. Cambridge Associates was primarily represented by Ms. Anne Spence who had an M.A. from Harvard and an M.B.A. from the Stanford University School of Business and who had significant experience as a financial analyst and consultant in organizational administration and strategy.

On October 26, 1988, Mr. Stubing formally announced his plan to resign as Director effective December 31, 1989 or at an

earlier time that was mutually agreeable. He said that this decision would enable the Committee on Strategic Planning and the
Council to consider the impact of the proposals they were weigh-
ing without concern for any consequences they might have on
him as the Director.

Dr. Mary Ann Payne completed her term as President on December 31, 1988, but continued her role with the Committee on Strategic Planning and reported on its activities at the Council meeting of
January 25, 1989. "There was a strong consensus within the Committee," she said, "the mission of the Academy remains essentially
unchanged." That mission, she continued, "is to improve the public's health through education—education of the medical and allied health professions; education of legislators, and education of
the public. The Library is maintained, seminars and conferences
are offered, and statements are issued to improve the public health.
As the location of the Academy is in New York City, the Academy's primary focus would be on the urban health problems and
issues relating to the New York metropolitan area."[54]

Dr. Payne commented that the proposals under consideration
do not constitute a "strategic plan" but, rather, they address major
structural changes.

## REPORT ON GOVERNANCE

At the Council meeting of March 22, 1989, Dr. Payne introduced
Ms. Spence who presented her report.[55] In preparing it, she had
interviewed members of the Council, members of the Committee
on Strategic Planning, and leaders of other prestigious membership
organizations, such as the Council on Foreign Relations, the American Academy of Arts and Sciences, the American Philosophical
Society, and the American College of Physicians. Her findings, she
said, suggested that more "activity is needed in the Academy, and
greater opportunity for the membership to fulfill its purpose of
improving the public's health." There was also a need to improve
the focus of the Academy's activities. She described "intermingling

of management, governance and membership" as a result of which "[M]anagement lacks the clear authority to solve problems." With the financial problems confronting the Academy, she said, there is the possibility that, within the next ten years, it would cease to exist.

The major conceptual point of the Report was her emphasis on a distinction between "governance" and "management." By governance, she referred to the oversight function of the Board of Trustees which has a fiduciary relationship in an organization with an endowment. The Academy had three tasks to face: "the improvement of its governance; the translation of its mission statement into specific courses of action; and the recruitment of a successor to Mr. Stubing whose resignation would become effective at the end of the year."

The urgency of the restructuring of the Academy was emphasized by the consideration that, without major changes, the recruitment of a promising successor to Mr. Stubing would be seriously compromised. Incidentally, it was reported, Mr. Stubing and several members of the Committee on Strategic Planning expressed the view that these changes would be accomplished more easily if his successor was a physician.

Ms. Spence said that the blurring of the distinction between governance and management was a structural fault often found in many membership organizations as they grow in financial assets and in staff. Clearly, her Report emphasized, there was an urgent need for a Chief Executive Officer who could provide responsible management and end the process of drawing down the Academy's financial assets as had been the case for the last fifteen years. The endowment was no longer capable of supporting the Library and the full range of committee activities, it pointed out. "If too many persons are responsible, including the membership, the Council, the standing committees, etc., then no one is responsible."[56]

The Report repeated the sobering news about the financial condition of the Academy. In the past fifteen years, it pointed out, "the purchasing power of the Academy endowment declined almost by half." Meanwhile, during this period, the major drain on the resources of the Academy had been the expenditures of the Library which had increased by 178 percent, a marked contrast to the 46 percent increase in expenditures for all other Academy programs (figures not adjusted for inflation). The Report projected that, if there were no growth in market value of the investment portfolio and no increase in resources through fund-raising, and expenditures continued at the current rate, the recently experienced deficits would be continued. As a result, the Report predicted that, by the year 2000, the endowment would have declined to a nominal value of $5 million while the cumulative deficit would have reached $9 million.

The Report recommended fourteen major changes. Perhaps the most fundamental was that the Academy should change its dominant governance characteristic from its current form as a "membership organization" to that of a "nonprofit institution" in which members have a role but, as in other major endowed institutions, do not govern the organization. Remaining to be determined was the delineation of just how much authority would be given to the "membership basis of the Academy."

The Report recommended the creation of a Board of Trustees as the single governing body in place of the current Council and Board of Trustees, whose size would be reduced from the current twenty-one Trustees to not more than fifteen. It also recommended the appointment of a full-time salaried President who would serve as the Chief Executive Officer with clear-cut managerial responsibilities. The President would serve at the pleasure of the Board while the Board would be headed by an elected Chairman having no management responsibilities. The Chairman's term would be no shorter than three years with a renewal option. He or she would appoint all committee chairmen and members, and would be involved in fundraising and the recruitment of new trustees. Most important, the Chairman would discuss "key policy issues" with the President establishing thereby "a close working relationship" between them.

It is clear, however, the Report pointed out, that it is not practical for a Board which meets once a month to involve itself in the details of management, even though the Chairman may speak to the Director almost daily.

Another major structural change was modification of the role and authority of the Academy's committees. The Report noted that "currently there are over 50 committees or subcommittees that are directly or indirectly involved in the governance or management of the Academy. Over 40 of these are subcommittees of the regular standing committees. Total membership on the standing committees alone ranges from 150 to 180 individuals, as specified in the By-laws. Adding the members on the Council and Board of Trustees and the committees they create, the total committee membership may reach over 250; this number does not include all subcommittee members."[56] The Report labeled this "extraordinary" and recommended that no committee should have more than twelve members, each of whom should serve no longer than three years.

The Report made a distinction between committees of the Board of Trustees and committees of the membership. Trustee committees, which should be chaired by a Trustee, are to discuss governance issues while the membership committees, which have no governance or management responsibilities, consider issues relating to programs, studies and projects.

To clarify the distinction between governance and management, the Report drew an analogy between the Academy and a museum. In a museum, "the Trustees govern, the professional president manages an internal staff, and the members enjoy certain rights and privileges provided through the efforts of the staff. These institutions also, of course, fulfill an obligation to the public. Even in a membership organization, the rights and privileges of the membership do not necessarily include governance, except as it is delegated to the Board of Trustees. Indeed, many membership organizations with a public mission have discovered that effective management can be achieved only through delegation of governance to the Board of Trustees."

There was some feeling that placing members of the Academy in the same role as museum members was not a particularly felicitous way of expressing the implications of the proposed changes. Clearly, museum members have very little involvement in the conduct of the affairs of the organization. They are primarily seen as supporters or patrons of the activities in return for which they may receive certain privileges, but they have little decision-making power.

The Report recommended merging the Committee on Public Health and the Committee on Medicine in Society. Indeed, it suggested that a single program committee review the activities of the Library, and conduct both the medical education programs and the programs related to public health issues.

The Trustee committees should include a nominating committee, a budget committee, a portfolio committee, a building committee, a development committee, a strategic planning committee, a committee on awards and fellowships, and a publications committee. With a Board of only fifteen members, an executive committee would not be needed.

The governance function, the report suggested, deals with "big picture items, such as strategic and policy issues while management deals with "nuts and bolts" items. As an example, the Report calls a decision about prices to be charged for room rentals a management issue that need not be brought before the Board. On the other hand, "a decision to reduce significantly the space available for rentals should be brought to the Building Committee and thence to the Board as a whole." It is the task of the President, the Report suggested, to define the issues, employ analytic skills to determine how and by whom they should be resolved. and solicit the support of the Trustees when deciding to bring the matter before that body.

It was noted that the Board at that time was made up almost exclusively of Fellows, leading to the suggestion that its membership be diversified to include individuals from the business and philanthropic communities. Such diversification, it was suggested, might open the door to possible augmentation of funding.

The decline of the past fifteen years in the value of the endowment, the Report warned, forces the Academy to choose between reducing expenses or increasing funds for programs, The latter, the report says, is a task that the Academy "has pursued with some success."

In addition, the Report advised, the Academy should embark on a capital campaign, an activity in which the President and the Chairman of the Board should take the lead. In a footnote, it suggested that the sale or lease of property rights or the addition of some public revenue such as City support for the Library, warrants consideration.

The discussion of the Report was continued at the April 26, 1989 meeting of the Council. Dr. Payne indicated that in individual discussions with most of the members of the Council, all but one (Dr. Duncan Clark) had indicated approval. She then presented a summary of what she described as the "core" of the proposals:

- Replacement of the bicameral form of governance with a single Board of Trustees (elected by the membership of the Academy), which would have full governance but no management responsibilities; and
- Provision for a full-time, salaried President with complete management responsibilities to replace the Director and honorific President.[57]

The discussion that followed was described in the minutes as "broad" and one in which every Council member present took part. Dr. Duncan Clark expressed "dissatisfaction with the process which had been followed thus far by the Committee on Strategic Planning. He had anticipated a comprehensive report with a written statement of goals and objectives and identification of strategic issues. He had found the mission statement inadequate and felt no opportunity for discussion had been provided. He expressed discomfort with what he perceived as the "hierarchical structure" proposed. In his opinion, the changes proposed would "disenfranchise the membership and radically change the nature of the organization."

Others said that "the process had been a good one, appropriately employing competent consultants" and noted that it "had received considerable debate and revision before ever reaching the

Council." Those taking a prominent position in supporting the proposed changes were such long-time Academy stalwarts as Drs. Mary Ann Payne, Martin Cherkasky, Norbert Roberts, Bernard Pisani, and Joseph Addonizio.

Assurances were sought that the membership would continue to play a major role in the affairs of the Academy. This concern was assuaged by a statement that the possibility of additional changes was not foreclosed.

A question of whether the Committees would continue to exist evoked the answer was that "the Committee structure would relate to the priorities agreed upon by Academy members and their elected leaders. The nature and number of committees were open to debate and could only be resolved as the organization's priorities were defined."

Dr. Mary McLaughlin, former Commissioner of Health of the City of New York and Chair of the Subcommittee on Options and Priorities, stressed the need for flexibility and emphasized that the By-laws must allow for change. She also voiced expressed concern about increasing the proportion of nonphysicians in the Fellowship and on the Board of Trustees.

Finally, although differing views were expressed, the requirement that only a physician could serve as President was approved.

The proposals, put forth by Dr. Payne in the form of motions to have a Board of Trustees replace the Council and Trustees and to have a full time President, were adopted with dissents by Drs. Duncan Clark and Campbell Moses, Chairman of the Committee on Medical Education.

On August 7, 1989, a Special Meeting of the Fellows was held, with President Dr. Joseph Addonizio in the chair. Only a relatively small number of Fellows attended, but more than 1,000 ballots were cast by proxy, and the proposed changes for a major restructuring of the Academy were approved by an overwhelming margin.

Shortly after presiding at the Fellows meeting, and in the midst of his term of office as President, Dr. Addonizio died. His passing was mourned greatly: Mr. Stubing and the Academy officers, Trustees and staff had warm memories of Dr. Addonizio's collegial approach to his associates. He was replaced by Vice President Cherkasky, who was named Acting-President. Dr. Cherkasky, the able long-term President of Montefiore Medical Center, who had retired several years earlier, had been very active in City and State health circles and was strongly committed to the reorganization of the Academy. In January 1990, when the new By-laws became effective, he became Chairman of the Board of Trustees and served in that role until the end of the year.

The final Report of the Committee on Strategic Planning was issued on October 11, 1989.[58] It formed the basis for the most profound changes in the Academy since its establishment in 1847.

## NOTES

1 [Anonymous]. William Charles Stubing named Director of the New York Academy of Medicine. 1986 *Newsnotes,* Spring 1986, pp. 1, 4.

2 Council of the New York Academy of Medicine. 1986 Minutes of meeting of April 16, 1986.

3 Payne MA. 1986 Presentation of the Academy Plaque to Duncan W. Clark, M.D. *Bulletin of the New York Academy of Medicine.* 62: 791–724.

4 Joseph SC, Schultz S, Stonebrenner R and Clarke P. 1987 AIDS policy and prevention. *Bulletin of the New York Academy of Medicine.* 63:659–672.

5 Committee on Public Health. 1986 Statement and resolution concerning the AIDS epidemic among intravenous drug abusers. *Bulletin of the New York Academy of Medicine.* 62–1033–1035.

6 [Anonymous]. 1964 Career scientist program. *Bulletin of the New York Academy of Medicine.* 40:63–64.

7 Committee on Public Health. 1988 Report to the Council. In: Council of the New York Academy of Medicine. Minutes of the meeting of January 28, 1988: Addendum I.

8 Committee on Honorary Fellowship. 1988 Report to the Council from the Committee on Honorary Fellowships: The Nomination of Anatoly Koryagin. January 11, 1988.

9 Pellegrino ED. 1990 The medical profession as a moral community. *Bulletin of the New York Academy of Medicine.* 66:231–232.

10 Reinhardt U. 1987 How to change the health care system. *Bulletin of the New York Academy of Medicine.* 63:7–19.

11 [Anonymous]. 1986 Current trends: The effectiveness of school health education. *MMWR* 35:593–595.

12 Kirn TF. 1988 Prevention starts in kindergarten in New York City. *Journal of the American Medical Association.* 259:2516–2517.

13 Federal Register. Nov. 5, 1986. 51:40211–40232.

14 Council of the New York Academy of Medicine. Minutes of the meeting of March 25, 1987.

15 Davis K. 1988 Health care and the nation's economic and social agenda. *Bulletin of the New York Academy of Medicine.* 64:5–14.

16 Etzioni A. 1990 Policy implications of socioeconomics. *Bulletin of the New York Academy of Medicine.* 66:5–17.

17 Committee on Medicine in Society. Minutes of the meeting of June 20, 1988.

18 Committee on Public Health. 1986 Statement and resolution on tobacco and health. *Bulletin of the New York Academy of Medicine.* 62:1086–1032.

19 Boreali v. Axelrod, 1987, 518 N.Y.S. 2d 443, 130 AD2d 07. Affirmed 71 NY 2d 1, 517 NE 2d 1350.

20 *McKinney's Consolidated Laws Annotated.* 1990 Article 13-E, New York State Public Health Law. St. Paul, MN: West Publishing Company.

21 S. 6189-A; A.8259-A. 1987 Hospital Reimbursement Bill.

22 Louis Harris Associates. 1987 *The Future of Information Systems for the Medical Sciences.* New York: New York Academy of Medicine.

23 Huth E. 1989 The information explosion. *Bulletin of the New York Academy of Medicine.* 65:647–661.

24 Food and Drug Administration. 1987 Food labeling: Public health messages on food labels and labeling. *Federal Register,* August 4, 1987. 52:28843–28849.

25 Committee on Public Health. 1987 Statement and resolution regarding proposed revision of Food and Drug Administration regulations concerning disease-related health claims on labels. *Bulletin of the New York Academy of Medicine.* 63:410–416.

26 Forbes AL. 1994 National nutritional policy, food labeling and health claims. In: Shils ME, Olson JA and Shike M, Eds. *Modern Nutrition in Health and Disease,* Eighth Edition. Philadelphia: Lea and Febiger. Vol. 2, pp 1626–1657.

27 Harris D. 1988 Symposium on Motor Vehicle Injuries: Welcome and introduction. *Bulletin of the New York Academy of Medicine.* 64:609.

28 Moynihan DP. 1988 Tribute to William Haddon, Jr., MD *Bulletin of the New York Academy of Medicine.* 64:606–607.

29 Moynihan DP. 1988 Symposium on Motor Vehicle Injuries: Keynote address. *Bulletin of the New York Academy of Medicine.* 64:610–616.

30 Moynihan DP 1959 Epidemic on the highways. *Reporter,* April 1959.

31 Walsh JD. 1989 Drug testing in the private and public sectors. *Bulletin of the New York Academy of Medicine.* 65:166–172.

32 Committee on Public Health. 1989 Symposium on science in society: Low level radioactive waste. *Bulletin of the New York Academy of Medicine.* 65:423–554.

33 Hall RJ. 1989 Radiation and life. *Bulletin of the New York Academy of Medicine.* 65:430–438.

34 Harris D 1989 Symposium on Nutrition and Children: Welcome. *Bulletin of the New York Academy of Medicine.* 65:1011.

35 Cuomo MR. 1989 New York State's initiatives in child nutrition. *Bulletin of the New York Academy of Medicine.* 65:1014–1019.

36 Winick M. 1989 The role of early nutrition on subsequent development and optimal future health. *Bulletin of the New York Academy of Medicine.* 65:1020–1025.

37 McGinnis JM. 1989 Nutrition and public policy. *Bulletin of the New York Academy of Medicine.* 65:1168–1174.

38 Committee on Public Health. 1989 Statement on Preservation of New York City's Drinking Water Quality. *Bulletin of the New York Academy of Medicine.* 65:898–904.

39 ibid., pp. 903–904.

40 ibid., p. 904.

41 Legato, M. 1986 The doctor, the patient and the third party payer: Three begins to make a crowd. *Bulletin of the New York Academy of Medicine.* 62:956–963.

42 Baehr G. 1962 Citation and presentation of the Academy Medal to Paul Klemperer, M.D. *Bulletin of the New York Academy of Medicine.* 38:240–244.

43 Rogers DE. 1986 Medical education and the doctor of tomorrow: An agenda for action. In: Josiah Macy Jr. Foundation National Seminar on Medical Education. *Clinical Education and the Doctor of Tomorrow.* New York: New York Academy of Medicine. pp. 109–113.

44 Council of the New York Academy of Medicine. 1989 Minutes of the meeting of February 22, 1989.

45 Relman AS. 1988 The purposes and prospects of the general medical journal. *Bulletin of the New York Academy of Medicine.* 64:875–880.

46 Jimenez F. 1988 Presentation of the 500,000 volume for the library. *Bulletin of the New York Academy of Medicine.* 64:891–892.

47 Committee on Library. 1987 *Guidelines on Fellows Library Privileges.* New York: New York Academy of Medicine.

48 New York Academy of Medicine 1996 *Library Services to Academy Fellows.* New York: New York Academy of Medicine.

49 Pascarelli AW. 1989 Guest editorial: Will libraries exist in the year 2000? *Bulletin of the New York Academy of Medicine.* 65:849–865.

50 Houbeck RL Jr. 1987 If present trends continue: Responding to journal price increases. *Journal of Academic Librarianship.* 13:214–220.

51 Cambridge Associates, Inc. 1987 *Investment Planning for the New York Academy of Medicine.* May 13, 1987.

52 Council of the New York Academy of Medicine. 1987 Minutes of the meeting of October 28, 1987.

53 Committee on Strategic Planning. 1989. *Final report, October 11, 1989.* p. 1.

54 Council of the New York Academy of Medicine. 1989 Minutes of the meeting of January 25, 1989.

55 Spence A. 1989 *Report on Governance, Second Draft.* Boston: Cambridge Associates, Inc. March 16, 1989.

56 ibid. p. 8.

57 Council of the New York Academy of Medicine. 1989 Minutes of the meeting of April 26, 1989.

58 Committee on Strategic Planning. 1989 *Final report.* New York: The New York Academy of Medicine October 11, 1989.

# Chapter 8
## *1991–1993*
## *President Barondess*

THE YEARS FROM 1990 on were truly momentous for the Academy as the changes recommended by the Committee on Strategic Planning and approved by the Board of Trustees and the Fellowship at large were implemented. When considered from a distance, these changes appear to be profound and cataclysmic but, in reality, they resulted from a slow, painstaking process of consultation, discussion, and modification as the Academy's officers, staff and a good portion of the Fellowship pondered their potential impact on the areas and/or activities in which they were particularly interested. While all this was transpiring, projects, committee activities and collaborative arrangements were being continued with little or no impediment to either their quality or their time-frame. A useful analogy would be attempting the internal reconstruction of a majestic home including taking down and putting up walls, doors and windows, rebuilding the plumbing, electrical and heating systems, and rearranging the furnishings, while the residents continued to live and work in it without interruption. It was truly a monumental undertaking that paved the way for the celebration of the 150th anniversary of the Academy and the extension of its mission into the fast-approaching new millennium. One hopes that, when the next in the series of Academy histories is written fifty or one hundred years hence, the architects and builders will receive appropriate recognition for this accomplishment.

When William Stubing, the last Director, left the Academy on December 31, 1989, to become President of the Greenwall Foundation, Dr. Shervert H. Frazier became the interim Executive Officer. Dr. Frazier, an eminent psychiatrist, was former Director of the National Institute of Mental Health who had held important positions in psychiatry at the Mayo Clinic, at Columbia, Harvard, and Baylor Universities, and at the MacLean Hospital in Boston. He had been a member of the Academy Board of Trustees for several years and also served as a member and as chairman of the Salmon Lecture Committee which sponsors the prestigious lecture in psychiatry presented annually at the Academy.

At the same time, Dr. Martin Cherkasky moved from his position as Acting President to become Chairman of the Board of Trustees. Together, they would carry the responsibility for handling the transition to the new regime and, for the next six months, would maintain the stability of Academy programs and staffing arrangements while the process of selecting and installing the new full-time President was going on.

## THE ACADEMY'S FINANCIAL STATUS

The Board of Trustees reviewed the details of the Academy's financial status as presented in a memorandum by Business Manager Daniel J. Ehrlich. He reminded them that the investment planning study presented in May, 1987 by Cambridge Associates, Inc. had recommended that, in order to gain financial equilibrium (i.e., to protect the long term value of the Academy's endowment), annual expenditures should not exceed 5.5 to 6 percent of the corpus of the endowment. He then reported that the expenditure rates for both the 1989 and 1990 budgets were 8.5 percent. To reduce the 1990 rate to the recommended 6 percent would require a reduction of expenditures budgeted for 1990 by about one-third. Otherwise, he warned, the Academy would be eating into its endowment at the rate of $1 million a year. The Academy would have to reduce programs unless it could increase the endowment, procure more and larger grants to support the programs, and/or make the programs income producing. Failure to achieve any of these alternatives would lead to a bleak future for the Academy.

Mr. Ehrlich then turned his attention to the Library. He reiterated the perennial concern that the cost of books and journals was rising faster than inflation and noted that holding 1990 purchases to the approximately $630,000 level of 1989 had been made possible only by modifying the collection policy and cutting back on subscriptions and book purchases. Further, he noted, without a major change in the operations of the Library, more space would be required for additional offices and stack areas. while climate (temperature and humidity) controls were still needed to deal with elevated summer temperatures in the book stacks. Also, he reported, the elevator in the old stacks would have to be replaced to comply with the building codes, a project that would require much rebuilding.

He reminded the Board of Trustees of the need to refurbish the meeting rooms, which had not been touched for over twenty years. Finally, he pointed to an accumulation of requirements which, although individually relatively small, added up to a very significant total. These included such items as new carpeting for Hosack Hall, replacement of chairs in the reading rooms, and some major plumbing repairs.

In the discussion that followed this report, Dr. Cherkasky noted that, according to the preliminary figures, the 1989 expenditures had been slightly under the budgeted amount but he acknowledged that the endowment continued to be eroding. The discussion continued to focus on the Library as a source of budget problems with one Trustee stressing the importance of the Library to the Academy. It was agreed to authorize some minor capital improvements, but replacement of the stack elevator was deferred.

To gain further insight into this problem a Committee to Study the Library was appointed. Dr. Vartan Gregorian, an Academy Trustee and President of the New York Public Library, who was soon to become President of Brown University, was named to chair it but the study was actually conducted by Dr. Thomas Q. Morris, former President and Chief Executive Officer of the Presbyterian Hospital who continued as Professor of Medicine at the Columbia University College of Physicians and Surgeons (*vide infra*).

## DR. JEREMIAH A. BARONDESS AS PRESIDENT

On February 8, 1990, the Presidential Search Committee headed by Dr. Martin Cherkasky with Ms. Margaret Mahoney, and Drs. Saul J. Farber, Ralph O'Connell, Mary Ann Payne, Thomas Q. Morris and Bernard J. Pisani as members, reported to the Executive Committee of the Board of Trustees that Dr. Jeremiah A. Barondess was their unanimous selection for the new post of President.[1] That selection was endorsed unanimously and, one week later, at a special meeting of the full Board of Trustees, it was again unanimously approved.

Dr. Jeremiah A. Barondess, who was to become the Academy's first full-time President on July 1, 1990, was born on June 6, 1924 in New York City. His father was a lawyer and his grandfather, Joseph Barondess, was a prominent labor leader on the Lower East Side of Manhattan.

After one year at Hofstra College and another at Pennsylvania State College, Dr. Barondess entered the armed forces during World War II and was assigned to Wayne State University and the University of Michigan under the Army Specialized Training Program, and then to the Johns Hopkins University School of Medicine, where he graduated as class valedictorian in 1949. He had an internship and an assistant residency on the Osler Medical Service of the Johns Hopkins Hospital, followed by two years with the US

Public Health Service as a Research Fellow in the Department of Virology at the University of Pennsylvania.

In 1953, he joined the staff of the New York Hospital as Assistant Resident in Medicine, and later Chief Resident, and on completion of his residency, began a distinguished career as a practicing physician and faculty member at the New York Hospital and Cornell University Medical College. In 1986, he was named the Irene F. and I. Roy Psaty Distinguished Professor of Clinical Medicine, and later held the William T. Foley Distinguished Professorship in Clinical Medicine. A man of great energy, he was the author or co-author of almost 100 contributions to the medical literature.

Dr. Barondess had played leading roles in some of the major national medical organizations. He served as President of the American College of Physicians in 1977–1978 and took pride in his success in directing that organization to a new emphasis on health policy and in getting the various medical subspecialty societies to work together.

He served as President of the American Osler Society and of Alpha Omega Alpha, the honorary medical society, and was a charter member of the Institute of Medicine of the National Academy of Sciences. There he chaired committees on alternatives to the medical negligence system and on medical technology assessment. A member of Phi Beta Kappa and Alpha Omega Alpha, he has received many honors. Among his closest friends, was Dr. David E. Rogers, whom he met while a student at Johns Hopkins.

With guidance from the Academy's counsel, Dr. Cherkasky negotiated a contract for the first five years of Dr. Barondess's Presidency which was ultimately unanimously approved by the Board of Trustees at its meeting of March 28, 1990. It stipulated that Dr. Barondess could continue to be involved in the academic community, but it was understood that he would give up his practice and his faculty chair and devote full-time to the Academy. It was agreed that other than in his participation in professional societies, any service on corporate or other boards of trustees would require "the advice and consent of the Board of Trustees."[2]

At the February 8, 1990 meeting of the Executive Committee, it has been recognized that the Academy's budget would have to be revised in light of the appointment of the new President and the need for additional staff for the newly-expanded office of the President, and, at a special meeting of the Board of Trustees on February 15, a supplemental allocation of $500,000 for the year 1990 was approved for that purpose. Later, on recommendation of the Committee on the Office of the President, chaired by Ms. Margaret Mahoney with Ms. Joyce Bove and Drs. Robert J Haggerty, Ralph A. O'Connell, John W. Rowe, and Thomas H. Meikle as members, it was agreed to commit an additional $5 million from the Academy's reserves to support the new structure over the next five years. This would dictate a full appraisal of the Academy's current activities. It would also cover the organization of a "convocation" in the fall at which the new President would be "appropriately unveiled to a new audience."

At the March 28 meeting of the Board of Trustees, at which the details of the agreement with Dr. Barondess were approved, he thanked the Board of Trustees for their confidence in him and indicated his strong belief in the enormous potential of the Academy. He said that he had been meeting with senior staff and had been looking into issues relating to medical education, urban health, medical ethics, biomedical research in New York City, and maternal and child health, and was very excited about the challenge he was undertaking. He indicated that he was supporting Dr. Rowe in preparation of a proposal to the Carnegie Corporation of New York for a study of the status of biomedical research in New York City based on findings indicating that research funding appeared to be shrinking. Dr. Barondess also reported that he was interviewing candidates for a Vice-president for Programs and a capital campaign manager, and announced that Dr. David E. Rogers had agreed to serve as Senior Advisor to the Academy to provide guidance on "program development and grant support."[2]

On June 11, 1990, Dr. Barondess convened a group of advisors at the Academy for a meeting to discuss future program possibilities. Participants included: Drs. D.A. Henderson, Dean of the Johns Hopkins School of Hygiene and Public Health; Stephen C.

Joseph, former New York City Commissioner of Health; Nathan G. Kase, President of the Associated Medical Schools of New York and Dean of the Mount Sinai School of Medicine; Paul Marks, President of the Memorial Sloan-Kettering Cancer Center; and David E. Rogers, Walsh McDermott University Professor of Medicine at the New York Hospital-Cornell Medical Center. Also present were: Reneé Fox, Professor of Sociology at the University of Pennsylvania; Gerald Laubach, Ph.D. President of Pfizer, Inc.; Mr. Laurance Rockefeller; and Bruce C. Vladeck, Ph.D. President of the United Hospital Fund. The Board of Trustees was represented by Drs. Martin Cherkasky, Bernard J. Pisani, Saul J. Farber, Paul D. Kligfield, Mary McLaughlin, and Mary Ann Payne. Seven observers from the Academy staff brought the total attendance to thirty-six. Extended discussion led to the conclusion that the future programmatic emphases of the Academy should be on urban health issues, medical education, health policy, and the health of the biomedical enterprise. In emphasizing issues of urban health, Dr. Barondess was echoing a recommendation of the Subcommittee of the Board of Trustees that had reviewed the mission of the Academy.

On assuming the Presidency, Dr. Barondess made presentations to each of the Standing Committees and to the Board of Trustees in which he discussed his plans.[3]

## THE BARONDESS AGENDA

Dr. Barondess outlined an agenda that would "be designed to lead to a substantial Academy program composed of multiple projects." It would include the 1990 Annual Health Conference sponsored by the Committee on Medicine in Society on *The Changing Agenda for Health Care in the Nation's Cities,* that would be followed by another in 1991 to be sponsored by the same Committee that would address *Pediatric Poverty and Health.* Additional efforts would deal with the problems of the municipal hospitals with particular emphasis on the affiliation contracts of the medical schools, with AIDS, and with the "precursors of major urban health problems such as substance abuse, sexually transmitted diseases and teenage pregnancy." Health policy projects and other areas to be considered included a one-day meeting on the genome project, and a meeting on the impact of New York State's new regulations on the hours of service and the supervision of hospital residents.

Dr. Barondess separated medical education programs from continuing education in clinical care. Under the former he cited a program to assist advisors of college premedical students in improving their counseling on careers in medicine. Under the latter, he spoke of continuing education programs for physicians that would address "cutting edge issues in bioscience and medicine."

## THE PRESIDENTIAL CONVOCATION

On October 18, 1990, a convocation was held to celebrate the inauguration of Dr. Barondess. Hosack Hall was full for this occasion as Fellows eagerly awaited word on the new directions the Academy would take. In opening the session, Chairman Martin Cherkasky described the origins and growth of the Academy. Although, he said, the Academy had been true to its goals of working to improve the health of the public, providing valuable educational experiences to the profession, and more specifically in working to foster public health activities, recent years seen the emergence of

massive problems in the distribution of medical care, with efforts to contain the ever-rising costs of health care, with the unsatisfactory health statistics of our country, particularly in our large urban centers, and with major shifts in the causes of disability and death, . . . . especially, and sadly, concentrated in our great cities. These causes include . . . expressions of urban malaise, such as substance abuse, teenage pregnancy, violence, and AIDS.[4]

Dr. Cherkasky said that it was in response to these problems that the reorganization of the Academy was undertaken by its Board of

Trustees "to move aggressively into the fields of urban health, health policy, medical education, and public health." He devoted a substantial portion of his address to the selection of Dr. Barondess as President: "The New York Academy of Medicine is fortunate to have this great new opportunity to make new contributions to this great City and to the State of New York. We are also fortunate to have as our first President in this new era a man of Dr. Barondess' intelligence, drive, and dedication."[4]

Dr. Louis Sullivan, US Secretary of Health and Human Services was the major speaker. He noted that he had received his training in internal medicine at New York Hospital-Cornell Medical Center and that he had in the process "learned a great deal from Dr. Barondess."

The message he delivered on behalf of the Bush administration was one of concern for the health problems of urban areas, including AIDS and drug abuse. Dr. Sullivan reported with pride that President Bush and he had asked Congress for the "largest increase in Head Start funding in history," and pledged that he would continue the expansion of Medicaid to cover more people with incomes as high as 185 percent of the federal poverty level, then ineligible for Medicaid. The Department of Health and Human Services, he reported, was undertaking a study of public and private health and long-term care financing whose goal was to make "access to care easier, control costs, maintain quality, and increase personal responsibility in promoting health and preventing disease."[5]

Dr. Barondess's response, entitled *The New York Academy of Medicine: Prospects and Opportunities,* compared and contrasted differences in the relevant "terrain" at the time of the Academy's founding and 1990.[6] The major agents of change leading to greater complexity included: "First, medicine has become enormously more effective, chiefly because of the development of a genuine research capacity that has given clinical care a scientific base for the first time in history. . . . ." The second change involves "the distribution, the availability, of the capacities of modern health care to our population" which raises questions of "finding equity in our social structure as it targets health care." The third change relates to the fact that "health care has become exceedingly expensive." With health care spending then at 12.5 percent of the gross national product, and projections showing that costs would approach $1 trillion in the year 2000, government would be forced to make major efforts to contain costs.[6]

The issues before medicine, he said, reveal that there are "multiple parties at interest." The situation can be described a "triangular field: at one angle of the triangle lie biomedical science, technology, and health care; at the second are social justice, equity, and the necessity of a moral basis for the manner in which we deploy our resources; and at the third are found the influences exerted by law and public policy." The analogy of the triangle emphasized the fact that a problem at one angle of the triangle will inevitably affect and be affected by the others. Selection of items for the future agenda of the Academy, Dr. Barondess said, "would be based on a set of clear parameters: they should be meaningful, that is, they should have some capacity, if moved in the direction of resolution, to improve the status quo; they should be 'doable,' capable, with appropriate inputs of energy and imagination, of coming to reasonable fruition; they should be drawn from a broad interpretation of our mission, enhancing the health of the public, seen as extending from basic biomedical research at the one extreme, through clinical investigation, patient care, and public health activities, to health policy formulation and execution at the other; and they should represent a mixture of cooperative efforts with elements of both the public and private sectors."[7] The agenda would address four major areas: recruiting and educating for the health professions; urban health; the health of the medical enterprise itself; and the medicine/science/society interface. He then enumerated a series of future projects, some of which were already underway.

Dr. Barondess quoted one of the Latin inscriptions on the facade of the Academy building, "He who shall be born a thousand ages hence will not be barred from his opportunity of adding something further," and concluded, "We are not barred either. I believe that, with the help of the Academy Fellowship, of the public and private sector elements addressing broad issues in health, and of the public, the Board of Trustees and staff of The New York Academy of Medicine can give new expression to those words."[8]

## THE NEW MANAGEMENT TEAM

Dr. Thomas Q. Morris, who would continue as Clinical Professor of Medicine at the Columbia University College of Physicians and Surgeons, was appointed Vice President for Programs. Dr. David E. Rogers, University Professor of Medicine at Cornell University Medical College and former President of the Robert Wood Johnson Foundation joined the staff as Senior Advisor, and Mr. Steven Pelovitz, a lawyer who was formerly chief of staff of the New Jersey State Department of Human Services and a former official of the Federal Health Care Financing Administration, was appointed Vice President for Fiscal Affairs and Management. It was noted that, in addition to his expertise in management and finance, Mr. Pelovitz had extensive experience in health policy formulation and implementation which would be particularly beneficial in the Academy setting. Mr. Daniel Ehrlich, the Business Manager, was invited to remain in that position, but he elected to retire.

## THE NEW BOARD OF TRUSTEES

The first action at the meeting of the new Board of Trustees on January 24, 1992 was the election of the slate of officers proposed by Dr. Mary Ann Payne as Chair of the Nominating Committee: Dr. Martin Cherkasky as Chair; Ms. Margaret Mahoney as Vice-Chair; Dr. Robert J. Haggerty as Secretary; and Dr. Ralph O'Connell as Treasurer.

The Board of Trustees agreed to postpone any changes in the structure and membership of the standing committees pending the installation of the new President. They also reaffirmed the charges to these committees. They authorized the Executive Committee to approve statements on behalf of the Academy when circumstances precluded waiting for action by the full Board, and left unchanged the procedures for the election of new Fellows and the designation of recipients of Honorary Fellowships and the Academy awards and fellowships.

## THE BOARD RETREAT

Early in January 1993, after the newly elected Trustees were seated, the Board of Trustees and the senior staff of the Academy held a two-day retreat to "address the Academy's mission, scope of activities, governance and financing."[9] Preparatory materials were made available prior to the retreat, at which discussions ranged widely over the changes that had been taking place in the two and a half years since the reorganization and those that were in progress; amendments of the By-laws that would be required; and long-term financial and capital needs. As intended, the resultant specific recommendations and actions were developed through explorations and discussions during the following year.[10] To facilitate and focus these discussions, Chairman Dr. Farber appointed an Ad Hoc Committee on the Retreat which he would chair and whose members were Ms. Margaret Mahoney, Mr. Theodore Sorenson and Drs. Margaret C. Heagarty, Charles Hirsch, Ralph A. O'Connell, and Jeremiah A. Barondess (ex officio). The results that eventuated were overwhelmingly approved by the Fellows at the Annual Business Meeting of December, 1993.

One item that received attention was the role of the President in priority setting and as spokesperson for the Academy. It had been the practice, for the most part, for formal statements addressed to the public and developed by a relevant unit of the Academy, to go for review by the Board of Trustees in a timely manner, and then be forwarded to the President for dissemination. Dr. Barondess reported that, on a number of occasions, he had received inquiries about the Academy's position on a particular issue that had not yet been reviewed by the Board of Trustees, and when there was no time to formally solicit their views. On such occasions, particularly when the matter was sensitive or controversial, he said, he consulted with the Chairman of the Board before responding.

Dr. Barondess noted that statements might occasionally be issued by entities working under the aegis of the Academy such as the Council of the Directors of the Designated AIDS Centers. These groups could speak in their own name, with a clear indication that, although the group might meet at the Academy, it did not speak for it.

Mr. Sorensen called to mind instances when the President is called to testify before legislative or other public bodies. Here, he said, the Board of Trustees must be given an opportunity either to have some input or at least to review what is proposed to said in the name of the Academy. Dr. Barondess indicated that this is way such situations were handled.

The upshot of these discussions was an agreement on the relationships among the President, the Board of Trustees and the public. The Board of Trustees, it was decided, should appoint the President, set policy for the Academy and assure its proper implementation, and exercise fiduciary responsibility. The President should serve as Chief Executive Officer, act as chief spokesman, manage activities of the Academy, and report on progress to the Board of Trustees.[10] In essence, this agreement ratified the existing practices and was an expression of support for the work of Dr. Barondess and his leadership team.

The discussion also clarified the issue of setting program priorities. Priorities, it was said, might not necessarily be determined by the issues themselves but rather by the feasibility of the program or its mode of operation. It went on to say, "A further consideration is that not everything needs to be prioritized against the same set of criteria, or necessarily by the same groups. Thus, projects originated by or occurring in the Library or in the Sections, or in the structure of research fellowships and awards, need not meet standards that might apply to issues in health policy. Matters pertaining to health policy should be explored with the Board of Trustees as appropriate, preferably early. A procedure that is satisfying to all in each instance may not be possible."[10]

One of the results of the retreat was the development of a list of requests from the Board of Trustees for analyses and possible actions by the staff. Many of these related to internal structure and function issues. They included recommendations for setting the cost of Life fellowship and establishing a new fee structure; criteria for new categories of membership such as medical students, resident physicians, individuals affiliated with academic institutions and learned societies, international corresponding Fellows and Honorary Fellowships; changes in the size of committees and the terms of service on them with explanation of the benefits of any proposed changes; potential cost savings through changes in such operational items as telephone usage, elevators, engineering survey, utility rates, and investment advisory fees; the advisability of a change of address; the solicitation and handling of testamentary gifts; links with the New York Public Library; and mechanisms to encourage greater involvement by the Fellows in Academy activities. Finally, there was a request for a review of current health care reform proposals as they relate to urban health.

## NEW SECTIONS

In 1993, two additional Sections were added to the programs of the Academy: one on Emergency Medicine and the other on Nuclear Medicine. Emergency Medicine, it was said, was "at the center of urban health care issues because it epitomizes many of the problems inherent in urban health care. Individuals without adequate access to health care utilize Emergency Rooms for basic health care, although care could be more effectively and efficiently delivered in other ambulatory care facilities. Additionally, trauma, due especially to violence, makes heavy demands on emergency rooms, making it both costly and difficult to deliver other emergency services."[11] The rationale for the Section on Nuclear Medicine, it was stated, was its status as a rapidly growing field of practice which had seen dramatic innovations in technology that had revolutionized the diagnosis and treatment of many disorders.

## ACADEMY FINANCES

In 1993, Mr. Pelovitz left the Academy and was replaced by Ms. Patricia Volland, who had been trained as a social worker, but also had an M.B.A. degree. She had been Director of Social Work at the Johns Hopkins Hospital in Baltimore and, before coming to the Academy, had been Vice-President for Management at the Long Island College Hospital in Brooklyn.

At the end of that year, Ms. Tova D. Friedler was appointed Director of Development. She was assigned responsibility for writing funding proposals, drafting the annual report, and preparing informational newsletters. An experienced development officer, she was asked to revivify and professionalize these affairs at the Academy. Over the next two years, she succeeded in intrducing the Academy programs to a range of new funders, among them Mr. Samuel Jacobs, whose grant provided the computer center that enhanced the ability of the public to research health questions in the Library, and Mrs. Geraldine Coles, who donated the collection of gold medals depicting the history of the Jewish people to the Academy. In addition, Ms. Friedler initiated the series of annual galas that produce substantial support of the operating budget.

## ACADEMY PUBLICATIONS

*Bulletin of the New York Academy of Medicine*

In 1993, with the retirement of Dr. William D. Sharpe after fifteen years as Editor, the Bulletin was revamped to become the *Bulletin of the New York Academy of Medicine: A Journal of Urban Health,* a publication dealing with both clinical and policy issues in that important arena. Initially, there would be only two numbers a year but, to make up for the reduction in the number of issues, arrangements were made to send the Fellows and other subscribers copies of the excellent *Newsletter* produced by the United Hospital Fund.

Dr. Robert J. Haggerty, an active Fellow of the Academy, a Trustee and the retired President of the William T. Grant Foundation, was named the new Editor with the understanding that he would work from his retirement home in Rochester, N.Y. A new nationally drawn Editorial Board was appointed; it included Robert Blendon, Sc.D., Karen Davis, Ph.D., David Mechanic, Ph.D., Susan Wolf, J.D., and Drs. David Blumenthal, Christine Cassell, Bernard Guyer, Margaret A. Hamburg, and Philip R. Lee.

In his first issue, Dr. Haggerty announced that the Bulletin will serve as a vehicle for articles relevant to urban health issues which

have both a clinical and a policy focus. For instance, large urban areas, such as New York City, Los Angeles, Chicago, and San Francisco, are the epicenters of the AIDS epidemic, the problems revolving around resurgent tuberculosis and resistant bacterial strains connected with it, substance abuse, violence, and injuries. We intend to publish articles relevant to the clinician dealing with these new or re-emergent clinical health problems. At the same time, there are special, although not unique, health policy issues related to urban populations: the large number of uninsured, problems in dealing with multiple cultures and languages of immigrant populations, the larger role of the public hospitals and public health departments, and the special needs for outreach and follow-up for disadvantaged populations. It is clear that urban health issues are complicated especially by the high frequency of social problems: poverty, violence, substance abuse, and cultural diversity. These considerations only emphasize the point that all medicine must integrate biological and social factors into patient care more than was done in the past.[12]

## THE LIBRARY

As noted earlier, due largely to concern over its impact on Academy expenditures, the Board of Trustees appointed a Committee to Study the Library, chaired by Dr. Vartan Gregorian, President of the New York Public Library, that was charged to produce a report that defined "a mission and program in order to develop a five and ten year strategic plan."[13] At the suggestion of Dr. Gregorian, the

Committee engaged a panel of expert library consultants which included Richard De Gennaro from the New York Public Library; Jay W. Lucker from the Massachusetts Institute of Technology; Patricia Battin from the Columbia University Libraries and the Commission on Preservation and Access; Donald Lindberg from the National Library of Medicine; and Richard A. Lyders from the Houston Academy of Medicine/Texas Medical Center Library.

The consultants visited the Library on July 30–31, 1990. They noted that it was one of the world's largest current and historical biomedical collections, with more than fourteen miles of shelved materials, including 680,000 catalogued works and 275,000 illustrations and portraits, supplemented by the Rare Book Room collection of some 49,000 volumes devoted to the history of medicine, science and other health-related disciplines. Approximiately 32,000 of these are raw materials dating from 1700 BC to 1800 AD, in which medical Americana and classic works in the history of Western European medicine and public health are especially well-represented. Primary source materials include over 2,000 manuscripts, photographs and artifacts, including the Edwin Smith Surgical Papyrus, which dates back to 1700 BC. Secondary sources include an extensive history of medicine reference collection and almost 100 subscriptions to current journals on the history of the health sciences. In addition, the collection also houses the archives of many health-related institutions and organizations, which serve as a primary resource for the history of health administration, public health, medical education and medical practice in New York.

The consultants felt that, in light of its mission, the Library was underfunded, particularly with respect to staff salaries and the need for computer equipment and software. In fact, they urged that construction of a new building be considered. They validated continuation of the Library's "leadership role" in the Regional Medical Library Program. As the only medical research library in New York City, they recommended expansion of services to the corporate community, but advised against the continued provision of consumer health information. That is a responsibility, they believed, that the public library system should undertake. They said that the historical collection should be maintained but not expanded, and suggested a major preservation effort for the nineteenth century materials.

In July 1990, Brett Kirkpatrick, the Librarian, left to become Director of the Library of the University of Texas Medical Branch in Galveston, and, in November, Ms. Anne Pascarelli, who had been appointed Acting Librarian, left to become Director of the Sheppard Library and Division of Instructional Resources at the Massachusetts College of Pharmacy and Allied Health Sciences in Boston. Mr. Arthur Downing was named Librarian. A summa cum laude graduate of Rutgers College with a Master of Library Services degree from Rutgers, he had joined the Library in 1985 as Head of the Bibliographic Services Unit. Because of his success in expanding the Library's fee-based research and document delivery services, he had been promoted to Associate Librarian in 1990. His expertise in managing information systems and databases represented a valuable asset.

The Library had pursued a policy of maintaining and enhancing its visibility in the library community by participating in consortia. Since 1966, for example, it had served as a medical information and referral resource in the New York State Interlibrary Loan Network and, in 1991, it joined METRO, the New York Metropolitan Reference and Research Agency. Also, since 1969, the Library had been awarded successive five-year contracts by the National Library of Medicine to serve as a Regional Medical Library, coordinating health science library resource sharing and providing on-line literature searching for librarians and health professionals in twenty-two eastern states. The most recent five-year contract for $5.5 million had been awarded in May 1991.

In 1990 the National Library of Medicine awarded a grant to the Library for the preservation department to remount the Edwin Smith Surgical Papyrus and to conserve forty-nine early American imprints. In 1991, the Library completed a two-year contract with the State of New York under which the Preservation Department completed a project to preserve the collection of almost 8,000 portraits of eminent physicians, in photographs, engravings and other prints. The Library also achieved its long-standing goal of putting its preservation efforts on a sound basis through a grant to establish the Gladys Brooks Book and Paper Conservation Laboratory in a large space on the fifth floor of the Academy Building. The room houses the equipment needed for rebinding books on the verge of disintegration and custom-building folders and boxes to house them. In addition to maintaining the Library's leadership in the conservation of priceless historical materials, the Laboratory provides training in the art and science of preservation.

After considerable deliberation at its meeting on March 20, 1991, the Board of Trustees unanimously approved the statement of directions for the future submitted by the Committee to Study the Library. It said that the Library should "preserve, enhance, and extend the historical collection and develop a programmatic effort within it; redefine the current core collection to support the mission and activities of the Academy; and continue and maintain the Regional Medical Library Program."[14] Further, in implementing this directive, the Library would "acquire core materials in clinical medicine and collect more comprehensively in areas corresponding to programs and interests of the Academy, such as urban health, medical education, health policy and the history of medicine. In order to insure access to a rapidly expanding body of medical literature with limited resources," the Library would work toward "toward greater sharing of resources among health science libraries as well as exploring electronic means of document retrieval."[15]

In 1992, the Library launched a Rare Book Adoption Program under which donors may underwrite the costs of conservation and cataloguing of particular items in the collection. In that same year, the Greenwall Foundation, whose President is William C. Stubing, the former Director of the Academy, funded a grant to the Academy to conserve the manuscript collections of three important figures in nineteenth century medicine: Frederick Dennis, Willard Parker and Lewis Albert Sayre. And, also in 1992, a generous bequest for the purchase of books on the history of medicine was received from the estate of Dr. Leonard Ciner.

During the same year, the Library initiated publication of the *Malloch Room Newsletter* to publicize the activities of the Rare Book Room to Fellows, Friends of the Rare Book Room and medical historians.

## Radium Samples

Among the historic artifacts in the Library collection, were fifteen radium samples from the work of Drs. Marie Curie, and Robert Abbe. These had been stored in various spaces within the Academy, most recently in the basement of the Academy building, and concern had arisen over the possibility that they had not been adequately shielded to eliminate the hazard of harmful radiation exposure. In September 1993, Dr. Barondess informed the Board of Trustees that these materials, which had never been properly displayed to the public, were being presented to the National Museum of American History of the Smithsonian Institution in Washington, DC. Arrangements for their transfer were handled by Dr. Thomas Q. Morris.

## The "Fellows' " Room (Hartwell Room)

In 1993, the Hartwell Room, also known as the "Fellows' " Room, which contains a 5,000 volume browsing collection on the history of medicine, was rededicated in a special ceremony that featured an address by William F. Bynum of the Wellcome Institute in London.

## THE COMMITTEE ON PUBLIC HEALTH

### Pregnancy and Substance Abuse

On March 22, 1990, as a follow-up to the statement issued in October 1989, the Committee on Public Health, in collaboration with the Medical and Health Research Association of New York City, the Columbia University School of Public Health, the Maternal and Child Health Program of the New York County Medical Society, the Greater New York March of Dimes, and the Agenda for Children Tomorrow, held a Symposium on *Pregnancy and Substance Abuse: Perspectives and Directions.* The program committee which arranged the symposium was chaired by Ms. Lucille Rosenbluth, President of the Medical and Health Research Association. In his introductory remarks, Dr. David Harris, Chairman of the Committee on Public Health and Commissioner of Health of Suffolk County, stated that the US standing in relation to infant mortality

has slipped to 20th place among the nations of the world. In large areas of our great cities, infant mortality rates are recorded which compare unfavorably with those of impoverished and underdeveloped nations. Explicable only as a lack of national will, the United States of America has failed to do what is commonplace in almost all other developed countries: we still do not guarantee each pregnant woman the prenatal and maternity services required for the successful outcome of her pregnancy.[16]

In her overview of the national policy perspective, Dr. Martha Falco, then a Visiting Fellow at the Cornell University Medical College, argued that the heavy reliance of the Reagan and Bush Administrations on the use of the criminal law strategy in the "War on Drugs" was not succeeding and that a greater emphasis on treatment is needed. "Experience of the past several decades," she said, "demonstrates that law enforcement as a dominant policy response has not succeeded in reducing drug abuse or drug related crime. Instead, the encouraging declines in overall drug use have resulted from personal health concerns and increased social disapproval of use."[17]

Following the Symposium, the Committee issued a statement on *Drug Use in Pregnancy: An Urgent Problem for New York City,* which recommended that experts be convened "to explore new approaches to the treatment of substance abuse during pregnancy and that these approaches be subject to rigorously designed clinical trials."[18] In addition, it was recommended that there be an increase in the number of treatment slots, greater publicity about the availability of services, amendments of State law to mandate the offering of preventive services to families where mothers are at risk of losing custody of their children because of drug abuse, and the development of training in parenting.

### The Committee as an Advocate

During 1990 and 1991, the Committee registered its views on a number of public health problems confronting the City. For example, in 1990, it conducted a workshop on drinking water quality in the greater New York area, and in 1991, it issued statements on *HIV Initiative in New York City Drug Treatment Settings* and on *Allowing Non-Prescription Possession and Sale of Hypodermic Needles and Syringes.* It addressed letters to key officials and organizations advocating increased access to maternal and child health services, to the *New York Times* pointing to the importance of social structures and community services as adjuncts to public housing, and to Peter Vallone, Speaker of the New York City Council, in support of the Tobacco Regulation Act.

### Tribute to Dr. David Axelrod

On October 23, 1991, a symposium to honor Dr. David Axelrod, the former Commissioner of Health of the State of New York, was held by the Academy with co-sponsorship by the New York State Department of Health and the Josiah Macy, Jr., Foundation. Originally Director of the Laboratory of the State Department of Health, Dr. Axelrod had served as Commissioner since 1979, almost thirteen years, before being stricken by a massive stroke and prolonged disability which forced him to relinquish his position as the leading public health official in the State and probably in the nation.

Through all these years, his powerful and controversial leadership epitomized New York State's approach to health: strong direction, a high degree of regulation, and concern for the disadvantaged. He served two Governors, Hugh Carey and Mario Cuomo, and was a brilliant and committed public servant who earned an enviable reputation for his unimpeachable integrity and his patience in withstanding attacks on positions he had taken in the public interest.

Throughout Dr. Axelrod's career with the State Department of Health he had a particularly warm relationship with the Academy. Unlike the Medical Society of the State of New York, which attacked his positions on more than one occasion, the Academy had been supportive of many of Dr. Axelrod's initiatives. He was always willing to meet with Academy committees and to address Academy meetings, and there were many instances in which the Academy and the State Department of Health collaborated in joint programs. On a personal level, he was gracious to Academy Fellows and staff, and his capacity for friendship was legendary. The symposium, presided over by Dr. Alfred Gellhorn, his close associate, was marked by presentations from many of Dr. Axelrod's colleagues at the Health Department.

On behalf of the Academy Board of Trustees, Fellows and staff, Dr. Thomas Q. Morris presented a citation to Dr. Axelrod which read, "His career has been marked by intellectual brilliance, forthrightness and courage. . . . Under his leadership, the Department of Health has introduced important initiatives bearing on the control of health care costs, improving access to health care, monitoring health care quality, and the conditions of postgraduate medical education." The citation also mentioned Dr. Axelrod's commitment to the struggle against HIV infection and his initiatives to broaden access to health care for all New Yorkers.[19]

## Noise and Health

In 1991, the Committee published a monograph on noise and health, edited by Thomas Fay, Ph.D., Professor of Clinical Audiology and Speech-Language Pathology in the Department of Otolaryngology at the Columbia University College of Physicians and Surgeons and Director of the Speech and Hearing Department at the Columbia-Presbyterian Medical Center.[20] The monograph presented a comprehensive review of the world literature on the subject of the effects of noise on health. In an age of heavily amplified music, chain saws, leaf blowers and the din of traffic, the monograph focused attention on a frequently overlooked health hazard. Of special relevance was the discussion of workplace exposures to noise and the prevention of occupational hearing loss.

## Testing Health Professionals for HIV/AIDS

In 1991, the Committee convened the deans of the medical schools in the New York area and the presidents of the major New York City teaching hospitals in a meeting to challenge a ruling, proposed by the Centers for Disease Control, that would require all health workers to be tested for HIV/AIDS. From their discussion, a Statement was developed which emphasized that the risk of contracting the HIV/AIDS virus from diseased health professionals is minimal.[21] It said that functionally impaired physicians should be withdrawn from the care of patients regardless of the cause of their impairment, and stressed that the testing of health professionals would only deflect attention from the real risks of HIV infection: casual sexual relations and intravenous drug use. The Statement was published in the *Journal of the American Medical Association*[22] and played an important role in persuading the Centers for Disease Control to reconsider and ultimately withdraw this proposal. Dr. Barondess also testified on this subject before the New York State AIDS Commission, the National AIDS Commission, and a committee of the Office of Technology Assessment of the US Congress.

In 1991, the Academy, under Dr. Rogers's leadership, organized two Councils for discussion of HIV/AIDS issues: one involved the Directors of the AIDS Designated Care Centers of New York State;

and the other involved individuals engaged in basic research on HIV/AIDS. These have continued to meet to the present time.

## Sexual Abstention in the Prevention of AIDS

On September 3, 1992, Dr. Barondess sent a letter to the President of the Board of Education of the City of New York regarding its requirement that teachers sign an oath pledging emphasis on abstention in instruction regarding the prevention of HIV infection and AIDS. The letter acknowledged that

> no one argues that sexual abstinence is not the most effective way to prevent acquisition of the infection. At the same time, abundant evidence indicates that most of our adolescents are sexually active. Whatever any of us believes about the appropriateness, morality or degree of responsibility with which adolescent sexual activity is undertaken, we cannot escape the fact that it occurs. We owe to these young people the clearest, the most authoritative public health advice we can possibly mobilize, delivered so as to be most likely to engage their thoughtful consideration. Tying efforts to deliver scientific fact and dispassionate advice to morality places at substantial risk the relevance of our educational and public health programs in connection with HIV infection and threatens to truncate efforts to fortify our young people with enough information to protect themselves.[23]

## Tuberculosis

A major effort by the Committee on Public Health in 1992 dealt with a response to the reemergence of tuberculosis as a major threat to the health of the people of the City. There had been a threefold increase in cases of TB since 1980, with 4,500 cases in 1991. Many of the persons infected had contracted a multidrug resistant form of the disease and many cases were found in persons whose immune systems had been compromised by HIV infection.

The Committee conducted two courses on clinical and epidemiological aspects of tuberculosis, with more than 500 health care persons in attendance. In addition, the Committee sought to inform the public about the nature of the disease, its clinical manifestations, methods of transmission and modes of detection, extent of communicability, and means of prevention and treatment. With financial support from the New York State Department of Health, the Committee staff published 12,000 copies of a poster detailing this information in English, Chinese, Haitian French and Spanish. The posters were circulated to libraries, prisons, health clinics, religious institutions and other sites within the city.

A subcommittee chaired by David J. Rothman, Ph.D., of Columbia University, examined the idea of developing a hospital dedicated exclusively to serving tuberculosis patients. It concluded that it would be more cost-effective for tuberculosis patients to be treated in general hospitals.

The Subcommittee also explored the issue of confining in secure settings noncompliant tuberculous patients who failed to follow the regimens recommended for the treatment of their disease. "The threat that noncompliance poses to the public health, in terms of both the spread of the disease and the proliferation of multi-drug-resistant strains, is so great as to justify a curtailment of liberty," it said. The findings were included in a special report published by the United Hospital Fund.[24] Following the publication of this report, the Academy presented testimony to the Board of Health endorsing an amendment to the New York City Health Code that would allow the Department of Health to physically detain persons with tuberculosis who remain noncompliant and a range of interventions has proved to be unsuccessful. At the same time, it was emphasized that the civil rights of these recidivist patients should be protected.

In addition, the Academy, in collaboration with the Centers for Disease Control and the New York City Health and Hospitals Corporation, undertook efforts to ensure uniform collection of data on tuberculosis testing, made contact with the US Food and Drug Administration urging the accelerated development of new anti-tuberculosis drugs and new dosage and delivery forms, joined the American Lung Association and other organizations in urging additional funding for tuberculosis control, and participated in the National Coalition to Eliminate Tuberculosis.

## "Urgent Issues in Public Health"

The 1992 Anniversary Discourse, *Urgent Issues in Public Health,* was delivered by Dr. Margaret A. Hamburg, Commissioner of Health of the City of New York.[25] She painted a picture of progress in advancing medical knowledge and technology in the face of daunting threats to health from poverty, shortages of health workers, poor distribution of health services, and growing rates of violence. "Our gaps in knowledge about what works in health education and why are severely compromising our battle against major illnesses," she said. "Many of our most serious diseases are associated with such behavioral risk factors as smoking, alcohol and other substance abuse, poor nutrition, high-risk sexual behavior, and violent behavior." She concluded by noting that "perhaps the greatest threat for potential spread of undetected or previously insignificant disease-causing organisms to take hold and produce disease is complaisance about such public health practices and interventions as immunization, sanitation, and infection-control measures. For whatever reasons, it is clear that the pattern of emerging new diseases—infectious, environmental or other—is not likely to go away. If anything, it will worsen due to the increasing mobility and complexity of modern life. A better understanding of these issues and concerns—from basic science to practical intervention—clearly must be part of the public health agenda in the future."

## COMMITTEE ON MEDICINE IN SOCIETY

### Commission on the Future of Child Health in New York City

In 1989, the last year of his third term, Mayor Edward I. Koch, responding to a recommendation from Health Commissioner Dr.

Stephen Joseph, created the Commission on the Future of Child Health in New York City. It was chaired by Dr. Robert J. Haggerty, President of the William T. Grant Foundation, a Trustee of the Academy and a member of the Committee on Medicine in Society. It became apparent after the report was completed that the administration was having second thoughts about having it published but, in August 1989, it was leaked to the press. It said, "some of the most pressing health problems affecting New York City today are related to social, environmental, family and psychological factors. . . . The child health 'system' has not responded well to the new health problems of increasing social morbidity and poverty because of financial barriers for the uninsured, fragmentation and duplication in services, and insufficient comprehensive programs."[26]

While suggesting that "health services cannot cure the social conditions that are affecting health," the report held that "comprehensive health services can reduce the damaging consequences of poverty by identifying health and behavioral problems early, treating them appropriately and providing support and guidance to families. An improved child health system would provide poor and near-poor children with easy access to a range of health and social services that can make a major difference in their lives." The Commission recommended that a new entity in the Mayor's Office be created to try "to overcome fragmentation of health services, end competition among agencies and improve planning" with leadership from the Department of Health, the Health and Hospitals Corporation, the Board of Education and other constituencies.

The Committee established a subcommittee, chaired by Dr. James Curtis, Chairman of the Department of Psychiatry at the Harlem Hospital Center, to study the report. The Subcommittee endorsed the concept of a "Council on Child Health" in the Mayor's Office and recommended that it be seen as more than advisory and be given authority over health resource allocation. "The Council should be provided with a per capita allocation of funds based on the number of children in the City as a regular appropriation to support its planning and development function," the Subcommittee recommended, and it should "seek waiver authority from the federal Government to achieve greater flexibility in the allocation of resources for child health services."[27]

## Commission on Biomedical Research and Development

In 1991, prompted by a perceived decline in government funding and private support for biomedical research in the New York area, and having obtained the requisite funding from the Carnegie Corporation of New York and the New York Community Trust, the Academy established the Commission on Biomedical Research and Development. It was chaired by Dr. John W. Rowe, President of the Mount Sinai Medical Center and a member of the Board of Trustees, and co-chaired by Dr. Barondess; the members of its executive committee included representatives from the biomedical research community, universities and medical schools, pharmaceutical and other biotechnology firms, leaders in the banking and real estate industries, and State and City officials. Barbara Cutler, J.D., Director of Public Affairs and Assistant Director of Business Development at the law firm Kaye Scholer Fierman Hays and Handler, was appointed Executive Director.

Initial areas of study included recruiting and retention of faculty; promoting university/industry relationships to support research; a study by the Mount Sinai School of Medicine which examined the transfer of technology from academia to industry; and a study supported by the Commonwealth Fund which examined the attitudes of biomedical scientists toward working in the City.[28]

Perhaps most significant was a critical analysis of the economic impact of biomedical research in the New York metropolitan area conducted by Nancy Aries, Ph.D., of the Baruch College of the City University of New York, and Elliott D. Sclar, Ph.D. of the Graduate School of Architecture, Planning and Preservation of Columbia University.

Drs. Aries and Sclar had conducted an earlier study in 1990, on behalf of the Greater New York Hospital Association Foundation, which examined the funding of biomedical research in New York City from 1970 to 1987 using the growth rate of the budget of the National Institutes Of Health (NIH) as a benchmark. Although New York institutions had received increases in NIH funding during that period, the increments were consistently smaller than the growth of the NIH budget. They found that, if New York City had kept pace with this measure, more than $108 million in additional funding would have been received in the City in 1987 alone.[29]

The new study was intended to determine whether this disturbing trend was continuing and to expand the area covered by it to include the seventeen county regional New York-New Jersey biomedical complex developed by the Port Authority of New York & New Jersey. The report indicated that "the health care industry is the major employer in New York City, accounting for 17% of the labor force," and playing an important role in this industry was biomedical research; in this regard New York was second only to Boston.[30] The authors suggested that biomedical research not only had a major economic impact in the region, but that "there is a strong correlation between the quality of care, the competence of the care givers and the presence of a robust medical research enterprise."

The report described the substantial economic impact of the research effort in the voluntary sector: $1.15 billion per year in direct spending with over $1 billion in total wages and salaries; some 32,600 regional jobs, including indirect and induced job creation; and about $61 million of various forms of tax revenues generated as a result of biomedical research in the region.

The disturbing aspect of the study was that the New York region was seen as "a pre-eminent locus of biomedical research" but, if long-term trends were to continue, the region would fall behind. Between 1980 and 1987 total funding by the National Institutes of Health finding grew by 21 percent but its allocations to the New York City area only increased by 6 percent in contrast to 29 percent for Boston. This decline was partially offset by an increase in funding for research in drug abuse and AIDS from the Alcohol, Drug Abuse, and Mental Health Administration. Only four other major metropolitan regions had growth rates that were slower than New York's: Chicago, New Haven, Madison, Wisconsin, and Rochester, Minnesota. The picture within New York City proper was worse than that for the region as a whole.

To improve New York's performance in research and technology, the Commission advised, efforts would have to be made to deal with the problem of rapidly rising laboratory and maintenance costs, and the very high housing costs and other features of living in New York that discourage the recruitment of investigators.

On the recommendation of the Report, a Council on Biomedical Research and Development was established in 1995 as a permanent independent body to bring biomedical research interests, industry, governmental agency and other business leaders together to coordinate planning for a more effective response to the problem. The Council, housed in the Academy, is co-chaired by Drs. Barondess and Rowe. Its Executive Director is Mr. Robert M. Schiffer, principal of the consulting firm of RMS Associates and former Executive Vice President and Director of Special Projects of the Governor's Business Advisory Board. The Executive Committee includes the deans of local medical schools, hospital executives, leaders in commerce and industry and City officials. Its primary funding initially came from New York State supplemented by the dues paid by its members (medical schools, health science centers, free-standing research enterprises, pharmaceutical firms, etc.); efforts are being made to obtain contributions from individuals and foundations. On March 21, 1996, the Council sponsored the first annual symposium on technology transfer and intellectual properties, hosted by the Academy. It has also developed, in conjunction with KPMG-Peat Marwick Health Services Group, the Contract Research Organization for Mega Clinical Trials. Having completed a marketing study, a business plan for this organization is under development.

## The Human Genome Project

With the intent of examining the policy implications and potential impact of federally funded "big science" decisions, the Academy, in April 1991, conducted a major symposium on *The Human Genome Project: Science and Public Priorities*. The aim was to consider the monetary and social costs as well as the impact on investigator-initiated research projects. The program was moderated by Dean Leon E. Rosenberg of the Yale University School of Medicine, who saw the genome project "as another significant step in understanding human variations and their implications for health and disease."[31] The faculty of nationally known experts in the relevant fields included: science policy—James Watson, Ph.D., the Nobel Laureate from Cold Spring Harbor Laboratory, and Dr. Bernard Davis of the Harvard Medical School; social policy—Mr. George Annas, an attorney from the Boston University School of Medicine who had achieved prominence for his writings on bioethical issues, and Ms. Dorothy Nelkin, a sociologist at New York University; public policy—Mr. Mark A. Rothstein, a lawyer at the Health Law and Policy Institute at University of Houston, and Dr. Troyan Brennan, a health policy expert at the Harvard Medical School. The Conference summarizer was William C. Richardson, Ph.D., President of the Johns Hopkins University. The sessions focused on the science, social and public policy implications of the Human Genome Project, notably the potential abuse of genetic screening; it also touched on such issues in medical ethics as the use of animals in research, and the role of public support for medical education, basic and clinical research.[32]

## Human Rights Controversies

In 1991, Dr. Victor Sidel, Professor of Community Medicine at the Albert Einstein College of Medicine and Montefiore Medical Center, brought a controversial issue relating to an alleged threat to human rights before the Committee on Medicine in Society.

The Kansas State Board of Trustees of the Healing Arts, the state's licensing authority, had received a complaint regarding Dr. Yolanda Huet-Vaughan, a physician in the army reserve, who had refused to respond to orders requiring her to go with her unit to Saudi Arabia to take part in Operation Desert Storm. She had been convicted by a military court martial and was serving a sentence in a military prison. The pending proceedings before the Kansas Board could lead to the loss of her license to practice as a civilian.

After the Committee voted unanimously to consider the issue, Chairman Dr. Eugene Feigelson appointed a Subcommittee on Human Rights. with Dr. Peter Rogatz as Chair and Drs. Robert J. Haggerty, Michael R. McGarvey and Edmund Rothschild as members. Their report was presented at the April 20, 1992 meeting of the Committee.[33]

The issue as seen by the Subcommittee, was whether, assuming the appropriateness of the court martial verdict finding her guilty of disobeying a military order, her conduct was such as to warrant discipline by the state medical licensing authorities. The Subcommittee noted the increasing sensitivity of the Academy to human rights issues in the United States and elsewhere throughout the world, especially in the former Soviet Union. They recalled that, on a few occasions, the Council had been critical of abuse of the human rights of physicians who were political dissidents in the Soviet Union.

They also noted that the Committee on Medicine in Society had been reviewing issues of physician discipline for some ten years and had supported the strengthening of disciplinary procedures against physician misconduct. They felt, however, that the evidence presented in this case, especially the testimony by military chaplains, that Dr. Huet-Vaughan's opposition to this particular war was motivated by political reasons or grounds of conscience and might, therefore, warrant military discipline, had no relevance to her ability to practice medicine as a civilian. The Subcommittee also recommended that such issues of human rights be considered an appropriate concern of the Academy.

At that meeting, Dr. Feigelson reported that, at an informal meeting with Drs. Jeremiah Barondess, Thomas Morris, Peter Rogatz, and Marvin Lieberman, Dr. Barondess had indicated that, although he was receptive to having the Academy respond to human rights concerns, the Academy did not have the resources to deal with the details of this type of case.

Nevertheless, the Committee did approve a statement which said, "We believe that before conviction of a crime or an offense should have any consequences for a physician's right to practice medicine, there should be a showing that the matter directly relates to fitness or competence to practice medicine in some substantial manner. We agree with the Supreme Court decision in recent licensure cases involving lawyers that there must be a rational connection between the conduct complained against and the fitness of the person to practice."

The Committee endorsed the Subcommittee's view that the procedure to suspend Dr. Huet-Vaughan's license was not warranted, and recommended that The Academy involve itself in her case. The Committee also recommendesd that an activity on human rights be adopted by the Academy, and that material on the human rights activities of other organizations be forwarded to the President and Board of Trustees.

Chairman Dr. Saul Farber appointed an ad hoc subcommittee of the Board of Trustees to deal with the issues. It was chaired by Dr. Charles Hirsch, the Chief Medical Examiner of the City of New York, and its members were Dr. Shervert Frazier of Maclean Hospital and former Executive Officer of the Academy, and Mr. Theodore Sorensen. They reviewed the Committee's statement and concluded that it was not feasible for the Academy to deal with individual cases. They did, however, recommend that "it is appropriate for the New York Academy of Medicine to become involved in human rights issues, with a perspective that allows the Academy to remain focused on major national and international issues relating primarily to the preservation of health and delivery of medical care."[34] They also suggested that,

Issues of human rights involving an individual are an appropriate focus for the attention and action of the New York Academy of Medicine when the rights of the individual have been or are about to be egregiously violated (e.g., denial of due process). In considering the commitment of resources, the New York Academy of Medicine should take into account the existence, adequacy, and impartiality of a local forum to redress an individual grievance. The Academy may also take into account whether an individual grievance is particularly disadvantaged by race sex, sexual orientation, religion, economic circumstances, ethnic enmity, age, disability or matter of conscience in such a way as to make the proceeding fundamentally unfair.

The Board of Trustees voted to accept the guideline suggested by the Ad hoc Committee with the modification that the Board could act with a simple plurality instead of the recommended two-thirds majority. It also requested the Committee on Medicine in Society to submit guidelines on the involvement of the Academy in human rights issues.[35]

## Pediatric Poverty

At the suggestion of President Barondess, the 1991 Annual Health Conference sponsored by the Committee on Medicine in Society addressed *Children at Risk: Pediatric Poverty and Health.* This was not the first Annual Health Conference on this topic; three years earlier, in 1988, the Committee had convened a conference on *Child Health: One Hundred Years of Progress and Today's Challenges.*[36] Nevertheless, because of his great concern about this problem, Dr. Barondess suggested that this issue be revisited, with particular attention to policy development, research priorities and advocacy relating to the myriad of issues raised by the health needs of children growing up in poverty. In addition, he expressed the hope that the Academy would "derive from the conference . . . an array of programs in the general area of pediatric poverty and health" which the Academy could carry forward over a substantial period of time.[37]

A feature of this Conference was the Duncan W. Clark Lecture delivered by Dr. David Ellwood, Professor of Public Policy at Harvard University's John F. Kennedy School of Government. Dr. Ellwood commented that, in addressing an Academy audience, he was following in the footsteps of his father, Dr. Paul Ellwood, who is credited with coining the term health maintenance organization, and who had addressed an Academy seminar sponsored some twenty years earlier by the Committee on Social Policy for Health Care. Prof. Ellwood, who was later to join the Clinton administration in 1993 as an Assistant Secretary in the Department of Health and Human Services, described the plight of the working poor who "unless they can find a full-time job that pays six or seven or eight dollars an hour, with full medical benefits, will be better off on welfare than working."[38] Dr. Ellwood recommended that one way of dealing with poverty among children is to guarantee medical care for everyone. In addition, he suggested expansion of the earned income tax credit which would provide a tax refund to all workers earning less than a minimum income and called for an increase in the minimum wage. For single parent families, he urged strengthening the enforcement of child support agreements and insurance to provide minimum child support benefits. The last would replace welfare benefits which are often so low that many recipients must cheat in order to survive.

After the conference, Dr. Barondess vigorously pressed the Academy staff for suggestions of programs that the Academy might introduce that might provide an adequate response to pediatric poverty. Among the responses was a recommendation by Dr. Jacqueline Messite for a program in which medical students would work on community health problems as volunteers. This, she suggested, not only might be a useful way to deal with the problem but it also might foster a sense of mission among future physicians to serve the disadvantaged. This suggestion was based on the long-standing program at Cornell University Medical College in which medical student volunteers spent time in the community visiting families and neighborhood centers to assist training individuals to receive and comply with health recommendations. After study of this model by the Academy's senior staff, it was felt that the idea was worthwhile—the Urban Health Corps was the result.[39]

## The Urban Health Corps

In April 1991, a meeting on *Medical Education and Community Service* was held at the Academy to present the concept of an Urban Health Corps to an audience that included persons from medical schools throughout the country. The notion of a corps of student volunteers aroused considerable enthusiasm.

Accordingly, Ms. Holly Michaels Fisher, the Academy's Director of Program Development, who had originally been hired to staff the Commission to Review the Health and Hospitals Corporation (*vide infra*), was directed to prepare a proposal for a program in which students at the ten metropolitan area medical schools would be encouraged to volunteer for community service, especially in the disadvantaged neighborhoods near their schools. The goals of the program were: to offer students opportunities to learn about community-based medical programs; provide needed services; and encourage students to develop a sense of obligation to meet social needs. The program would seek to foster collaboration among the schools, local government and community agencies, and the medical students, and would encourage the development of community projects. It was intended that the students' commitment and accomplishments would be appropriately recognized by their schools. An advisory group held meetings with students and faculty at a number of schools, and identified students who were interested in becoming involved and, with funding from the Fan Fox and Leslie R. Samuels Foundation, the program was formally launched in 1993.

Professional Discipline

In July 1993, in response to a request from the New York State Education Department for the Academy's opinion of its proposal to simplify the discipline of professions other than medicine in the State, President Baroness appointed an ad hoc committee consisting of Drs. Martin Cherkasky, Arthur Aufses, Jr. and Joseph Post, with Marvin Lieberman, Ph.D., as staff.

The Committee viewed the legislative proposal as a major improvement over the very complicated process currently employed in that it gave the Department of Health jurisdiction over the discipline of physicians and physician assistants. It recommended further simplification of the appeals process which still remained unduly complicated, urging that the appeal process for all licensed professionals (e.g., accountants, nurses, engineers, and architects) should be the same as that for physicians. The recommendations were accepted but the Legislature did not act on the Department of Education proposal.

## COMMITTEE ON MEDICAL EDUCATION

### Advising The Premedical Student

The 1980s had seen a decade-long decline in the number of applications to medical schools while hospitals were facing a shortage of nurses approaching crisis dimensions and the available pool of biomedical researchers was shrinking. As a first step to confront this problem, the Academy, in October 1991, convened a one-day symposium on *Advising the Premedical Student*. Partially funded by a grant from the Robert Wood Johnson Foundation, the Symposium was aimed at helping premedical advisers in undergraduate colleges to become more effective in encouraging promising students from diverse backgrounds to consider a career in medicine. The keynote speaker was Dr. Robert G. Petersdorf, President of the Association of American Medical Colleges, and a major address on *Managing the Costs of Medical Education* was presented by Robert L. Beran, Ph.D., Assistant Vice President of that organization. Other speakers included Drs. Alvin Tarlov of the New England Medical Center and the Harvard School of Public Health, Antoinette F. Hood of Johns Hopkins University, and Stephen R. Smith of the Brown University Program in Medicine, Ruby Hearn, Ph.D., of the Robert Wood Johnson Foundation, and three medical students who described in positive terms their experiences at medical school. The symposium attempted to "consider how to provide [college students] with realistic, up-to-date and objective information about getting into medical school, financing medical education, preparing themselves academically and trying to see what the world ahead is going to be like, not alone for physicians but for patients as well."[40] The proceedings were published in an attractive paperback book which had a wide distribution.[41]

## Associate Members-in-Training

In 1992, a new category of membership called "Associate Members-in-Training" was approved by the Board of Trustees. The privileges of this category of membership include subscriptions to the *Bulletin,* eligibility to attend Academy programs free of charge and use of the Library free of charge. Associate Members-in-Training are not eligible to vote or to hold office in the Academy, but are encouraged to participate in Section activities. Eligibility for this membership is limited to not more than five years or the duration of education plus two years, whichever comes later. Members in this category should have the potential for the intellectual pursuit of medical careers or, if in fields allied to medicine, should display promise of appointment to positions in universities, hospitals or institutions allied to medicine. The hope in creating the new membership class was to make the advantages of professional organizations more apparent to students and residents.

Demise of the Committee on Medical Education

In 1993, it was decided to discontinue the meetings of the Committee on Medical Education. This decision reflected the feeling
among the Executive Staff that the Committee had long outlived
its usefulness as a forum for the discussion of issues in medical
education thanks to the proliferation of other bodies, such as the
Associated Medical Schools of New York and of New Jersey and
the Association of American Medical Colleges, which were addressing issues of undergraduate and graduate medical education.
For the Academy to do a creditable job of reviewing policy initiatives and having an impact in these areas, it would require a level
of resources which might not be justified in light of the more
pressing issues in urban health that the Academy was committed to
follow.


NITRIC OXIDE AND THE NERVOUS SYSTEM


A major meeting on November 2, 1992, organized by Dr.
Thomas Morris, featured an in-depth discussion of *The Role of
Nitric Oxide in the Nervous System*. Nitric oxide is a major
neurotransmitter, a vasoactive substance, and has a remarkable
set of functions in the brain and the nervous system as well as the
circulatory system. The participants in the symposium were especially distinguished. They included Salvadore E. Moncada, Ph.D.,
Research Director of the Wellcome Foundation Research Laboratories; Robert Furchgott, Ph.D., State University of New York,
Health Sciences Center at Brooklyn; Robert A. Marletta, Ph.D.,
from the University of Michigan; and Drs. Solomon H. Snyder
from the Johns Hopkins University, Eric Kandel from the Columbia University College of Physicians and Surgeons, and John
Garthwaite from the University of London. Over 200 persons
attended this symposium.

## THE COMMISSION TO REVIEW THE HEALTH AND
## HOSPITALS CORPORATION

The greater visibility of the Academy and its prestige resulted in a request from Mayor David N. Dinkins for Dr. Barondess to create and chair an independent Commission to review the structure and function of the New York City Health and Hospitals Corporation, and recommend changes that would improve the efficiency and quality of the health services it delivered. The Commission, which was administered by the Academy and housed in the Academy building, was supported by grants from the New York City Health and Hospitals Corporation, the Altman Foundation, the Carnegie Corporation of New York, the Commonwealth Fund, Morgan Guaranty Trust Company, the New York Community Trust, the Robert Wood Johnson Foundation and the United Hospital Fund. The Academy made in-kind contributions.

The Commission issued a report in November 1992 which concluded that the Health and Hospitals Corporation should be allowed to continue to fulfill New York City's historic commitment to assure that all persons would receive health care regardless of their ability to pay. It opposed the privatization of the Corporation, suggesting that the costs of this move would outweigh the benefits. However, it emphasized the great need to improve the quality of the care it being provided and recommended that an effective system to monitor and improve the quality of care be put in place. The Commission called for strengthening the affiliation contracts between the Corporation and the medical schools and academic medical centers, and suggested that an independent "affiliation oversight board" be created "to establish a dispute reconciliation mechanism available to the affiliates and the Health and Hospitals Corporation." The Commission also recommended that a "monitoring body should be put in place to oversee the manner and pace of the implementation of the recommendations of the Commission."[42] Although the Academy played a major role in the creation and deliberations of the Commission, neither its work nor its recommendations were reviewed by any body of the Academy—it was truly an independent Commission.

Members of the Commission who were close to the Corporation shared information about its deliberations with the appropriate Corporation officials and a number of its recommendations, particularly those relating to budgeting, were adopted even before the Report was completed. The Dinkins Administration and the Corporation were willing to implement some of the findings and recommendations of the report, but it became clear the City was not enthusiastic about setting up the recommended independent body to oversee the implementation of the report.

A hearing on the implementation of the Commission's report, at which Dr. Barondess testified, was conducted by the Health Committee of the New York City Council on March 23, 1993. At the Board of Trustees meeting on March 24, 1993, Mr. Theodore Sorensen suggested that the Editorial Board of the *New York Times* be approached to encourage them to identify as one of their major causes the establishment of the independent oversight body the Commission recommended. Dr. Barondess replied that he had written to the Deputy Mayor requesting consideration of this recommendation but had not received a reply. It was clear that neither the Mayor, nor the Corporation Board, nor the unions, nor the affiliated medical schools were interested in such oversight.

## 1992 DEMOCRATIC NATIONAL CONVENTION

In conjunction with the 1992 Democratic National Convention in New York City and in co-sponsorship with the Greater New York Hospital Association, the Academy presented a panel discussion of *American Health Policy for the 1990s and Beyond.* Held at the Hilton Hotel where many of the delegates were staying, it attracted more than 400 convention delegates and others. The program was chaired by Mr. Joseph A. Califano, Jr., the Secretary of Health, Education and Welfare during the Carter administration, and featured talks by Representative Henry Waxman of California, Chairman of the Subcommittee on Health and Environment of the House Energy and Commerce Committee, Governor John C. Waihee, III, of Hawaii, Mr. Richard J. Davidson, President of the American Hospital Association, Ms. Karen Ignani, Director of the Employee Benefits Department of the AFL/CIO, Mr. Walter Maher, Director of Federal Relations for the Chrysler Corporation, and Drs. Uwe Reinhardt, health economist from Princeton University, Arnold S. Relman, Editor Emeritus of the *New England Journal of Medicine,* James S. Todd, Executive Vice President of the American Medical Association, and Reed Tuckson, President of Charles R. Drew University.

The panelists agreed that the status quo could not be maintained and that significant reform of the health care delivery system is needed. No consensus was reached, however, on the kinds of reforms needed to achieve the goals of universal coverage, control of costs and enhancement of the quality of care. The discussion was very lively and there were interesting questions and comments from the audience. The program was later televised over a cable TV medical network. Its primary intent, presenting the issues for the delegates, was achieved. Efforts to extend the format to the Republican convention in Houston were unsuccessful.

## OFFICE OF SPECIAL POPULATION PROJECTS

In 1993, at the suggestion of Dr. David E. Rogers, the Office of Special Population Projects was created to serve as a focus for Academy activities in relation to HIV infection and AIDS. The Office was funded by the New York State AIDS Institute. It created the Council of AIDS Program Directors, comprised of the directors of Designated AIDS Centers recognized by the New York State AIDS Institute and their counterparts in public hospitals, and the New York AIDS Forum, which brought together leaders in HIV/AIDS research and the AIDS clinical directors to improve communication between those conducting research, clinical care givers and community leaders active in the fight against AIDS. The Council of AIDS Directors has been particularly concerned about how managed care programs have responded to the needs of persons with AIDS. Also functioning under the auspices of this Office are the Council of HIV Long-Term Care Clinical Directors and the Council of HIV Ambulatory Care Clinical Directors. The Office was initially headed by Ms. Ellen Rautenberg, former Assistant Commissioner for AIDS Program Services in the New York City Department of Health. When she left in 1944 to become Vice President of the Medical and Health Research Association of the City of New York, the Office was headed by Ms. Ellen Parish, a registered nurse with an M.P.H. from Tulane University who had established the Designated AIDS Center at the Lenox Hill Hospital, and Mr. Gary Stein, a lawyer and social worker who had been Policy Director of the Orphan Project at the Fund for the City of New York which focuses on policy relating to the children of parents lost to AIDS.

## CELL SIGNAL TRANSDUCTION

The Academy held a major basic science program on *Cell Signal Transduction* on October 4, 1993. This was a cutting edge program that was attended by over 400 Fellows, physicians, students and researchers from institutions around the country. The Conference Chairman was Dr. Joseph Schlessinger of the New York University Medical School, and the speakers included Drs. Alex Ullrich of the Max Planck Institut für Biochemie, David Baltimore of Rockefeller University, and Richard Axel, of the Columbia University College of Physicians and Surgeons. The Conference focused on new knowledge of the cellular and molecular biology of highly conserved pathways in signal transduction and on mutational events that lead to alterations in signaling molecules that may underlie various developmental disorders and diseases.

## VIOLENCE: A MAJOR PUBLIC HEALTH PROBLEM

In April 1994, the Academy issued a statement on *Firearm Violence and Public Health: Limiting the Availability of Guns* which called for restrictions on the availability of firearms and encouraged educational and other initiatives to curb the epidemic of violence. This statement was endorsed by leaders in health care throughout the New York Metropolitan Area, including the deans of all of the medical schools and heads of the major hospitals. It was published in the *Journal of the American Medical Association.*[43]

This statement was released at a press conference held at the Academy that was addressed by Dr. Margaret Hamburg, New York City Commissioner of Health, Dr. Mark Chassin, New York State Commissioner of Health; Ms. Maria Mitchell, Special Advisor to the Mayor, and Mr. Kenneth E. Raske, President of the Greater New York Hospital Association. A special resource panel, which included Dr. Charles S. Hirsch, Chief Medical Examiner of the City of New York, Dr. Cheryl Heaton, Associate Dean of the Columbia University School of Public Health, and Drs. Barbara Barlow and Arthur Cooper, trauma surgeons, was on hand to answer questions from the press. The conference received both local and national news coverage and was the springboard for launching the Health Coalition Against Violence.

Health Coalition Against Violence

The Health Coalition Against Violence, based at the Academy, brought together representatives of community-based organizations such as the Children's Aid Society, medical specialty societies, the City and State Departments of Health, and the New York County District Attorney's Office in a cooperative effort to advocate for violence prevention initiatives, set a research agenda, and define a proactive role for the health care community. It joined with the Task Force on Violence of the American College of Physicians to develop a survey instrument to probe the attitudes of physicians toward gun control, and worked with the Handgun Epidemic Lowering Plan, a Chicago-based national organization, to develop unified public service messages against handgun violence.

## Hearings on the Media Role in Violence

In October 1994, the Academy joined the New York State Martin Luther King, Jr. Commission and Institute for Nonviolence in a legislative hearing on *Media's Social Responsibility In an Era of Epidemic Societal Violence* that focused on the depiction of violence by the media and its impact on society. In addition to more than thirty students, parents, church and community leaders, testimony was presented to a panel of legislative leaders and government officials by Governor Mario Cuomo, former Mayor David Dinkins, and Senior Vice President Dr. Alan R. Fleischman, who reiterated the Academy's strong support for gun control measures.

## Violence in the Workplace

In March 1995, Dr. Messite organized an all-day *Seminar on Workplace Violence: Preventive and Interventive Strategies.* It examined the workplace as a special microcosm in which employees, employers and government as the stakeholders have special opportunities for intervention and prevention that may be applicable more widely. Speakers included: Dr. Linda Rosenstock, Director of the National Institute for Occupational Health and Safety and Ms. Lynn Jenkins, Acting Chief of its Injury Surveillance Section, Michael Benjamin, Executive Director of the Institute for Mental Health Initiatives, Bill Borwegen, Director of the Occupational Health and Safety Department of the Service Employees International Union, Jeffrey Fagan, Ph.D., of the Rutgers University School of Criminal Justice, Jay W. Malcan, Ph.D., Crime Prevention Policy Analyst at the Virginia Crime Prevention Center, Representative Charles Schumer (Dem/NY), a staunch advocate of federal gun control legislation, and Drs. Edward Anselm then Corporate Medical Director of the Executive Health Group, Jeffrey P. Kahn, President of the Academy of Organizational and Occupational Psychiatry, Herbert D. Kleber, Professor of Psychiatry at the Columbia University College of Physicians and Surgeons, Gerald A. Kraines, President and CEO of the Levinson Institute of Waltham, Massachusetts, Philip Landrigan, Chairman of the Department of Community Medicine at the Mount Sinai School of Medicine, James Melius, Director of Occupational Health and Environmental Epidemiology at the New York State Department of Health, David H. Reid, III, National Medical Director at US Postal Service Headquarters in Washington, DC, Kenneth Tardiff, Director of the Section of Epidemiology of the Department of Psychiatry at the Cornell University Medical College, Carol Wilkinson, Program Director at IBM Corporation, and, representing the Academy, President Jeremiah A. Barondess and Senior Vice President Alan R. Fleischman.

The speakers agreed that violence is pervasive in the workplace, as it is in society in general. Homicides were reported to be a major cause of death among workers, mainly as the result of violent crimes, but their impact and cost are considerably outweighed by the prevalence of near misses, physical assaults, abusive behavior and threats of violence, most of which go unreported and unrecognized. Violence, it was said, is not just a criminal justice problem nor just one involving aberrant behavior attributable to alcohol, drugs or mental illness. Violence is often predictable and preventable, it was emphasized. The speakers, assisted by comments and suggestions from the large and interested audience, reviewed a number of measures that might be taken to deal with workplace violence and called for a concerted effort on the part of workers, employers, occupational health professionals and other relevant specialists to develop a coherent set of strategies for prevention and intervention. A summary of the proceedings was published in the *Journal of Occupational and Environmental Medicine.*[44]

## NOTES

1 Executive Committee, Board of Trustees, New York Academy of Medicine. 1990 Minutes of the meeting of February 8, 1990.

2 Board of Trustees, New York Academy of Medicine. 1990 Minutes of the meeting of March 28, 1990.

3 Board of Trustees, New York Academy of Medicine. 1990 Minutes of the meeting of September 26, 1990.

4 Cherkasky M. 1991 Introductory remarks at the Presidential Convocation of the New York Academy of Medicine, October 19, 1990. *Bulletin of the New York Academy of Medicine.* 67:105–107.

5 Sullivan LW. 1991 Meeting the need: Government partnership in service to mankind. *Bulletin of the New York Academy of Medicine.* 67:108–112.

6 Barondess JA. 1991 The New York Academy of Medicine: Prospects and opportunities. *Bulletin of the New York Academy of Medicine.* 67:113–118.

7 ibid. p. 116.

8 ibid. p. 118.

9 Board of Trustees, New York Academy of Medicine. 1992 Minutes of the meeting of September 23, 1992.

10 Ad Hoc Committee on the Retreat. 1993. Report to the Board of Trustees, New York Academy of Medicine. Presented at the meeting of March 24, 1993.

11 New York Academy of Medicine. 1993 *Annual Report* p. 13.

12 Haggerty RJ. 1993 The Bulletin—A new focus, a new look. *Bulletin of the New York Academy of Medicine.* 70:4–7.

13 Board of Trustees, New York Academy of Medicine. 1990 Minutes of the meeting of January 24, 1990.

14 Board of Trustees, New York Academy of Medicine. 1991 Minutes of the meeting of March 20, 1991.

15 New York Academy of Medicine. *1991 Annual Report.* p. 8.

16 Harris D. 1991 Symposium on Pregnancy and Substance Abuse: Perspectives and Directions: Introduction. *Bulletin of the New York Academy of Medicine.* 67:191–192.

17 Falco M. 1991 Drug abuse: A national perspective. *Bulletin of the New York Academy of Medicine.* 67:196–200.

18 Committee on Public Health. 1990 Statement on drug use in pregnancy: An urgent problem for New York City. *Bulletin of the New York Academy of Medicine.* 66.193–197.

19 Morris TQ. 1992 Welcome. *Bulletin of the New York Academy of Medicine.* 68:174–175.

20 Fay T. 1991 *Noise and Health.* New York: New York Academy of Medicine.

21 Committee on Public Health. 1991 Statement on the risk of contracting HIV infections in the course of health care. *Bulletin of the New York Academy of Medicine.* 67:184–186.

22 New York Academy of Medicine. 1981 Statement on the risk of contracting HIV infections in the course of health care. *Journal of the American Medical Association.* 265:1872–1873.

23 Barondess JA. 1992 *Letter to the President of the New York City Board of Education.* October 22, 1992.

24 United Hospital Fund 1992 *The Tuberculosis Revival: Individual Rights and Societal Obligations in a Time of AIDS.* New York: United Hospital Fund.

25 Hamburg MA. 1993 Urgent issues in public Health *Bulletin of the New York Academy of Medicine.* 69:14–22.

26 Mayor's Commission on the Future of Child Health in New York City. 1989 *Report* p. 5.

27 Committee on Medicine in Society. 1990 Minutes of the meeting of February 26, 1990.

28 Commission on Biomedical Research and Devepment. 1993 *Report.* New York: New York Academy of Medicine.

29 Aries N. 1990 *The Status of Biomedical Research in New York City.* New York: The Greater New York Hospital Foundation, Inc.

30 Aries N and Sclar ED. 1991 *Report on the Economic Impact of Non-Profit Sector Sponsored Biomedical Research in the Metropolitan New York Region.* New York: New York Academy of Medicine.

31 Rosenberg LE. 1992 The human genome project. *Bulletin of the New York Academy of Medicine.* 68:113–114.

32 Davis BD, Annas GJ, Nelkin D, Rothstein MA, Grennan TA, Richardson WC, et al. 1992 The Human Genome Project, an agenda for science and society. *Bulletin of the New York Academy of Medicine.* 8:115–170

33 Subcommittee on Human Rights. 1992 *Report on the Case of Dr. Yolanda Huet-Vaughan.* Presented to the Committee on Medicine in Society, April 20, 1992.

34 Ad hoc Committee on Human Rights. 1992 Memorandum to the Board of Trustees, June 29, 1992.

35 Board of Trustees, New York Academy of Medicine. 1992 Minutes of the meeting of July 22, 1992.

36 [Multiple authors] 1989 Child health: One hundred years of progress and today's challenges. *Bulletin of the New York Academy of Medicine.* 65:255–418.

37 Barondess JA. 1992 Conference on pediatric poverty and health: Introductory remarks. *Bulletin of the New York Academy of Medicine.* 68:5–7.

38 Elwood D. 1992 Impact of poverty on children. *Bulletin of the New York Academy of Medicine.* 68:8–16.

39 Fisher, HM. 1995 Community service as an integral component of undergraduate medical education: Facilitating student involvement. *Bulletin of the New York Academy of Medicine.* 72:76–86.

40 Barondess JA. 1993 Introduction. In: Anonymous, *Advising Premedical Students.* New York: New York Academy of Medicine. pp. 1–2.

41 [Anonymous]. *Advising Premedical Students* New York: New York Academy of Medicine.

42 Mayoral Commission to Review the Health and Hospitals Corporation. 1992 *Report.* New York: New York Academy of Medicine.

43 New York Academy of Medicine. 1994 Firearm violence and public health: Limiting the availability of guns. *Journal of the American Medical Assoication.* 271:1281–1283.

44 Warshaw LJ and Messite J. 1996 Workplace violence: Preventive and interventive strategies. *Journal of Occupational and Environmental Medicine.* 38:993–1006.

# Chapter 9
## 1994–1997
## The New Academy

New Staff
JUNIOR FELLOWS PROGRAM
TASK FORCE ON HEALTH CARE REFORM
PUBLIC SERVICE ANNOUNCEMENTS
THE LIBRARY
    Museum Mile Program
    Lectures, Readings and Exhibits
    Interlibrary Linkages
    History of Medicine Program
    Symposium to Honor Dr. Saul Jarcho
    The Samuel Jacobs Health Information Center
    NYAM Website
    The Medallic History of the Jewish People
HIV/AIDS
    HIV Professional Development Project
    HIV/AIDS Information Outreach Project
OFFICE OF SPECIAL POPULATIONS PROJECTS
CENTER FOR URBAN EPIDEMIOLOGIC STUDIES
HARM REDUCTION IN DRUG ADDICTION
CAPITAL PUNISHMENT
THE URBAN HEALTH INITIATIVE
DOMESTIC VIOLENCE
THE MARGARET E. MAHONEY SYMPOSIA
INSIDE URBAN HEALTH
THE DIVISION OF PUBLIC HEALTH
SECTION ON HEALTH CARE DELIVERY
DIVISION OF HEALTH AND SCIENCE POLICY
NEW OFFICERS OF THE BOARD OF TRUSTEES

OFFICE OF SCHOOL HEALTH PROGRAMS
Death of Dr. John Waller
Program Progress
Careers in the Health Professions Program
EVIDENCE-BASED MEDICINE PROGRAM
REAPPOINTMENT OF DR. BARONDESS
THE 150th ANNIVERSARY CELEBRATION
NOTES

B Y THE END OF 1994, the new divisional structure of the Academy was beginning to emerge. The By-laws changes approved in 1989 continued to mandate a Committee on Nominations and a Committee on Admission. The Committee on Medical Education had already been abolished while the other previously mandated standing committees (Medicine in Society, Public Health and the Library) were allowed to continue at the discretion of the Board of Trustees.

An April 1994 document circulated by Dr. Barondess described the committee structure which had existed for many years as "characterized by loci for program origination, development and management, executive directors attached to each, serving essentially as stewards of the committees, open enrollment for interested Fellows, a laissez-faire or lay executive tradition, little or no extramural funding, products largely in conferences or statements published in the *Bulletin of the New York Academy of Medicine*. This structure has served the Academy well in the past but needs to be altered and expanded."[1]

The document then continued to describe the new governance/management structure which had begun to be implemented in 1990. The changes included programming assembled around a centralized Academy agenda devoted primarily to issues in urban health; more focused programming; increasing the number and diversity of the constituencies served; increasing complexity of the issues addressed; more interaction with other organizations and with policy makers; more interaction with academic centers and the hospital environment; an expanded full-time staff; program initiation and management now largely generated by full-time staff; and bringing diverse interested parties into the programming.

The document suggested that the committees be merged into a formal structure of three divisions: Public Health; Medicine and Public Policy; Library, Information Resources and Management. Each would have full-time staff responsible for program development that would lead to "increased and expanding effectiveness." The committees would continue as part of the divisions and provide expertise in program development. The document reiterated the expectation that substantial proportion of the costs of the divisions would be provided from outside sources.

The Division of Public Health would have responsibility for maternal, child and family health, communicable diseases, environmental health, mental health and addictions, biostatistics, epidemiology and surveillance, special populations and related issues (e.g., homelessness, violence, etc.). The Division of Medicine and Public Policy would be concerned with health care systems and organization, health care economics, health care financing and reimbursement, health manpower planning, health care practice, undergraduate and graduate training for the health professions, science policy, biomedical research policy and training. The Division of Library, Information Resources and Management would be responsible for communication with Fellows, relations with the public and with the medical, educational and bioscience communities, Regional Medical Library functions, electronic information linkages, the history of medicine program, the scholars in residence, graduate education, and fellowship programs, and interinstitutional linkages (museums, historical societies, etc.).

Certain activities and programs would primarily be centered in the Office of the Senior Vice-President: programs, Section activities, new Section development, research fellowships and other endowed awards, special lectures, school health activities, health career programs, basic science programs, and ad hoc program oversight. Some activities might engage more than one division:

e.g., AIDS, tuberculosis, the effects of homelessness and pediatric poverty, and substance abuse.

Legislative and executive branch liaison would be informed by divisional efforts. Further there would be "para-divisional" structures: the Center for Epidemiological Studies, the Council on Biomedical Research and Development, and the Nutrition Center.

The implementation of the divisional structural was handled with great care by Dr. Barondess. He addressed meetings of the committees and met with their key members to respond to questions and solicit comments. He provided assurances that the committees would continue to function, although with altered responsibility: instead of the committees taking the lead with support being provided by the staff, the staff would be charged with program development, with the committees providing support and expertise. This reversal of roles was balanced by the prospect of obtaining new resources.

## New Staff

On July 1, 1994, Dr. Alan R. Fleischman joined the staff of the Academy as Senior Vice President, replacing Dr. Thomas Morris who remained at the Academy as Senior Advisor to the President. Dr. Fleischman, a pediatrician and neonatologist, and an expert in medical ethics, continued his affiliation at the Albert Einstein College of Medicine as Clinical Professor of Pediatrics and Clinical Professor of Epidemiology and Social Medicine, and continued as a Fellow of the Hastings Center. At the Academy, he assumed responsibility over programmatic functions, including medical education, public health, and urban health initiatives. In addition, he provided supervision to the standing committees during the interregnum.

Ms. Holly Michaels Fisher left the Academy in 1994 to join the staff of the Visiting Nurse Service of New York. She was succeeded by Julie Hantman, M.P.H., who served as Project Director of the Urban Health Initiative until March, 1996.

On December 31, 1994, Dr. Jacqueline Messite retired as Executive Director of the Committee on Public Health, but continued at the Academy as a Consultant for another year.

On the same date, Dr. Marvin Lieberman retired as Executive Director of the Committee on Medicine and Society and, in anticipation of the 150th anniversary in 1997, accepted the assignment of updating the history of the first hundred years of the Academy, produced in 1949 by Dr. Philip Van Ingen.

In July 1995, James G. Spellos, formerly Director of Meeting Services of the Society of Nuclear Medicine, joined the Academy staff as Director of Medical Education and served in that position until November 1996. Adam Margolis, who had been hired as a member of his staff in September 1995, was promoted to Associate Director of Medical Education in December 1966.

In July 1996, Maureen G. Leness, formerly Assistant Director for Development of the New York Downtown Hospital, became Director of Development. She is a member of the Advisory Board of the Long Island Chapter of Save the Children, and of the Turtle Bay Music School in New York City.

Edward Morman, Ph.D., has been appointed Associate Librarian for Historical Collections and Programs. He is responsible for the Rare Book Room and for creating scholarly research programs, outreach, and planning lectures and exhibitions on the history of medicine. He served as Librarian of the Institute for the History of Medicine and as Lecturer in the History of Science, Medicine and Technology. He holds master's and doctoral degrees from the Department of History of the University of Pennsylvania and in the sociology of science

At the Stated Meeting of June 27, 1994, Dr. Barondess presented his friend, Dr. David E. Rogers, with the John Stearns Award for Lifetime Achievement in Medicine. The entire Academy community was saddened when Dr. Rogers died on December 5, 1994, after a long illness. A memorial service in his honor was held on March 30, 1995 in Hosack Hall. In addition to Dr. Barondess, tributes to Dr. Rogers and his distinguished career were presented by Dr. Morton D. Bogdonoff, Professor of Medicine at the New

York Hospital-Cornell-Medical Center, Dr. Robert Heyssel, President Emeritus of the Johns Hopkins Health System, Dr. Robert Blendon from the Harvard School of Public Health, Mr. Thomas Maloney, President of the Institute for the Future, Ms. Margaret Mahoney, former President of the Commonwealth Fund and Vice Chair of the Academy Board of Trustees, Dr. Dennis P. Whalen, Executive Deputy Director of the New York State Department of Health, Mr. Terrance Keenan, Special Program Consultant at the Robert Wood Johnson Foundation, Bruce Vladeck, Ph.D., Administrator of the Health Care Financing Administration, and Dr. Philip R. Lee, Assistant Secretary for Health at the US Department of Health and Human Services.

## JUNIOR FELLOWS PROGRAM

The Junior Fellows Program: A Science and Medicine Initiative for New York City Public High Schools, launched in January 1996 under the auspices of the Academy Office of School Health Programs and the Library, in collaboration with the Mount Sinai Medical Center, is aimed at introducing selected middle school students to career opportunities in science, medicine and research. This program brings the students into contact with mentors in the various fields and provides experiences in laboratories, clinics and medical centers as well as inculcating library research skills and computer literacy.

The initial program commenced on January 25, 1996, when twenty-six middle school students from Community School District 26 in Queens were inducted into the Academy as Junior Fellows by Dr. Barondess in the first of a series of eleven sessions which culminated in a formal graduation ceremony on June 3rd. Each student was assigned a mentor—a resident or intern from Mount Sinai Medical Center—with whom research ideas in such focal areas as infectious diseases, cancer, cell physiology and aging, alternative medicine, and embryology and genetics were developed. Community school district personnel, including science teachers and library media specialists, assessed and coached the students between the sessions and assisted in their research. The program was coordinated by Leslie Goldman and Freya Kaufman of the Office of School Health Programs and Rhonna Goodman of the Library staff. It was funded in part by the Lounsbery Foundation, the Morris Foundation and Community School District 26.

In further outreach efforts to young people, over 2,000 students from over 100 of New York City's public, private and parochial high schools attended seminars on *Career Opportunities in Medicine, Career Opportunities in Nursing,* and *Career Opportunities in Medicine and Science,* while a fourth seminar for 100 middle school guidance counselors provided information about career opportunities in health care, academic requirements and the financing of health-related education.

## TASK FORCE ON HEALTH CARE REFORM

The Anniversary Discourse presented at the June 1994 Spring Stated Meeting by Mr. James R. Tallon, Jr., President of the United Hospital Fund and an Academy Trustee, addressed *Health Reform: The New York Reality.* In it, he described the pressures on the health care delivery system in coping with the convergence of the federal, state and municipal changes in health care policies and financing.

That set the stage for the initiation of the Task Force on Health Care Reform, a twenty-six-member group that included several members of the Board of Trustees: Drs. Saul Farber and Martin Cherkasky and Mr. Tallon, as well as Dr. Michael R. McGarvey, Senior Vice President for Health Industry Services at Blue Cross and Blue Shield of New Jersey, and also an Academy Trustee. Dr. McGarvey chaired the group, which was staffed by Ms. Fisher. To distinguish the Academy from the many other organizations reacting to the health care reform proposals of the Clinton Administration, the Task Force focused on the "urban perspective," that is, the impact of proposed reforms on lower-income, inner city communities, a perspective to which, it was felt, not enough attention was being paid.

The Task Force described the relatively poor health status of these communities, demonstrated by such indices as high rates of infant morbidity and mortality, epicenters of HIV/AIDS prevalence, tuberculosis case rates, and the epidemic proportions of violence. While it lauded reforms which would improve access to health care services, such as universal coverage, adequate benefits, and incentives for providers to serve in underserved communities, the Task Force emphasized the need for attention to the underlying social factors that directly affect health, such as poverty, inadequate housing, poor educational opportunities, lack of jobs, family disintegration, and violence. Unless these are addressed, the Task Force said, the nation would continue to experience excessively high levels of preventable morbidity and mortality. "Attacking these underlying causes of poor health in our society." The Task Force said in its Report, "must continue to be the long-term public policy agenda."[2]

The report of the Task Force was unanimously endorsed by its members and was presented to the Board of Trustees. In discussing it, several Trustees suggested that it was not sufficiently rigorous in its references to the fiscal constraints that should be considered in the design of a health reform package but, in the end, the Board accepted the position of the Task Force. The report was published to provide a template against which health care reform proposals could be assessed in relation to the health needs of the nation's cities. Copies were sent to a large number of federal and state legislators.

## PUBLIC SERVICE ANNOUNCEMENTS

In 1994, the Academy entered into an agreement with Bloomberg Information Radio to air public service announcements on health information. The announcements, each of which runs for a month, are aired several times each day. They are written for a lay audience and include a toll-free telephone number to call for further information. They cover topics suggested by a designated group of Fellows, who also review them for quality control. The Library reference staff provides information and data as needed. Among the subjects covered are: advance directives for health care decision-making; childhood and adult immunizations; lead screening for toddlers; coping with domestic violence; strokes; hospice care; bicycle helmets;, slips and falls in the elderly; blood donation; exercise; depression; and glaucoma. Their impact is attested to by the receipt of several hundred telephone requests for additional information.

## THE LIBRARY

### Museum Mile Program

In 1994, as in previous years, the Library participated in the Museum Mile program, in which many of the cultural institutions on upper Fifth Avenue open their doors to the public. In 1994, it was estimated, more than 200 persons toured the Library on that day and were provided with information about the collections and the history of the Academy. Books and surplus items from the collections were offered for sale and complimentary bookmarks were distributed. Persons who chose not to tour the building were able to have questions about the Academy answered by staff members stationed in the building lobby.

### Lectures, Readings and Exhibits

In 1994, the Section on Historical Medicine, assisted by funding from the New York State Council on the Humanities, presented a successful series of lectures on *Race and Ethnicity in American Medicine: An Historical Perspective.* The lectures included *The Maliocchio Versus Modern Medicine: The Challenge of Italian Health Traditions to Public Health in New York City a Century*

*Ago,* by Alan Kraut, Ph.D.; *Making a Place for Ourselves: The Development of Black Hospitals, 1890–1920,* by Dr. Vanessa Gamble; and *Averting a Pestilence: The 1892 Typhus Epidemic and the Quarantining of East European Jews on New York's Lower East Side,* by Dr. Howard Markel. More than 250 persons attended the lectures and had an opportunity for discussion with the speakers during the receptions that followed.

Among the continuing cultural programs is the popular series of Clinical Readings by prominent physician authors and other writers on medical topics. The 1994 series included Susan Sontag who read from her *Illness as Metaphor* and *AIDS and Its Metaphors;* Dr. Sherwin B. Nuland, who read from his prize-winning best seller, *How We Die;* and Dr. Marc D. Straus, a popular poet who read from his *Poetry and Medicine,* a book in which he examined the clinical encounter and its implications. In 1996, Lance Morrow, a senior writer and essayist for *Time* magazine, read from his book, *Heart, a Memoir,* in which he described his experience in having two myocardial infarctions, and Dr. Ethel Person, Professor of Clinical Psychiatry at the Columbia University College of Physicians and Surgeons, reading from her book, *By Force of Fantasy, How We Make Our Lives,* provided a thought-provoking description of fantasy as a central component of mental life.

The Library continues to mount exhibitions from its collection and from materials loaned to it or from traveling exhibitions. For example, in 1994, there was an exhibit of artifacts relating to the assassination of President Abraham Lincoln, and another on *The Legacy of Dioscorides: Pharmacy from Antiquity to Enlightenment,* which featured rare books and manuscripts tracing the history of pharmacy from ancient Greece to the eighteenth century, including the herbals of Dioscorides and the first official Pharmacopoeia of the United States. An exhibit of *Treasures of New York Academy of Medicine Library* featured displays of the ninth-century Apicius manuscript cook book and the 1543 first edition of Vesalius' *De Humani Corporis Fabrica,* as well as a traveling exhibit organized by the State University of New York at Binghamton and sponsored by the Oskar Diethelm Library of the Department of Psychiatry at the New York Hospital-Cornell University Medical Center on *Madness in America: Cultural and Medical Perceptions of Mental Illness before 1914.*

In April 1996, the Library presented the first in a series of six exhibits devoted to the Academy's role in public health over the past 150 years and into the future. This exhibit, *Public Health and the Changing Urban Landscape,* focused on the influence that the field of public health had on the development of New York City, as well as the Academy's contributions in this regard.

Interlibrary Linkages

A major advance in service to the public was the Library's provision of unlimited free access to the databases of the National Library of Medicine, the only medical library to provide this service in New York City. In addition, the linkage with the New York Public Library, through which its patrons are referred to the Library for materials and information services that would otherwise be unavailable, was continued.

As a Regional Medical Library, the Library continued to support resource sharing activities among the 694 health sciences libraries in the Middle Atlantic States. Outreach to health professionals on the use of libraries and databases was pursued through demonstrations at meetings of such professional organizations as the Clinical Laboratory Management Association, the American Medical Women's Association, the American Academy of Psychology and the Radiological Society of North America. In addition, the Library added a new program providing information services to twenty community-based organizations serving the HIV/AIDS community.

An important cooperative relationship has been established with the New York Public Library, the Office of Library Services at the City University of New York and the New York Reference and Research Library Agency's (METRO) Hospital Library Service Program. It provides NOAH (New York Online Access to Health

Information), a bilingual Internet gateway to consumer health information on the World Wide Web. The project is funded by the US Department of Commerce National Telecommunications and Information Administration through its Telecommunications and Information Infrastructure Assistance Program and by matching funds.

NOAH is available at public libraries in Manhattan, the Bronx and Staten Island, the METRO hospital libraries and the Academy Library. It provides access to the health information resources on the World Wide Web which are not available to persons without access to the Internet. Since most of the World Wide Web is in English, a machine-translation program is used to make the material available in Spanish. In addition to such useful providers of health information as the Gay Men's Health Crisis, the March of Dimes, the National Cancer Institute, and the New York City Department of Health, NOAH offers access to such health information databases as ONCOlink of the University of Pennsylvania and those of the National Institutes of Health and the National Library of Medicine.

In April 1996, it was announced that the National Library of Medicine had renewed for five years, through 2001, the Academy contract to serve as the Regional Medical Library for the Middle Atlantic Region, In addition, the Eastern On-line Training Center, a program provided at the Academy, became the National On-line Training Center for all of the United States. Although a few classes will be given at the National Library of Medicine, all on-line training in MEDLARS databases will be coordinated through the National On-line Center at the Academy. The two five-year contracts total $6.3 million.


History of Medicine Program


Building on the magnificent collection of materials on medical history in the Library, the scholarly interests of the Fellows, and the growing interest in medical history on the part of the university community in Greater New York area, the Academy announced in 1995 the formation of a History of Medicine Program, designed to promote scholarship in the history of public health and medical practice through a graduate program, fellowships, and a series of lectures.

It includes the Interuniversity Consortium, a graduate program in the history of health, medicine and society, offered jointly by the departments of history of Columbia University, the City University of New York and the State University of New York at Stony Brook. This joint program will enable those interested in the history of medicine and public health to obtain a graduate degree in the field. An initial orientation seminar is held in the Fellows Room of the Library and the participants have access to the Rare Book Room and the historical collections. Part of the program is the endowed Klemperer Fellowship which supports short-term research using the collections of the Library; in 1996, Dr. Russell Viner was named the first Fellow, and he will study the life and works of Dr. Abraham Jacobi, the great pioneer in pediatrics who was President of the Academy from 1885 to 1888, and who, in 1860, founded the first pediatric clinic in the country at the New York Medical College.

## Symposium to Honor Dr. Saul Jarcho

As part of the History of Medicine Program, the Academy hosted an all-day symposium in June 1995 to recognize the accomplishments of Dr. Saul Jarcho, one of the preeminent medical historians of the current era. A magna cum laude graduate of Harvard University, he earned an M.A. degree in Roman Literature from Columbia University before graduating from the Columbia University College of Physicians and Surgeons. During World War II, he was Chief of the Analysis Branch of the US Army Medical Intelligence Division. A Fellow since 1940, his contributions to the Academy include service as Chairman of the Section on Historical and Cultural Medicine from 1947 to 1948, Editor-in Chief of the *Bulletin* from 1967 to 1975, and Chairman of the Committee on the Library from 1977 to 1978. Many of his over 500 scholarly articles have appeared in the *Bulletin*.

Speakers at the Symposium, among whom were Daniel M. Fox, Ph.D., President of the Milbank Memorial Fund, Dr. Gert H. Brieger of Johns Hopkins University, and Gerald Grob, Ph.D., of Rutgers University, lauded Dr. Jarcho's career as a medical historian, as a paleopathologist, a researcher in cardiology and public health and, above all, as a distinguished physician. A highlight of the Symposium was the presentation to Dr. Jarcho of the George Urdang Medal of the American Institute of the History of Pharmacy.

### The Samuel Jacobs Health Information Center

Through a generous grant from Mr. Samuel Jacobs, one of the founders of Star Industries, Inc., a major New York City wholesale liquor distributor, the Library has created the Samuel Jacobs Health Information Center, which is designed to provide easy access to electronic information in health and medicine to the general public. Located in the reference area of the main Library, the Center offers eight computer work stations including large color monitors, printers, and headphones for listening to audio files. They are connected to a network of resources, including those on the Internet and the over forty biomedical databases produced by the National Library of Medicine. In addition to searching the holdings of the Library as well as other medical libraries around the world, users may browse collections of current and historical medical images, consult full-text virtual libraries in subject areas such as HIV/AIDS and the history of medicine, and locate consumer health information produced by voluntary health agencies, government agencies and community-based organizations. Access is provided through a user-friendly graphical interface, and reference librarians are always available to provide assistance.

NYAM Website

The addition of a website at the Academy has provided an opportunity to disseminate information about programs and services to a global audience. The uniform resource locator (URL) for the Academy home page on the World Wide Web is http://www.nyam.org.

In addition to descriptions of Academy programs and upcoming events, the home page offers the full texts of several Academy publications, such as the *HIV Professions Newsletter* and the *Malloch Room Newsletter*. The Library home page allows searching of the on-line catalog which includes medical journals, books published since 1950 and 15,000 items from the rare book collection. The website also includes a link to NOAH (New York On-line Access to Health), a consumer health information system developed jointly by the Library, the City University of New York, the New York Public Library, and METRO, a local library consortium.

The Medallic History of the Jewish People

Thanks to a generous donation from Geraldine H. Coles in memory of her husband, Dr. Jerome S. Coles, Chairman of the Board of Trustees of New York University Medical College from 1976 to 1985, the Library has acquired a set of solid gold medals entitled *The Medallic History of the Jewish People*. One of only five sets issued in 22-karat gold with an appraised value of $125,000, the medals consist of 120 subjects honoring the lives of the men and women who have contributed to the Jewish identity for over four thousand years. Subjects were selected by a board of advisors of distinguished Jewish historians headed by the late Cecil Roth, and the production of the medals over a period of five years starting in 1969 by the Judaic Heritage Society marks the first time that medallic art has been used to describe the physical, cultural and spiritual dimensions of the Jewish heritage.

HIV/AIDS

HIV Professional Development Project

With support through the federal Ryan White Program, the Academy created the HIV Professional Development Project in 1994. Its purpose is to encourage the recruitment of health and social work professionals for the battle against HIV/AIDS, enhance their professional development, and provide support to address caregiver burnout. It is headed by Gary Stein. Based on a needs assessment conducted by the Columbia University School of Public Health, the Hunter College Center on AIDS, Drugs and Community Health, and the Division of Health Resources Development of the New York State Department of Health, the Project conducted a series of interdisciplinary professional and site specific focus groups to which more than eighty health care and social service professionals working in the HIV/AIDS arena contributed their expertise. This led to the formation of an Advisory Council comprising forty-five community leaders in HIV/AIDS services.

To help counteract loss of qualified staff due to burnout, the Project places psychologists and clinical social workers in forty community-based HIV/AIDS organizations and hospitals to conduct staff support groups that provide health professionals with essential emotional support and the skills needed to cope with the stress of dealing with this devastating disease

The Project also started a summer intern program that placed medical, nursing and social work students in hospitals and community-based organizations in the City and Westchester County, where they were indoctrinated in the knowledge, skills, and attitudes needed for the provision of HIV/AIDS care. It also designed an advanced, innovative HIV/AIDS-focused curriculum for the City's academic medical centers, and began to publish *HIV Professions,* a newsletter and employment clearing house for HIV care providers.

In March 1995, the Project conducted a one-day forum on *Perspectives in HIV Care: A View from the Front Lines,* which featured an overview of the epidemic and the problems of the professionals working to control it. The speakers eloquently discussed the professional and personal impacts of over ten years of HIV/AIDS care including ethical issues, the problems of special populations, and policy perspectives of the Congressional approaches to the disease. One speaker, Dr. Paul Scoles, of Ardmore, Pennsylvania, in discussing the plight of HIV-infected health workers, poignantly described how his own career as a surgeon was effectively ended when it became known that he was HIV-positive. The proceedings of this forum were published in the *Bulletin* and attracted much attention.[3]

### HIV/AIDS Information Outreach Project

The HIV/AIDS Information Outreach Project has been creating a number of pages for New York City AIDS service organizations as part of the Academy Internet website. The pilot group in the project, located at < http://www.aidsnyc.org >, is the AIDS Treatment Data Network, which has published a very extensive set of information on the treatments and clinical trials available for persons with HIV/AIDS. This network site receives an average of more than 10,000 visits each week. Sites have also been established for the National AIDS Treatment Advocacy Project, which provided same-day reports from the Third Conference on Retroviruses and Opportunistic Infections sponsored by the Infectious Diseases Society of America and the National Institutes on Health in January 1966, as well as for the clinical materials form the New York State AIDS Institute.

### OFFICE OF SPECIAL POPULATIONS PROJECTS

Under the aegis of the Office for Special Population Projects, the Council of AIDS Program Directors, the medical directors of the Designated AIDS Centers in the State, continued to meet regularly to discuss such issues as state funding for care and the ability of managed care to deal with the disease. Under the auspices of the New York AIDS Forum this Council joined representatives of the local research community in sponsoring joint meetings intended to enhance communications between the two professional arenas. At one of these meetings, Drs. William Paul, Director of the Office of AIDS Research, and Bernard Fields, of Harvard University, discussed the future of HIV/AIDS research and the role of basic science in it.

The Council of HIV Long-Term Care Clinical Directors discussed the problem of HIV-positive patients who continue to use intravenous drugs, the management of tuberculosis in AIDS patients, and the potential effects of proposed changes in Medicaid reimbursement.

Along with the HIV Ambulatory Care Directors Group, these Councils meet regularly at the Academy to share experiences and information and to develop strong policy positions of advocacy for the patients they serve. By circulating informational materials to State and City legislators, giving testimony, and providing personal contacts, they help to highlight the needs of individuals with AIDS and their caregivers. Also, in concert with Dr. Barbara DeBuono, the New York State Commissioner of Health, they urged the maintenance of adequate health and social services for New Yorkers with HIV/AIDS, and joined in publicizing the need to reauthorize and fully fund the federal Ryan White CARE Act which allocates funding to the State and the City for programs of HIV/AIDS services.

Finally, the Project created a Curriculum Development Advisory Committee, co-chaired by Dr. Stanley Yancovitz, Chief of Chemical Dependency at the Beth Israel Medical Center, and Celestine Pulchon, Ph.D., Director of Psycho-Social Training in the Social Medicine Program at the Montefiore Medical Center. This Committee designed *Identifying, Engaging and Managing the Active Substance User in the Primary Care Setting,* an innovative curriculum for a two-day course for primary care practitioners that features skills-building sessions as a supplement to didactic lectures.

CENTER FOR URBAN EPIDEMIOLOGIC STUDIES

Originally developed by Drs. Jeremiah Barondess, Margaret Hamburg and David E. Rogers, the Center for Urban Epidemiologic Studies began to take shape in 1994 as a public-private partnership between the Academy and the New York City Department of Health. It was designed as a multi–institutional, multidisciplinary instrument to improve the health status of urban populations, especially the residents of inner cities, with participation by all of the local medical schools and the Columbia University School of Public Health. Appointed to head it was Dr. Stuart Bondurant, formerly Dean of the University of North Carolina School of Medicine and, before that, Dean of the Albany Medical College. Dr. Bondurant, a graduate of the Duke University Medical School who had practiced as a cardiologist, had also been President of the American College of Physicians as well as Chairman of the Association of American Medical Colleges.

Funding was provided initially by grants totaling more than $1.7 million from the Carnegie Corporation of New York, the Metropolitan Life Foundation, the New York Community Trust and the Robert Wood Johnson Foundation. Subsequently, additional grants were provided by Pfizer, Inc., Pharmacia & Upjohn, and the Aaron Diamond, Equitable, and Overbrook Foundations.

The organizational strategy involved housing the core research and administrative staff at the Academy with additional staff located at the collaborating institutions. A Management Advisory Committee was established, to include the Director of the Center, the Academy President, the New York City Commissioner of Health and a senior representative from each of the participating institutions. A Scientific Advisory Committee was appointed, comprising three nationally-recognized experts in public health epidemiology and policy: Gordon deFriese, Ph.D.; Gilbert S.Omenn, M.D., Ph.D.; and Leon Gordis, M.D.

Early in 1996, Dr. Bondurant announced that compelling personal reasons required him to resign his position as Director of the Center and return to his home in North Carolina, and in November 1996, Ezra Susser, M.D. Ph.D. became the Director. A psychiatrist and epidemiologist, Dr. Susser's experience includes service as Director of the Division of Epidemiology and Community Psychiatry at the New York State Psychiatric Institute, Associate Director of that Institute's HIV Center for Clinical and Behavioral Studies, and Co-Director of the Psychiatric Epidemiology Training Program at the Columbia University School of Public Health. Additions to the staff included Mary Bassett, M.D., M.P.H., a medical epidemiologist who is also Director of the Harlem Prevention Center; Bruce Levin, Ph.D., Nancy Scholer, M.Sc., an epidemiologist; and Sonia Montiel as Administrative Assistant and Grants Manager. Wendy Wisbaum, formerly Associate Project Officer in the Health Group at UNICEF, was appointed Executive Officer.

A signal early accomplishment of the Center was the establishment of a strong working relationship with the US Centers for Disease Control and Prevention (CDC). The CDC is providing expert consultation and has assigned Theresa Diaz, M.D., MPH, a senior level research epidemiologist, to work full-time at the Center. (The CDC is also assisting in the replication of the Center model in Detroit and Seattle.)

Bruce Levin, Ph.D., an experienced biostatistician, has started work to improve the accessibility and utility of the epidemiologic databases maintained by the New York City Department of Health and other private and public agencies to facilitate the tracking of health care problems of the underprivileged who are the prime targets of the Center's research.

In 1996, an additional number of projects was already underway:

- A study of risk behaviors and HIV infection in young injecting drug users, involving collaboration with the New York City Department of Health, the Columbia University School of Public Health, and the Albert Einstein College of Medicine/Montefiore Medical Center. This study is supported by a $1.3 million grant from the Centers for Disease Control and Prevention.
- A Working Group on Asthma, co-chaired by Drs. Diaz and Hamburg.
- Research on violence that will address such issues as the determinants

and antecedents of weapons acquisition among urban school children, and data needs for the development of intervention programs to reduce school-based violence. This effort has received a $20,000 planning grant from the William T. Grant Foundation.

- A study of HIV risk reduction that will involve analysis of the results of *Sex, Games and Videotapes,* an HIV prevention intervention for homeless men with mental illness, supported by an $80,000 grant from the New York City Department for Homeless Services.
- Investigation of the development of a more sophisticated index of the risk of HIV transmission.

## HARM REDUCTION IN DRUG ADDICTION

In March 1995, the concept of treating drug addiction primarily as a medical and public health issue was revisited through a Symposium on *Harm Reduction Policies and Practice: International Developments and Domestic Initiatives,* held at the Academy with support from Beth Israel Medical Center and Montefiore Hospital. The program focused on foreign experiences with harm reduction strategies in dealing with drug addiction. Playing leading roles in organizing the meeting were Dr. Ethan Nadelmann of the Lindesmith Center on Drug Policy, supported by the Soros Foundation, Dr. Ernest Drucker of the Department of Community Medicine at the Albert Einstein College of Medicine, and Ms. Julie Hantman. The speakers included Colin Brewer, MB, MRCS, DPM, MRC Psych, from the United Kingdom, Dr. Giel Van Brussel from the Netherlands, Dr. Robert Haemmig from Switzerland, and Dr. Alex Wodack from Australia.

Harm reduction objectives were defined as the attempt to: "refine and revise our understanding of addiction, in light of developments in neuroscience, clinical practice, and public health; to develop better treatment methods, including substitution drugs, as well as new ways to organize the delivery of existing methods; and to explore how new models for distributing controlled substances may reduce harms."[4] Harm reduction methods in other countries

are much more flexible in the way they handle methadone maintenance compared to the United States and, it was suggested, "Foreign programs to provide drugs to long time users, under medical
supervision, are sensitive to addicts' needs and preferences, and
proffer alleviation of social harms caused by the illicit drug trade."

During 1995 and 1996, the harm reduction concept was studied
by the Committee on Medicine in Society through presentations by
a variety of experts in the field of addictions and their treatment,
by wide-ranging discussions by the Committee members, and by
research by Dr. Alan R. Fleischman, Ms. Julie Hantman and Mr.
Gary Stein of the Academy staff.[5] After many revisions, a Statement was approved by the Committee in November 1996 and
forwarded for consideration by the Board of Trustees.[6]

While cocaine and other abused substances were mentioned, the
Statement focused on heroin, due largely to the availability of
methadone as a management tool and the desire to impact initially
on areas of urgent, immediate concern. It reiterated the basic principles set forth in earlier Academy documents:

- "First, drug treatment should be accessible to all drug users seeking
  care, including those who are incarcerated. . . . and the medical community should be prepared to commence treatment when users request it;
- Second, addiction is a complex, chronic, relapsing illness for which
  various inpatient, residential and outpatient treatments are used depending on the substances involved, the intensity and duration of the
  addiction, the characteristics and tolerances of the patient, and the
  circumstances involved; and,
- Third, whether users are in treatment, are waiting for a treatment slot
  to become available, or are not yet ready for treatment, steps need to be
  taken to reduce the health-related harms associated with injecting drug
  use.

The Statement offered a series of recommendations including:
expansion of heroin treatment programs; methadone treatment
programs guided by generally accepted medical standards and indi-
vidualized treatment plans; special efforts directed to treatment for
pregnant women who use drugs and for incarcerated substance

abusers; education and specialized training programs for medical students, residents and generalist physicians; inclusion of reimbursement for drug treatment in the health care coverage by insurers and managed care entities; and, finally, adequately funded research directed at improving the effectiveness of addiction treatments. Recommendations specifically targeted to harm reduction included: support and expansion of current State-funded needle exchange programs; rescinding the ban on using federal funds for such programs and research; and changing the law to allow pharmacies to sell hypodermic syringes and needles without prescription and decriminalizing their distribution and possession.

## CAPITAL PUNISHMENT

At the January 25, 1995 meeting of the Board of Trustees, Dr. Barondess suggested that, since it was likely that New York State would shortly reinstate the death penalty, it would be appropriate for the Academy to consider the ethics of physician involvement in legal executions. After extensive discussion, a provisional statement prepared by Dr. Alan Fleischman and endorsed by the Committee on Medicine in Society was presented at the February 22, 1995 meeting of the Executive Committee of the Board. The statement echoed the views of other medical organizations in opposing the involvement of physicians in executions. It stated that, "The primary duty of physicians is to benefit the patient directly by alleviating pain and suffering and where possible to maintain and restore health. Indeed the most fundamental principle of medicine, *'primum non nocere'*, (first, do no harm), requires that physicians attempt to heal with care and compassion and avoid all actions that decrease the well-being of an individual patient. . . . .Guided by these principles, the New York Academy of Medicine believes that it is inappropriate for physicians to be involved in the conduct of capital punishment."[7]

This issue continued to be discussed at great length by both the Committee on Medicine in Society and the Board of Trustees, and at its September 27, 1995 meeting, the Board reviewed a revised statement in which disciplinary action against any physician participating in capital punishment was proposed. By this time, the Legislature had approved and the Governor had signed the bill reinstating the death penalty.

The activities in question range from designing the procedures and participating in the administration of fatal doses of drugs to monitoring the status of executed individuals to pronounce death. Since individuals sentenced to death could not be executed if they were mentally incompetent, there was also the problem of the ethics of psychiatric evaluations and treatment that would improve an individual's mental status sufficiently to allow him or her to be executed.

It was reported that the American College of Physicians, the American Medical Association, the American Nurses Association, and the American Public Health Association had issued a statement which included the following: "We also call all health care professional societies to ensure that their members know and understand that participation in an execution is a serious violation of ethical standards. Professional societies should impose disciplinary actions on those members who do participate in executions."[8]

A number of those involved in the discussions were troubled by the requirement of disciplinary action if a physician were involved in an execution. It was generally agreed that that participation in capital punishment is unethical, but since it was now legal, there was discomfort with the wording regarding physician discipline. In addition, Dr. Charles Hirsch, the City's Chief Medical Examiner, pointed out that, since the law required autopsies in all fatalities among prisoners, the proposed statement would subject a pathologist to disciplinary action for performing his or her duty. In the end, the Statement was modified to declare that "physician involvement in capital punishment is unethical" without defining the specifics of the involvement, and it was approved by the Board.[9] It was distributed to a large number of political figures, including the Governor, the Commissioners of Health and Social Services, and members of the Legislature.

## THE URBAN HEALTH INITIATIVE

During 1995, more than 250 volunteers from 10 medical schools worked on over 60 projects, bringing the total of participants since the program was initiated in 1993 to more than 750. The volunteers provided HIV/AIDS education, developed health services in shelters for the homeless, and engaged in youth violence preventive and mentoring efforts. The success of the Urban Health Initiative (UHI) attests to the interest of medical students in serving in disadvantaged communities and to the dedication and skill of the Academy staff and the cooperating faculties. Ms. Julie Hantman served as Executive Director of the program until 1996.

The UHI offered grants of $500 each to encourage students' special projects and provided technical assistance in project development. It provided workshops in health education skills in which Ms. Leslie Goldman, Executive Director, Deputy Director Joanne De Simone Eichel and the staff of the Office of School Health Programs played a prominent role. It published a quarterly newsletter, and conducted a number of symposia on such urban health issues as drug abuse, treating people with AIDS, careers in public health and preventive medicine, and homelessness in New York City. In April 1995, the UHI conducted a half-day meeting that included presentations on human rights, the homeless and domestic violence, and featured a keynote address on *Health Activism at Home and Abroad* by Dr. Jim Yong Kim, a physician and anthropologist who is Executive Director of Partners in Care. Another half-day forum in October 1995 reviewed current developments in managed care.

## DOMESTIC VIOLENCE

In April 1994, the Academy organized the Health Coalition Against Violence to bring together health professionals, health educators, and representatives of government agencies, professional organizations and community-based organizations to develop and implement health-related strategies to control and prevent violence. Dr. Jacqueline Messite played a leading role in this effort, which was funded by a $25,000 grant from the Altman Foundation.

On June 27, 1995, a meeting of the Coalition was held at the Academy to discuss possible intervention strategies by health care institutions in the community that might be effective. Dr. Stephen G. Lynn, Director of Emergency Medicine at the St. Luke's-Roosevelt Hospital Center, described the work of the Domestic Violence Surveillance Project, which deals with abuse and rape and focuses on preventing domestic disputes from leading to violence. Also discussed was another interesting model of intervention that has proved quite successful: the Harlem Hospital Injury Prevention Program, conducted since 1988 under the auspices of its Department of Pediatrics. This program, which conducts a little league for baseball, dance classes, gardening projects and other activities aimed at channeling youthful interest and energy into nonviolent areas, has resulted in a 44 percent reduction in violence-related-injuries among youngsters in Central Harlem.

## THE MARGARET E. MAHONEY SYMPOSIA

In 1995, with the co-sponsorship of the Commonwealth Fund, the first annual *Margaret E. Mahoney Symposium on the State of the Nation's Health* was held at the Academy.[10] Ms. Mahoney had retired in 1994 as president of the Commonwealth Fund after a distinguished career as a Foundation executive including work at the Robert Wood Johnson Foundation and the Carnegie Corporation of New York. As a member and later as Vice Chair of the Board of Trustees, she played a major role in many Academy activities, including the reorganization that was started in 1990.

The keynote speaker was Dr. Philip R. Lee, Assistant Secretary for Health in the US Department of Health and Human Resources. A roundtable chaired by Dr. Samuel Thier, President of the Massachusetts General Hospital, discussed issues in child health, health insurance, the evolution of managed care, and future public health initiatives. It featured presentations by Dr. Richard Behrman, Managing Director of the David and Lucille Packard Foundation, Mr. Willis Gradison, President of the Health Insurance Association of America, Dr. Joseph Dorsey, Senior Medical Director of the Harvard Community Health Plan, and Lawrence D. Brown, Ph.D. Director of the Division of Health Policy and Management at the Columbia University School of Public Health.

In addition, Dr. Karen Davis, who had succeeded Ms. Mahoney as President of the Commonwealth Fund, and members of her staff, presented progress reports of four major programs that had been initiated by Ms. Mahoney: minority health, patient-centered care, women's health initiatives, and managed care. The proceedings were summarized by Dr. Stuart Bondurant, Director of the Center for Urban Epidemiologic Studies at the Academy.

A second Margaret E. Mahoney Symposium was held on May 13, 1996. Speakers included Dr. Karen Davis, Dr. Barbara DeBuono, New York State Commissioner of Health, and Uwe Reinhardt, Ph.D., Professor of Political Economy at the Woodrow Wilson School of Public and International Affairs at Princeton University. Bruce C. Vladeck, Ph.D., Administrator of the Health Care Financing Administration, received the Margaret E. Mahoney Award in recognition of his distinguished contributions to public service and the advancement of the health of the public.

## INSIDE URBAN HEALTH

In November 1995, the Academy joined the Institute of Medicine in hosting an all-day symposium on *Inside Urban Health* to commemorate the twenty-fifth anniversary of the establishment of Institute of Medicine of the National Academy of Sciences. Dr. Kenneth Shine, President of the Institute, delivered the Keynote Address, in which he noted that the urban health focus reflected the Academy focus on urban populations and recognition of the fact that 80 percent of Americans now live in metropolitan areas.

Mayor Rudolph Giuliani delivered the luncheon address on *The*

*Role of Governments in Combating Urban Health Problems,* in which he presented the case for privatizing the City's public hospital system. The Mayor argued that government would be more effective in contracting with others for health services than in operating them. Too much of the municipal hospital system, he said, is dedicated to providing jobs for municipal workers. Privatizing the system would lead to the removal of a major financial burden from the city and would also lead to better care for indigent New Yorkers.

Perhaps the most eloquent and effective address made at the meeting was the presentation by Dr. Margaret C. Heagarty, Director of Pediatrics at Harlem Hospital and a Trustee of the Academy. She spoke movingly about the continued need for the City to commit itself to providing services to disadvantaged children, expressing grave doubts that the negative impact on children of the proposed cuts in welfare and Medicaid had been fully understood by the proponents of these reductions. Also participating in the celebration was Dr. Barbara De Buono, Commissioner of Health of the State of New York.

## THE DIVISION OF PUBLIC HEALTH

In 1995, the Division of Public Health was created as a venue for convening a variety of players in the field of public health to support the public health community as it addresses such issues as infectious disease prevention, environmental health and community health promotion in the wake of current changes in health care, and to foster greater collaboration between public health and medical practice. The Division dovetails neatly with the Academy's tradition as an independent organization that deals both with policy and performance in health care and will share the focus of the reorganized Academy on issues relating to the at-risk and underserved urban populations. Its goal is to provide the public health community with meaningful support as it attempts to reposition itself in an environment characterized by distrust of government, fiscal constraints, cultural diversity, multifactorial health problems and the emergence of managed care. It plans to accomplish this goal by:

- Improving access of the public health community to useful existing information (e.g., hooking up health departments to the resources of the National Network of Libraries of Medicine through the Internet);
- Generating user-friendly knowledge bases to fill unmet needs (e.g., creating an interactive electronic inventory of experiences around the country to provide health officials with up-to-date information relevant to their local conditions);
- Filling critical gaps in policy analysis and health systems research (e.g., assessing the impact of Medicaid managed care on the financing, organization and delivery of population-based public health services); and
- Establishing a broad-based platform for dialogue and partnerships (e.g., linking traditional public health with other stakeholders who are having an increasing role in carrying out the public health mission).

Dr. Roz Diane Lasker was appointed Director of the Division. An internist and endocrinologist, she came from the US Department of Health and Human Services where she had been Deputy Assistant Secretary for Health Policy Development, making major contributions in reorienting federal data policies in support of population health and in the restructuring of public health programs to promote federal/state collaboration and accountability. She had also served as Principal Policy Analyst for the Congressional Physician Payment Review Commission.

As a means of introducing herself and her plans for the Division, she addressed the Committee on Public Health in November 1995 on *Condition Critical? The Health of the Public Health System in an Environment of Rapid Change.*[11] Her goal, she said, was to focus "as much attention on the health of the public health system as on the health of the populations that the system is intended to serve."

She described the challenges to the public health systems in the country stemming from changes in the overall health care system and noted that her main concern was to resolve differences between medicine and public health. The picture was not entirely bleak, she said, "because in some parts of the country, departments of public health were indeed attempting to strengthen the public health infrastructure."

Dr. Lasker described *Public Health and Medicine: Partnering to Improve Community Health in the 21st Century,* a project, for which a substantial grant has been received from the Robert Wood Johnson Foundation, that would "explore how changes in the current environment create both the need and opportunity for these two sectors to overcome past differences and work together to improve community health." This project will engage experts with a broad range of perspectives in the production of a monograph that would "clarify the roles that medicine and public health can play in improving community health, present a sound rationale for forging a partnership between the two in the current health environment, document the benefits that could be achieved through such a partnership (to the population at large as well as to health professionals), offer concrete examples of synergistic partnerships in action, and identify the incentives, tools and skills that are required for such constructive collaboration." The American Medical Association and the American Public Health Association, working in conjunction with the Academy, have committed to distribute 250,000 copies of the monograph to practitioners, educators, students and researchers in both fields.

Dr. Lasker depicted the Committee on Public Health as playing a "vital advisory role, helping to shape the overall agenda for the Division," with its members invited to play a role in the design and implementation stages of projects. She said that the Committee could also play a role in "identifying and pursuing its own initiatives."


## SECTION ON HEALTH CARE DELIVERY

In late 1995, a new provisional Section on Health Care Delivery was formed with the purpose of developing educational programs on the delivery, policy, and economics of health care and on health care management and administration, and providing a framework for the Fellows to help the Academy develop strategies in health policy. Its first Chair was Ms. Ellen Rautenberg, Vice-President of the Medical and Health Research Association of New York City. The first activity of the Section was the development of *The Culture of Managed Care in New York State: A Health Policy Seminar Series,* four seminars conducted in 1995 and 1996 at which authoritative speakers from community medicine, patient advocacy groups, medical practice, academia and the managed care industry addressed the impact of managed care on patient populations, practicing physicians and health care institutions. The first in the series featured a presentation by Dr. Karen Schimke, Deputy Commissioner of the New York State Department of Health on *Policy Directions of Managed Care in New York State.* The second series of educational seminars on *The Future of Health Policy in New York State: the Debate over NYPHRM (New York Prospective Hospital Reimbursement Methodology),* presented In the Spring of 1996, included programs on *Framing the Debate: NYPHRM 1966, Uncompensated Care,* and *Graduate Medical Education.*

## DIVISION OF HEALTH AND SCIENCE POLICY

The Division of Health and Science Policy was created in 1996 to become the focal point for the Academy's research activities pertaining to the organization and financing of health care. It is directed by Bradford H. Gray, Ph.D., who came to the Academy in September 1996 from Yale University where he was Adjunct Professor of Research in Public Health and Director of the Institution for Social and Policy Studies and the Program on Non-Profit Organizations. He was previously a senior staff member and study director at the Institute of Medicine, and a staff member of both the National Commission for the Protection of Human Subjects of Biomedical and Behavioral Research and the President's Commission for the Study of Ethical Problems in Medicine and Research. During this period, he was also a faculty member at the University of North Carolina at Chapel Hill.

The Committee on Medicine in Society will support and extend the work of the Division which will carry out empirical research, sponsor conferences on important health policy issues, and collaborate with other parts of the Academy, particularly the Division of Public Health and the Center for Urban Epidemiologic Studies, and with other organizations on projects relevant to its mission.

The Division will be responsive to the enormous changes that are occurring in health care delivery in New York and the country. Its initial research agenda will emphasize three topics: the operation and impact of managed care; the implications of the growing role of for-profit entities in health care, and the changing conditions of medical professionalism. Of particular concern are developments that affect the urban poor and the professionals and institutions that serve them, ways of enhancing the trustworthiness of medical care in the managed care era, and the community impact of managed care organizations.

## NEW OFFICERS OF THE BOARD OF TRUSTEES

On December 15, 1995, Dr. Saul Farber presided at his last meeting as Chairman of the Board. He was succeeded on January 1, 1996 by Mr. Stanley Brezenoff, President of Maimonides Medical Center, who had been a Trustee since 1992. Mr. Brezenoff had become familiar with health care issues as an executive of the Ford Foundation and through successive appointments by Mayor Koch as Administrator of Human Resources, President of the New York City Health and Hospitals Corporation, and Deputy Mayor. On leaving the City, he became Executive Director of the Port Authority of New York and New Jersey.

At the same time, Ms. Margaret Mahoney was succeeded as Vice Chair by Dr. Ralph O'Connell, Dean and Provost of the New York Medical College. A psychiatrist at St. Vincent's Hospital and

Medical Center, Dr. O'Connell had served for many years as the Academy's Treasurer, a post that was assumed by Mr. Richard Menschel, a limited partner of the Goldman Sachs Group and Co-Chair of the Board of the Hospital for Special Surgery. Mr. Paul Kligfield continued as Secretary.

New 1966 Board members included Dr. Richard Rifkind, Chairman of the Sloan-Kettering Institute at Memorial Sloan-Kettering Cancer Center, Dr. Victor Alicea, President of Boricua College in New York, and Mr. Dean O'Hare, Chairman, President, and Chief Executive Officer of the Chubb Corporation.

## OFFICE OF SCHOOL HEALTH PROGRAMS

### Death of Dr. John Waller

The Office suffered a grievous loss on June 5, 1995 with the death of Dr. John Waller who had founded and so skillfully nurtured the School Health Program. A moving memorial service to recall the many contributions of this singularly gracious and highly regarded physician was held in the Rare Book Room of the Library.

### Program Progress

The Office of School Health Programs continues to be headed by Executive Director Leslie Goldman. Ms. Joyce Bove of the New York Community Trust is Chair of the Management Committee with Mrs. Anne Waller, Dr. Waller's widow, who has long been active in such community health projects as the Maternity Center Association, serving as Vice Chair. It continues to be funded by grants from the Board of Education with matching funds from the private sector. Although the former were reduced by 30 percent, this gap in its current annual budget of $600,000 was made up by increased funding from private sources.

The goal of the programs is to help students develop the skills, attitudes and knowledge needed to lead and maintain healthy lives. Since the inception of the Program in 1979, "Growing Healthy," the program for elementary schools, has trained over 6,250 teachers in 627 of the City's 632 schools, and reached over 500,000 youngsters. In addition, it offers workshops for teachers of special populations, such as the staff development program for the New York State School for the Deaf.

"Being Healthy," the program for middle schools, has involved the training of more than 500 middle school teachers, counselors, health services personnel and parent leaders. In 1966, this program was being used in nearly half of the City's 181 middle schools.

In 1995, to complete the range of school-based heath education programs from kindergarten to grade 12, the Office launched "Staying Healthy," a comprehensive initiative for high school students. This program addresses the needs of teenagers and includes such topics as feelings and handling emotions; how to avoid harmful behaviors such as smoking, drinking and drugs; building stronger relationships with families and friends; prevention of violence; and prevention of sexually transmitted diseases, including HIV/AIDS.

The Office is at the cutting edge of the technology of health education. It tailors its programs to meet the needs of individual local school districts and is developing *Health Education in Partnership with Parents,* a training program for parents. To help health professionals working in classrooms make a significant impact on students, it conducts workshops for physicians, scientists and medical students doing community service in schools. These workshops focus on student-centered health education strategies, how to deal with sensitive issues, and classroom management techniques.

The Office, which is staffed by experienced teachers, administrators and professional health educators, also establishes linkages with non-profit organizations that work with schools, providing program design, curriculum and staff development. For example, it has received a grant from the American Skin Association to prepare educational modules on skin health for children, and it has become part of a national network disseminating information on health education.

Most important, the Office works with other departments of the Academy. As the Academy activities become more focused on the community, it helps to relate them to the school system. It has moved into health and science education and educational technology training, and is working with medical students involved in the Urban Health Initiative to enable them to relate more effectively to young children.

## Careers in the Health Professions Program

In furtherance of its belief that exposure to the possibility of future health careers is part of comprehensive health education, the Office has undertaken the Careers in the Health Professions Program. This program has a number of elements which include the following:

- Seminars on *Career Opportunities in the Health Professions* that are open to middle and high school students and which provide opportunities to meet informally with physicians, researchers, nurses, technicians and other health professionals;
- *Scientists in the Schools,* which places scientists in school classrooms;
- *Medical Students in Service to Schools,* which places medical students in classrooms to assist teachers in conveying health information to students; and
- *The New York Academy of Medicine as a Learning Center,* which includes visits to the Library, the Rare Book Room, and the Preservation Center to view books and artifacts and to interact with librarians and preservationists.

## EVIDENCE-BASED MEDICINE PROGRAM

In the fall of 1996, the Academy, in conjunction with the New York Chapter of the American College of Physicians, presented a two-part, four-day course for those who teach residents on *Teach-*

*ing Evidence-based Medicine.* "Evidence-based medicine is the conscientious, explicit and judicious use of current best evidence in making decisions about the care of individual patients....... integrating individual clinical expertise with the best available external clinical evidence from systematic research."[12] The course, oversubscribed by teaching internists and academic health science librarians, marked the beginning of an ongoing effort in New York to support the practice of evidence-based medicine and to provide the resources needed for such practice.

The Academy has agreed to be the site of an Evidence-based Medicine Resource Center which will be cosponsored by the New York Chapter of the American College of Physicians. The Center can be reached at its Internet address, < http://www.nyam.org/library/eblinks.htm >. In addition, the Academy will support hospital librarians' needs and will be available for small group and individual on-site teaching in the use of these electronic resources.[13]

## REAPPOINTMENT OF DR. BARONDESS

By the Spring of 1996, over six years had elapsed since the restructuring of the Academy began to be implemented in accord with the By-Laws revision implemented as of January 1, 1990. On July 1, 1996, Dr. Barondess completed six years as President of the Academy. His original contract as President was for a term of five years. At the end of 1995, he received a vote of confidence from the Board of Trustees, who extended the term for another five years. Under the new structure of the Academy and under its new leadership, the Academy has a more visible presence on the local, state and national health care scene than it had six years ago. Its financial condition has much improved, and it has embarked on and is continuing to plan programs to advance its mission as the organization begins its preparations to celebrate its 150th Anniversary in 1997.

THE 150th ANNIVERSARY CELEBRATION

The 1996 Spring Stated Meeting of the New York Academy of Medicine, which took place at the Academy on April 30, 1996, marked the commencement of the Academy's celebration of its sesquicentennial, focused on *150 Years of Leadership: Advancing Urban Health*. Stanley Brezenoff, Chairman of the Board of Trustees, presided. The Anniversary Discourse was presented by Witold Rybczynski, the Martin and Margy Meyerson Professor of Urbanism at the University of Pennsylvania. Prof. Rybczynski's topic was *City Planning and Urban Health*. Dr. Barondess, in greeting the audience assembled for the festive dinner served in the main reading room of the Library, noted that "during the Anniversary Celebration, the Academy would hold a series of meetings to fashion the *Urban Health Agenda,* a set of specific recommendations to advance knowledge and action addressing the health needs of the urban populations into the next millenium."

The Meeting also featured the presentation of three awards. The 1996 Academy Plaque for Service to the Academy was given to Saul J. Farber, M.D., Provost of the New York University Medical Center and Dean and Chairman of the Department of Medicine of the New York University School of Medicine. Dr. Farber had served as Chairman of the New York Academy of Medicine's Board of Trustees from 1991 through 1995. The 1996 Academy Medal for Distinguished Contributions to Biomedical Sciences was given to Eric R. Kandel, M.D., University Professor, Columbia University College of Physicians and Surgeons for his remarkable contributions to neurobiology. The John Stearns Award for Lifetime Achievement in Medicine, first given in 1991, was given to Joshua Lederberg, Ph.D., Sackler Foundation Scholar and President Emeritus of Rockefeller University.

Almost one hundred years ago, upon the occasion of the Academy's fiftieth Anniversary celebration on January 29, 1897 at Carnegie Hall, only 8 of the 184 physicians who founded the organization in 1847 were still living. Two of them spoke: Samuel S. Purple, whose gift of books founded the Library, and Lewis Sayre. In his address, Dr. Sayre said, "After fifty years of steady growth in membership, social influence, and in scientific advancement, the Academy stands as an efficient bulwark and protection to the public health, not alone of this City and State, but of the whole country."[14]

Although Dr. Sayre may have been unduly influenced by the fervor of the celebration to describe the Academy's "steady growth," and thus overlooked the setbacks, conflicts, and tensions which may confront any living organization, he was accurately expressing an aspiration that still governs the Academy today: to be an "efficient bulwark and protection to the public health." As it enters upon its sesquicentennial celebration, the Academy remains true to its long-term purpose: to "focus on how to advance knowledge and effectively address the health needs of urban populations." In adapting itself as an organization to its changing environment, the Academy has periodically redefined the critical tasks before it, and addressed them with more or less success. It has sought to remain true to a tradition of searching out new ways to promote the health of individual patients and populations. As Dr. Barondess noted in the Academy's 1994 Annual Report: "The forces acting on the health of individuals as well as the health of populations are always in a state of evolution: that is to say they are never stable and will never be so, since the pressures that act on human health shift continually. . . . . As it is with the health of individuals, and of populations; so it is with the health of organizations devoted to the health of individuals and populations."[15]

## NOTES

1 Barondess JA. 1994 Organizational Structure: Letter to Board of Trustees and Committee Chairs, April 19, 1994.
2 Task Force on Health Care Reform. 1994 *The Urban Perspective: Making Health Care Reform Responsive to the Needs of Urban America*. New York: New York Academy of Medicine.
3 [Multiple authors] 1995 Perspectives in HIV Care: A view from the

front lines. *Bulletin of the New York Academy of Medicine.* 72: 171–315.

4 Drucker E and Hantman JA. 1995 Harm Reduction Drug Policies and Practice: International Developments and Domestic Initiatives. *Bulletin of the New York Academy of Medicine.* 72:335–336.

5 Hantman JA. 1995 Research on needle exchange: Redefining the agenda. *Bulletin of the New York Academy of Medicine.* 72:397–412.

6 Committee on Medicine in Society. 1996 *Addiction Treatment: Promoting a Medical Approach to Substance Use.* November 22, 1996.

7 Executive Committee of the Board of Trustees, New York Academy of Medicine. Minutes of the meeting of February 22, 1995.

8 American College of Physicians, American Medical Association, American Nurses Association, American Public Health Association. 1994 *Health Care Professional Participation in Capital Punishment: Statement from Professionals Regarding Disciplinary Action.* March 23, 1994.

9 New York Academy of Medicine. 1966 *Statement on Physician Involvement in Capital Punishment.* Adopted February 1995; Revised March 1996.

10 Multiple authors] 1995 Margaret E. Mahoney Symposium: Proceedings. *Bulletin of the New York Academy of Medicine.* 72 Supplement: 550–662.

11 Lasker RD. 1996 *Condition Critical? The Health of the Public Health System in an Environment of Rapid Change.* Unpublished manuscript, November 6, 1995.

12 Sacket DL. Rosenberg WC, Gray JAM, Haynen RB and Richardson WS. 1996 Evidence-based medicine: What it is and what it isn't. *British Medical Journal.* 312:71–72.

13 American College of Physicians, New York Chapter. 1996 New York evidence-based medicine program launched. *ACP New York Chapter Newsletter.* November 1966, p. 4.

14 Sayre LA. 1903 *The Celebration of the Semi-Centennial Anniversary of the New York Academy of Medicine, January 29, 1897.* New York: New York Academy of Medicine. pp. 17–18.

15 New York Academy of Medicine. 1995 *The New York Academy of Medicine: 1994 Annual Report.* New York: New York Academy of Medicine. pp. 4–5.

# Afterword

As THIS RICH CHRONICLE TELLS US, over the years, The New York Academy of Medicine has been a singular institution, a place where research and policy analysis have focused on the important issues of the day in medicine, reflecting the perspective and interests of physicians as guardians of public health and patient welfare. That mission is as important today as it has been over the last one hundred and fifty years.

As the health care system is tranformed by managed care and contracting financial resources, issues like access and quality are being decided almost without debate. The role of the physician as the arbiter of care and advocate of patients is being called into question. We have reason to worry that the doctor's traditional relationship with the patient is in danger of turning into a business pact with insurance companies. Little attention is paid to developing standards to measure the effectiveness of managed care and to hold the plans accountable for the vast sums of public and private dollars involved. Impact on the poor and the uninsured of the dramatic changes in policy and delivery system is at best, an afterthought.

The Academy of Medicine must continue to be a center where these important health policy issues can be engaged with empirical research, scientific analysis, and informed debate. In recent years, the Academy has structured itself to serve precisely that role: the Center for Urban Epidemiologic Studies, the Division of Health and Science Policy, and the Division of Public Health are tackling the most compelling and difficult questions emerging in health policy. Their work gives me great confidence that the Academy's special past is prologue to a vital future role in shaping an agenda for health care in New York and urban America.

Stanley Brezenoff
Chairman, Board of Trustees
The New York Academy of Medicine
January 1997

# Appendix

## SPECIAL ACADEMY AWARDS

### The Academy Medal

For distinguished contributions in biomedical science.

| | |
|---|---|
| 1930 | Dr. Carl Koller |
| 1931 | Dr. David Marine |
| 1934 | Dr. Charles Norris |
| 1936 | Dr. Alfred Newton Richards |
| 1938 | Dr. Bela Schick |
| 1944 | Dr. Oswald T. Avery |
| 1947 | Dr. James A. Miller |
| 1953 | Dr. Rufus Cole |
| 1954 | Dr. Edward A. Parks |
| 1955 | Dr. Allen O. Whipple |
| 1956 | Dr. Eugene F. DuBois |
| 1958 | Dr. Alphonse R. Dochez |
| 1959 | Dr. Peyton Rous |
| 1960 | Dr. Eugene L. Opie |
| 1961 | Dr. E. V. McCollum |
| 1962 | Dr. Paul Klemperer |
| 1963 | Dr. Andre Cournand |
| | Dr. Dickinson W. Richards |
| 1964 | Dr. Gilbert J. Dalldorf |
| 1965 | Dr. Richard E. Shope |
| 1966 | Dr. Samuel Z. Levine |
| | Dr. Rustin McIntosh |
| 1967 | Dr. Donald D. Van Slyke |
| 1968 | Dr. Michael Heidelberger |
| 1969 | Dr. Harold W. Brown |
| 1970 | Dr. Harry Eagle |

1971    Dr. Solomon Berson
1972    Dr. James A. Shannon
1973    Dr. Rebecca Lancefield
1974    Dr. H. Sherwood Lawrence
1975    Dr. George Hirst
1976    Dr. Charles A. Ragan, Jr.
1977    Dr. Henry G. Kunkel
1978    Dr. Saul Krugman
1979    Dr. Maclyn McCarty
1980    Dr. Erwin Chargaff
1981    Dr. Karl Meyer
1982    Dr. Rene DuBos
1983    Dr. Edwin D. Kilbourne
1984    Dr. Vincent P. Dole
1985    Dr. Lloyd J. Old
1986    Dr. Irving S. Wright
1987    Dr. Thomas C. Chalmers
1988    Dr. Paul Cranefield
        Dr. Brian Hoffman
1989    Dr. Elvin A. Kabat
1990    Dr. Matthew Scharff
1991    Dr. Maria I. New
1992    Dr. Robert F. Furchgott
1993    Dr. John H. Laragh
1994    Dr. Harold S. Ginsberg
1995    Dr. William Trager
1996    Dr. Eric R. Kandel
1997    Dr. David Baltimore

## The John Stearns Award

For lifetime achievement in medicine.

1991    Dr. Lewis Thomas
1993    Dr. Maclyn McCarty
1994    Dr. David Rogers
1995    Dr. Donald A. Henderson

1996    Dr. Joshua Lederberg
1997    Dr. David Satcher


## The Academy Plaque

For exceptional service to the Academy.

1952    Dr. Orrin Sage Wightman
1953    Mr. John W. Davis
1954    Dr. Seth Minot Milliken
1955    Dr. Haven Emerson
1958    Dr. Malcolm Goodridge
1959    Dr. Montgomery B. Angell
1960    Dr. Shepard Krech
1961    Dr. George Baehr
1962    Dr. Robert L. Levy
1963    Dr. Asa Liggett Lincoln
1964    Dr. William Barclay Parsons
1965    Dr. Arthur M. Master
1966    Dr. Benjamin P. Watson
1967    Dr. Howard Reid Craig
1968    Dr. Claude Heaton
1969    Dr. Peter Marshall
1970    Dr. J. Burns Amberson, Jr.
1971    Dr. Samuel W. Lambert, Jr.
1972    Dr. Frank B. Berry
1973    Dr. Jerome P. Webster
1974    Miss Gertrude L. Annan
        Miss Janet Doe
1975    Dr. Albert C. Santy
1976    Dr. Paul Reznikoff
1977    Dr. Frank Glenn
1978    Dr. George A. Perera
1979    Dr. Saul Jarcho
1980    Dr. John L. Madden
1981    Dr. Edward E. Fischel

1982    Dr. Joseph Post
1983    Dr. Iago Galdston
1984    Dr. August H. Groeschel
1985    Dr. John V. Waller
1986    Dr. Duncan W. Clark
1987    Dr. Norbert J. Roberts
1988    Dr. Bernard J. Pisani
1989    Dr. Maurice E. Shils
1990    Dr. Fidelio A. Jimenez
1991    Dr. Mary Ann Payne
1992    Dr. Martin Cherkasky
1993    Margaret E. Mahoney
1994    William C. Stubing
1995    Dr. Robert J. Haggerty
1996    Dr. Saul J. Farber
1997    Dr. Thomas Q. Morris

## THE NEW YORK ACADEMY OF MEDICINE LECTURES AND AWARDS

### The Sylvia and Herbert Berger Lecture

To recognize contributions in clinical or basic sciences made by a distinguished educator, researcher, or clinician.

1983    George Wald, Ph.D
        Torsten N. Wiesel, M.D.
1985    Christian J. Lambertsen, M.D.
        Robert M. Winslow, M.D.
1986    Richard J. Kitz, M.D.
1987    Stephen M. Ayres, M.D.
1989    Jerold F. Lucey, M.D.
1992    Joshua Lederberg, Ph.D.
1994    James D. Watson, M.D.

The Millie and Richard Brock Lecture in Pediatrics

To honor commitment to the health needs of children.

1995    Gwendolyn Scott, M.D.
1996    Stephen Ludwig, M.D.


The Duncan Clark Lecture

For major contributions with regard to the social aspects of medicine.

1986    Uwe E. Reinhardt, Ph.D.
1987    Karen Davis, Ph.D.
1988    George A. Silver, M.D.
1989    Amitai Etzioni, Ph.D.
1990    Nathan Glazer, Ph.D.
1991    David Ellwood, Ph.D.


The Robert S. Coles Distinguished Lecture in Ophthalmology of
the Raymond and Beverly Sackler Foundation

To recognize outstanding achievement in the field of ophthalmology.

1987    Stephen J. Ryan, Jr., M.D.
1988    Charles L. Schepens, M.D.
1989    Manus C. Kraff, M.D.
1990    Bradley Straatsma, M.D.
1991    Frederick A. Jakobiec, M.D.
1992    M. Bruce Shields, M.D.
1993    Howard Fine, M.D.
1994    Robert B. Nussenblatt, M.D.
1995    Neil R. Miller, M.D.
1996    Alan H. Friedman, M.D.

# Appendix

## The Howard Fox Lecture

For notable contributions in the field of dermatology.

1962  V. Pardo-Castello, M.D.
1963  Arthur C. Curtis, M.D.
1964  Herman Pinkus, M.D.
1965  J. Walter Wilson, M.D.
1966  J. Graham Smith, Jr., M.D.
1967  Kurt Hirschhorn, M.D.
1968  Robert J. Gorlin, D.D.S., M.S.
1969  Urs W. Schnyder, M.D.
1970  Harvey Blank, M.D.
1971  Eugene M. Farber, M.D.
1972  James Trimble, M.D.
1973  Frances Pascher, M.D.
1974  Adolph Rostenberg, M.D.
1975  Walter B. Shelley, M.D.
1976  Harold O. Perry, M.D.
1977  Marion B. Sulzberger, M.D.
1978  Edward V. Zegarelli, D.D.S.
1979  Robert I. Goltz, M.D.
1980  Rees B. Rees, M.D.
1981  Eugene Van Scott, M.D.
1982  Thomas B. Fitzpatrick, M.D.
1983  John S. Strauss, M.D.
1984  Clarence S. Livingood, M.D.
1985  Orlando Canizares, M.D.
1986  Aaron B. Lerner, M.D.
1987  William L. Weston, M.D.
1988  Steven I. Katz, M.D.
1989  Eugene A. Bauer, M.D.
1990  Barbara Ann Gilchrest, M.D.
1991  Edward J. O'Keefe, M.D.
1992  Daniel M. Sauder, M.D.
1993  Madeleine Duvic, M.D.
1994  Joseph Jorizzo, M.D.

1995   John R. Stanley, M.D.
1996   Brian Berman, M.D.


## The Iago Galdston Memorial Lecture

To recognize distinguished scholars in areas of inquiry related to the historical, philosophical, and humanistic aspects of medicine.

1993   Daniel M. Fox, Ph.D.
1995   Jonathan D. Moreno, Ph.D.
1996   Daniel Callahan, Ph.D.


## The Glorney-Raisbeck Lecture and Award in Cardiology

For outstanding contributions to the field of cardiovascular disease.

1988   Milton J. Raisbeck, M.D.
1990   Anthony N. Damato, M.D.
1991   William Ganz, M.D.
1992   John W. Kirklin, M.D.
1994   Judah Folkman, M.D.
1994   Richard Gorlin, M.D.
1995   Russell Ross, Ph.D.
1996   Jan L. Breslow, M.D.


## The Paul Klemperer Award and Lecture

For exceptional scientific achievements and contributions to the study of connective tissues and their diseases.

1988   Jerome Bross, M.D.
1989   Frank J. Dixon, M.D.
1990   Stephen M. Kane, M.D.
1991   Morris Ziff, M.D.

1992   K. Frank Austen, M.D.
1993   Eng M. Tan, M.D.
1994   Hugh O. McDevitt, M.D.
1995   Charles G. Cochrane, M.D.
1996   John P. Atkinson, M.D.


## The John Kingsley Lattimer Lecture

To recognize significant contributions to research in the history of medicine.

1988   Thomas E. Cone, Jr., M.D.
1989   Allan M. Brandt, Ph.D.
1990   Kenneth M. Ludmerer, M.D.
1991   Dale C. Smith, M.D.
1992   Joel D. Howell, M.D., Ph.D.
1993   William F. Bynum, M.D., Ph.D.
1996   David Rosner, Ph.D.
1996   Ruth Macklin, Ph.D.


## The Charles H. May Memorial Lecture

To acknowledge distinguished scholars in the field of ophthalmology.

1946   W.J.B. Riddell, Ph.D.
1948   Adalbert Fuchs, M.D.
1950   Karl Safar, Ph.D.
1950   Kenneth C. Swan, M.D.
1951   Phillips Thygeson, M.D.
1952   T. Keith Lyle, Ph.D.
1953   H.B. Stallard, Ph.D.
1954   John Foster, M.D.
1955   Alan C. Woods, M.D.
1956   Edwin B. Dunphy, M.D.
1957   Alfred E. Maumenee, M.D.

| 1958 | Harold G. Scheie, M.D. |
|------|------------------------|
| 1959 | Frank B. Walsh, M.D. |
| 1960 | Wilbur C. Rucker, M.D. |
| 1961 | A. Gerard Devoe, M.D. |
| 1962 | Joaquin Barraquer, M.D. |
| 1963 | David G. Cogan, M.D. |
| 1964 | Lorenz Zimmerman, M.D. |
| 1966 | Sir Benjamin Rycroft, M.D. |
| 1967 | John M. McLean, M.D. |
| 1968 | Frank W. Newell, M.D. |
| 1969 | Alson E. Bradley, M.D. |
| 1970 | David Shoch, M.D. |
| 1971 | Renè Hugonnier, M.D. |
|      | S. Hugonnier-Clayette, M.D. |
| 1972 | Bernard Becker, M.D. |
| 1973 | Irving Leopold, M.D. |
| 1974 | Goodwin M. Breinin, M.D. |
| 1975 | Charles J. Campbell, M.D. |
| 1976 | Joseph A.C. Wadsworth, M.D. |
| 1977 | Claes H. Dohlman, M.D. |
| 1978 | Arnall Patz, M.D. |
| 1979 | Philip Knapp, M.D. |
|      | Keith M. Zinn, M.D. |
| 1980 | Donald M. Shafer, M.D. |
|      | Jerry A. Shields, M.D. |
|      | Lawrence G. Pape, M.D. |
| 1981 | D. Jackson Coleman, M.D. |
|      | Keith M. Zinn, M.D. |
|      | Frederick A. Jakobiec, M.D. |
| 1982 | George R. Merriam, M.D. |
| 1983 | Frederick Blodi, M.D. |
| 1984 | Charles L. Schepens, M.D. |
| 1988 | J. Donald Gass, M.D. |
| 1990 | Irving Leopold, M.D. |
| 1991 | Robert Ritch, M.D. |
| 1992 | Linn Murphree, M.D. |
| 1993 | Carmen A Puliafito, M.D. |
| 1994 | Jorge A. Alvarado, M.D. |

1995   Craig A. McKeown, M.D.
1995   Steven Podos, M.D.


## The Lewis Rudin Glaucoma Prize

For the most outstanding glaucoma research published during the previous year.

1995   Clive Migdal, M.D., FRCS., FRCOphth, Walter Gregory,
       Ph.D., and Roger Hitchings, FRCS, FRCOphth
1996   Harry Alan Quigley, M.D.
       Evan B. Dreyer, M.D., Ph.D.


## The Thomas William Salmon Medal

To honor notable advances in psychiatry, mental hygiene, and related fields.

| | | | |
|---|---|---|---|
| 1942 | Adolf Meyer, M.D. | 1970 | Oskar Diethelm, M.D. |
| 1945 | Joseph W. Moore, M.D. | 1970 | Roy R. Grinker, Sr., M.D. |
| 1963 | Earl D. Bond, M.D. | | |
| 1963 | Robert H. Felix, M.D. | 1970 | M. Ralph Kaufman, M.D. |
| 1965 | Lawrence Kolb, M.D. | | |
| 1966 | Kenneth E. Appel, M.D. | 1971 | John Whitehorn, M.D. |
| 1966 | Nathaniel Kleitman, Ph.D. | 1971 | David Shakow, M.D. |
| | | 1971 | S. Bernard Wortis, M.D. |
| 1967 | Stanley Cobb, M.D. | 1972 | Francis J. Braceland, M.D. |
| 1967 | David M. Levy, M.D. | | |
| 1967 | Karl A. Menninger, M.D. | 1973 | Lauretta Bender, M.D. |
| 1968 | Karl Bowman, M.D. | 1973 | H. Houston Merritt, M.D. |
| 1968 | Nolan D.C. Lewis, M.D. | | |
| 1969 | Franklin G. Ebaugh, M.D. | 1974 | Walter E. Barton, M.D. |
| | | 1974 | Leo Kanner, M.D. |
| 1969 | Clarence B. Farrar, M.D. | 1975 | David Blain, M.D. |
| 1969 | Titus Harris, M.D. | 1976 | David McKenzie Rioch, M.D. |
| 1969 | Harry C. Soloman, M.D. | | |

| 1977 | F.C. Redlich, M.D. | 1987 | Julius Axelrod, Ph.D. |
|---|---|---|---|
| 1977 | Joseph Zubin, Ph.D. | 1988 | Professor Sir Martin |
| 1978 | Robert A. Cohen, M.D. | | Roth |
| 1978 | John C. Eberhart, Ph.D. | 1990 | Daniel X. Freedman, |
| 1978 | Howard F. Hunt, M.D. | | M.D. |
| 1979 | George Tarjan, M.D. | 1991 | Shervert H. Frazier, |
| 1980 | Ewald W. Busse, M.D. | | M.D. |
| 1981 | Eli Robins, M.D. | 1992 | Gerald L. Klerman, |
| 1982 | Seymour S. Kety, M.D. | | M.D. |
| 1983 | Lawrence C. Kolb, M.D. | 1993 | Donald F. Klein, M.D. |
| 1984 | John Bowbly, M.D. | 1994 | Heinz Lehmann, M.D. |
| 1984 | John Romano, M.D. | 1995 | Leon Eisenberg, M.D. |
| 1985 | Erik Stromgren, M.D. | 1996 | Herbert Pardes, M.D. |
| 1986 | Jerome D. Frank, M.D., Ph.D. | 1996 | Melvin Sabshin, M.D. |

## The Thomas William Salmon Lecture

Honoring major contributions to the understanding of psychiatry, neurology, and mental hygiene.

| 1932 | Adolf Meyer, M.D. | 1944 | John Rawlings Rees, |
|---|---|---|---|
| 1934 | C. Macfie Campbell, M.D. | | M.D. |
| | | 1945 | Roy Graham Hoskins, |
| 1935 | William A. White, M.D. | | M.D. |
| 1936 | Samuel T. Orton, M.D. | 1946 | David Mordecai Levy, |
| 1937 | William Healy, M.D. | | M.D. |
| 1938 | David K. Henderson, M.D. | 1947 | Harold Dwight Lasswell, Ph.D. |
| 1939 | Edward A. Strecker, M.D. | 1948 | Torbjoern O. Caspersson, M.D. |
| 1940 | Nolan D.C. Lewis, M.D. | 1949 | Stanley Cobb, M.D. |
| 1941 | Robert Dick Gillespie, M.D. | 1950 | John Farquhar Fulton, M.D. |
| 1942 | Emilio Mira, M.D. | 1951 | Arthur H. Ruggles, M.D. |
| 1943 | Abraham Arden Brill, M.D. | 1952 | Franz Joseph Kallman, M.D. |

| | | | |
|---|---|---|---|
| 1953 | Ralph Linton, Ph.D. | 1974 | William Goldfarb, M.D., Ph.D. |
| 1954 | William Alvin Hunt, Ph.D. | 1975 | Walle J.H. Nauta, M.D., Ph.D. |
| 1955 | John C. Whitehorn, M.D. | | |
| 1956 | Horace W. Magoun, Ph.D. | 1976 | John Romano, M.D. |
| 1957 | David McKenzie Rioch, M.D. | 1977 | Solomon H. Snyder, M.D. |
| 1958 | Alexander H. Leighton, M.D. | 1978 | Isaac M. Marks, M.D. |
| | | 1979 | Michael L. Rutter, M.D. |
| 1959 | Curt Paul Richter, Ph.D. | 1980 | Robert N. Butler, M.D. |
| 1960 | Harry F. Harlow, Ph.D. | 1981 | Arvid E. Carlsson, M.D. |
| 1961 | Seymour S. Kety, M.D. | 1982 | Louis Sokoloff, M.D. |
| 1962 | Rene Dubos, Ph.D. | 1983 | Lee N. Robins, Ph.D. |
| 1963 | Joel Elkes, M.D. | 1984 | Mary Dinsmore Salter Ainsworth, Ph.D. |
| 1964 | Dana L. Farnsworth, M.D. | 1985 | Eric R. Kandel, M.D. |
| 1965 | Manfred S. Gutmacher, M.D. | 1986 | Albert J. Stunkard, M.D. |
| | | 1987 | Torsten M. Wiesel, M.D. |
| 1966 | Paul D. Maclean, M.D. | 1988 | Jerome Kagan, Ph.D. |
| 1967 | Theodore Lidz, M.D. | 1989 | Marvin Stein, M.D. |
| 1968 | Jose M.R. Delgado, M.D. | 1989 | Robert Ader, Ph.D. |
| 1969 | William C. Dement, M.D., Ph.D. | 1990 | Herbert Weiner, M.D. |
| | | 1991 | Floyd E. Bloom, M.D. |
| 1970 | Kenneth Keniston, Ph.D. | 1992 | Aaron T. Beck, M.D. |
| 1971 | Neal E. Miller, Ph.D. | 1993 | Joseph T. Coyle, M.D. |
| 1972 | Julius Axelrod, Ph.D. | 1994 | Philip S. Holzman, Ph.D. |
| 1973 | Lyman C. Wynne, M.D., Ph.D. | 1995 | Paul Greengard, Ph.D. |
| | | 1996 | Myron A. Hofer, M.D. |

## The Ferdinand C. Valentine Award and Lecture

For outstanding contributions to the art and science of urology.

| | | | |
|---|---|---|---|
| 1962 | Charles B. Huggins, M.D. | 1964 | Harry Goldblatt, M.D. |
| | | 1965 | Moses Swick, M.D. |
| 1963 | Meredith F. Campbell, M.D. | 1966 | Theodore McCann Davis, M.D. |

| 1967 | Alexander B. Gutman, M.D., Ph.D. | 1983 | John Kingsley Lattimer, M.D. |
|------|------|------|------|
| 1968 | Terence Millin, M.B., B.Ch. | 1984 | Hugh Judge Jewett, M.D. |
| 1969 | William Kolff, M.D. | 1985 | William Hardy Hendren, III, M.D. |
| 1970 | John H. Harrison, M.D. David M. Hume, M.D. John Merrill, M.D. Joseph E. Murray, M.D. | 1986 1987 | Pablo A. Morales, M.D. George R. Nagamatsu, M.D. |
| 1971 | Robert S. Hotchkiss, M.D. | 1988 1989 | Joseph J. Kaufman, M.D. Fathollah K. Mostofi, M.D. |
| 1972 | Rubin Flocks, M.D. | 1990 | Kurt Amplatz, M.D. |
| 1973 | Alfred Jost, M.D. | | Wilfrido R. Casteneda- |
| 1974 | Victor F. Marshall, M.D. | | Zuniga, M.D. Ralph V. Clayman, M.D. |
| 1975 | Sven I. Seldinger, M.D. | | Robert P. Miller, M.D. |
| 1976 | Reed M. Nesbit, M.D. | | Arthur D. Smith, M.D. |
| 1977 | Eugene Myron Bricker, M.D. | 1991 1992 | Thomas A. Stamey, M.D. Richard Turner-Warwick, |
| 1978 | David Innes Williams, M.B., B.Ch. | | D.M. Keith Waterhouse, M.D. |
| 1979 | Meyer M. Melicow, M.D. | 1993 | C. Eugene Carlton Jr., M.D. |
| 1980 | Willard E. Goodwin, M.D. | | John T. Grayhack, M.D. Jay Y. Gillenwater, M.D. |
| 1981 | William P. Didusch | 1994 | John P. Donohue, M.D. |
| 1982 | Willet Francis Whitmore, Jr., M.D. | 1995 1996 | Frank Hinman, Jr., M.D. Paul C. Peters, M.D. |

## The Nahum J. Winer Memorial Lecture

To recognize exceptional achievements in the field of cardiovascular disease.

| 1992 | Myron L. Weisfeldt, M.D. |
|------|------|
| 1993 | Mary Allen Engle, M.D. |
| 1995 | Jane Somerville, M.D. |
| 1996 | Gerald R. Marx, M.D. |

## ACADEMY PUBLICATIONS:
## HISTORY OF MEDICINE SERIES

Volumes Published Since 1947

No.

8. Van Ingen, Philip. 1949 *The New York Academy of Medicine: Its First Hundred Years.* New York: Coumbia University Press.

9. Gilbert, Judson Bennet. 1951 *A Bibliography of Articles on the History of American Medicine, Compiled from "Writings on American History" 1902–1937.* New York: The New York Academy of Medicine.

10. Lancisi, Giovanni Maria. 1952 *De aneurysmatibus, opus posthumum.* New York: Macmillan.

11. Lambert, Samuel, Willy Weigand and William Ivins, Jr. 1952 *Three Vesalian Essays to Accompany the Icones Anatomicae of 1934. New York:* Macmillan.

12. Teodorico, dei Borgognoni. 1952 *The Surgery of Theodoricus Borgognoni.* New York: Appleton-Century Crofts.

13. Morgagni, Giambattista. 1960 *The Seats and Causes of Diseases Investigated by Anatomy: in Five Books, Containing a Great Variety of Dissections, with Remarks. To Which Are Added Very Accurate and Copious Indexes of the Principal Things and the Names Therein Contained.* New York: Hafner.

14. Pinel, Phillipe. 1962 *A Treatise on Insanity.* New York: Hafner.

15. Rush, Benjamin. 1962 *Medical Inquiries and Observations upon the Diseases of the Mind.* New York: Hafner.

16. Corvisart des Marets, Jean Nicholas, Baron. 1962 *An Essay on the Organic Diseases and Lesions of the Heart and Great Vessels.* New York: Hafner.

17. Laennec, Rene Theophile Hyacinthe. 1962 *A Treatise on the Diseases of the Chest.* New York: Hafner.

18. Heberden William. 1963 *Commentaries on the History and Cure of Diseases.* New York: Hafner.

19. Charcot, Jean Martin. 1963 *Lectures on the Diseases of the Nervous System.* New York: Hafner.

20. Bowditch, Henry Ingersoll. 1963 *The Young Stethoscopist*. New York: Hafner.

21. Burns, Allan. 1964 *Observations on Some of the Most Frequent and Important Diseases of the Heart*. New York: Hafner.

22. Hales, Stephen. 1964 *Statistical Essays, Containing Haemastaticks*. New York: Hafner.

23. Ramazzini, Bernardino. 1964 *Diseases of Workers*. New York: Hafner.

24. Woodward, Joseph Janvier. 1964 *Outlines of the Chief Camp Diseases of the United States Armies*. New York: Hafner.

25. Esquirol, Etienne. 1965 *Mental Maladies, A Treatise on Insanity. With an Introduction by Raymond de Saussuere*. New York: Hafner.

26. Greisinger, Wilhelm. 1965 *Mental Pathology and Therapeutics*. New York: Hafner.

27. Garrison, Fielding H. 1966 *Contributions to the History of Medicine*. New York: The New York Academy of Medicine.

28. Puschmann Theodor. 1966 *The History of Medical Education*. New York: The New York Academy of Medicine.

29. Clossy, Samuel. 1967 *The Existing Works, With a Biographical Sketch*. New York: Hafner.

30. Bick, Edgar Milton. 1968 *History and Source Book of Orthopaedic Surgery*. New York: Hafner.

31. Bucknill, John Charles, Sir, and David H. Tuke. 1968 *A Manual of Psychologic Medicine*. New York: Hafner.

32. De Mirfield, Johannes. 1969 *Surgery*. New York: Hafner.

33. Kraepelin, Emil. 1968 *Lectures on Clinical Psychiatry*. New York: Hafner.

34. Meynert, Theodor. 1968 *1833–1892: Psychiatry; A Clinical Treatise on Diseases of the Fore-Brain Based upon a Study of its Structure, Functions, and Nutrition, Part I*. New York: Hafner.

35. Ray, Isaac. 1968 *Mental Hygiene*. New York: Hafner.

36. Smith, Stephen. 1973 *The City That Was: The Report of the General Committee of Health, New York City, 1806*. Metuchen, NJ: Scarecrow Reprint Corp.

37. Virchow, Rudolf Ludwig Karl. 1973 *Post-mortem Examinations and the Position of Pathology among Biological Studies*. Metuchen, NJ: Scarecrow Reprint Corp.

38. New York (City) Mayor's Committee on Marihuana. 1973 *The*

*Marihuana Problem in the City of New York*. Metuchen, NJ: Scarecrow Reprint Corp.

39. Duciaux, Emile. 1973 *Pasteur, the History of a Mind*. Metuchen, NJ: Scarecrow Reprint Corp.

40. Walker, Alexander. 1973 *Documents and Dates of Modern Discoveries in the Nervous System*. Metuchen, NJ: Scarecrow Reprint Corp.

41. Cranefield, Paul. 1974 *The Way In and the Way Out: Francois Magendie, Charles Bell and the Roots of the Spinal Nerves*. Mount Kisco, NY: Futura.

42. Ober, William B., Editor. 1973 *Great Men of Guy's*. Metuchen, NJ: Scarecrow Reprint Corp.

43. Barzun, Jacques. 1973 *Burke and Hare: The Resurrection of Men:* New York: The New York Academy of Medicine.

44. Dewhurst, Kenneth Eastham. 1974 *Ancient Physician's Legacy to his Country: Thomas Dover's Life and Legacy*. Metuchen, NJ: Scarecrow Press.

45. Mayo, Herbert. 1974 *Anatomical and Physiological Commentaries*. Metuchen, NJ: Scarecrow Press.

46. Farr, William. 1975 *Vital Statistics: a Memorial Volume of Selections from the Reports and Writings of William Farr*. Metuchen, NJ: Scarecrow Press.

47. *The Confederate States Medical and Surgical Journal (1864–1865)*. 1976 Metuchen, NJ: Scarecrow Press.

48. Cranefield, Paul. 1976 *Claude Bernard's Revised Edition of his Introduction a l'Étude de las Medecine Experimentale*. New York: Science History Publications.

49. Jarcho, Saul, Editor. 1976 *Essays on the History of Medicine, Selected from the Bulletin of the New York Academy of Medicine*. New York: Science History Publications.

50. Morgagni, Giambattista. 1986 *The Seats and Causes of Diseases Investigated by Anatomy, in Five Books, Containing a Great Variety of Dissections, with Remarks, To Which Are Added Very Accurate and Copious Indexes of the Principal Things and Names Therein Contained*. Mount Kisco, NY: Futura.

51. Jarcho, Saul. 1986 *Italian Broadsides Concerning Public Health: Documents fromj Bologna and Brescia in the Mortimer and Anna Neinken Collection*. Mount Kisco, NY: Futura.

52. Bertapaglia, Leonardo. 1989 *On Nerve Injuries and Skull Fractures*. Mount Kisco, NY: Futura.

# About the Authors
# Marvin Lieberman

Marvin Lieberman, a native New Yorker attended the City College of New York, where he received his Bachelor's degree with honors in Government and was elected to Phi Beta Kappa. After receiving a Master's degree in Political Science from Columbia University, he went on to New York University, where he received a J.D. from the New York University School of Law and a Ph.D. from the New York University Graduate School of Arts and Science.

After serving as a Public Administration Intern and Budget Aide with the New York State Division of the Budget in Albany, and completing military service, his experience included work with the New York City Department of Health and with the Blue Cross Association. With the help of a Career Scientist's Award form the Health Research Council of New York, he conducted studies on urban medical economics at the New York City Department of Health, the Hunter College Urban Research Center, and the New York Academy of Medicine.

His association with the Academy began in 1964, and in 1969, he was appointed Executive Secretary of the Committee on Medicine in Society, a position he retained until his retirement in 1995. From 1981–1982 he served as Acting Director of the Academy.

He has held faculty appointments at the Department of Community Medicine of the, Albert Einstein College of Medicine, the Columbia University School of Public Health, and the New School for Social Research, and is currently affiliated with the Advanced Management Program for Clinicians at New York University's Robert F. Wagner Graduate School of Public Service. He has been a consultant to many health-related organizations, including the Office of Economic Opportunity, the Committee for Economic Development, the National Institute of Mental Health, the National Multiple Sclerosis Society, the New York State Joint Legislative Committee on Health, and the Columbia University study of Prepayment Plans in New York State.

He has published or edited monographs and articles on the financing of urban health services, mental health funding issues, national health care financing, and legal and ethical issues in medicine.

He has served as President of the Public Health Association of New York City, as Chairman of the Board of the Fund for Aging Services attached to the New York City Department for the Aging, and on various committees of the Association of the Bar of the City of New York. He served as Chairman of the Committee on Public Affairs of Cancer Care, Inc., and as a member of the New York State Advisory Committee on Physician Recredentialing.

He and his wife, Purlaine, have three children and seven grandchildren.

# Leon J. Warshaw

Leon J. Warshaw, a native New Yorker, received an BA from Columbia College and, in 1942, an MD from the Columbia University College of Physicians and Surgeons, where he was elected to Alpha Omega Alpha. He was certified in 1953 by the American Board of Internal Medicine, and, in 1957, by the American Board of Preventive Medicine in Occupational Medicine. After completing an internship on the First Medical Division (Columbia University) at Bellevue Hospital, he pursued a number of interlocking and overlapping careers. For a time, he practiced internal medicine and cardiology in New York City, and held faculty positions at Columbia University and at New York University where he is currently Clinical Professor of Environmental Medicine. His hospital affiliations included more than a decade as Chief of the Cardiovascular Research Unit at Beth Israel Hospital.

He joined the medical department of the F.G. Shattuck Corporation, and then became Medical Director of Paramount Pictures Corporation, United Artists Corporation and the American Broadcasting Company. He was appointed Vice President and Chief

Medical Officer of the Equitable Life Assurance Society where, in addition to employee health and insurance medicine, he became involved in HMO start-ups around the country as well as other aspects of health care organization and financing.

He was appointed by Governor Carey to two terms on the Governor's Health Advisory Council. Governor Cuomo appointed him Chairman of the Advisory Council on Alcoholism and Alcohol Abuse Services, a post he has retained during the first years of the administration of Governor Pataki, During the first administration of Mayor Edward I Koch, he served for two and a half years as Deputy Director for Health Affairs of the Mayor's Office of Operations, a group of loaned executives from the private sector who attempted to improve the management of the City government and its many agencies.

On his retirement, he organized, and for twelve years directed, the New York Business Group on Health, a nonprofit coalition of some 300 organizations in the New York Metropolitan Area who joined in addressing issues relating to the availability, quality and cost of health care services and the impact of injury and disease on employees' well-being and productivity.

Dr. Warshaw has pursued research in clinical pharmacology, the treatment of heart disease, the effects of high altitude, cellular biology relating to tissue transplantation and carcinogenesis, and work stress. In the early phases of the space program, he served as a consultant on capsule configuration. In addition to the classic, *The Heart In Industry,* and a manual on *Managing Stress,* he has authored or co-authored over 300 journal articles and book chapters. He served as Associate Editor of the *Journal of Occupational Medicine,* and is Associate Editor of the 4th Edition of the *Encylopaedia of Occupational Health and Safety* which the International Labor Office will publish in 1997.

He was elected to Fellowship in the American College of Occupational and Environmental Medicine which, in 1992, presented him with the William F. Knudsen Award, its highest honor, given in recognition of a distinguished career in occupational health. He received an Honorary Fellowship in the Society of Occupational

Medicine of London. He also has been elected a Fellow of a number of organizations including the American College of Physicians, the American College of Cardiology, the American Public Health Association, the American College of Preventive Medicine, and the New York Academy of Sciences. He has served on the Board of Directors of the New York and the American Heart Associations, the New York and the National Safety Councils, the Health Systems Agency of New York City, and the Medical and Health Research Association.

He became a Fellow of the New York Academy of Medicine in 1960, served as Chairman of the Section on Occupational Medicine from 1964 to 1966, and, from 1977 to 1996, was a member of the Committee on Medicine in Society.

# Index